Progress in Drug Research
Fortschritte der Arzneimittelforschung
Progrès des recherches pharmaceutiques
Vol. 42

Progress in Drug Research
Fortschritte der Arzneimittelforschung
Progrès des recherches pharmaceutiques
Vol. 42

Edited by / Herausgegeben von / Rédigé par
Ernst Jucker, Basel

Authors / Autoren / Auteurs:
Michael J. Parnham · Vera M. Kolb · Shradha Sinha and Sudha Jain ·
A. Das, J. H. Wang and E. J. Lien · Berend Olivier, Jan Mos, Maikel
Raghoebar, Paul de Koning and Marianne Mak · H. Hugh Fudenberg
and Giancarlo Pizza · Giancarlo Pizza, Caterina de Vinci and H. Hugh
Fudenberg.

1994   Birkhäuser Verlag
Basel · Boston · Berlin

Editor:

Dr. E. Jucker
Steinweg 28
CH-4107 Ettingen
Switzerland

© 1994 Birkhäuser Verlag, P. O. Box 113, CH-4010 Basel, Switzerland
Softcover reprint of the hardcover 1st edition 1994
    Printed on acid-free paper produced from chlorine-free pulp

ISBN-13: 978-3-0348-7155-6   e-ISBN-13: 978-3-0348-7153-2
DOI: 10.1007/978-3-0348-7153-2

Contents · Inhalt · Sommaire

Foreword

Volume 42 of "Progress in Drug Research" contains seven reviews and the various indexes which facilitate its use and establish the connection with the previous volumes. The articles in this volume deal with organization and management of drug research; luteinizing hormone regulators; natural products as anticancer agents; flavonoids and their pharmacological activity; serenics in the control of mental disturbances; Transfer Factor and its application and with Transfer Factor in malignancy.

In the 34 years that "Progress in Drug Research" has existed, the Editor has enjoyed the valuable help and advice of many colleagues. Readers, the authors of the reviews, and last but not least, the reviewers have all contributed greatly to the success of this series. Although the comments received so far have generally been favorable, it is nevertheless necessary to analyze and to reassess the current position and the future direction of such a review series.

So far, it has been the Editors intention to help disseminate information on the vast domain of drug research, and to provide the reader with a tool with which to keep abreast of the latest developments and trends. The reviews in PDR are useful to the non-specialists, who can obtain an overview of a particular field of drug research in a relatively short time.

The specialist readers of PDR will appreciate the reviews' comprehensive bibliographies, and, in addition, they may even get fresh impulses for their own research. Finally, the readers can use the 42 volumes of PDR as an encyclopedic source of information.

It gives me great pleasure to present this new volume to our readers. At the same time I would like to express my gratitude to the authors who willingly accepted the task of preparing extensive reviews. My sincere thanks also go to Birkhäuser Verlag, and, in particular to Mrs. L. Koechlin and Mssrs. H.-P. Thür and A. Gomm. Without their personal commitment and assistance, editing PDR would be a nearly impossible task.

Basel, April 1994   DR. E. JUCKER

Vorwort

Der vorliegende 42. Band der Reihe «Fortschritte der Arzneimittel-forschung» enthält sieben Übersichtsartikel sowie die verschiedenen Register, welche das Arbeiten mit diesem Werk erleichtern und den Zugriff auf die vorhergehenden Bände ermöglichen. Die Artikel des vorliegenden Bandes behandeln – wie das Inhaltsverzeichnis zeigt – verschiedene aktuelle Gebiete der Arzneimittelforschung und ermöglichen es dem Leser, sich rasch einen guten Überblick über diese Gebiete zu verschaffen.

Seit der Gründung der Reihe sind 34 Jahre vergangen. In dieser langen Zeitspanne konnte der Herausgeber immer auf den Rat der Fach-kollegen, der Leser und der Autoren zählen. Ihnen allen möchte ich meinen Dank abstatten. In diesen Dank sind auch die Rezensenten eingeschlossen, denn sie haben wesentlich zum guten Gedeihen der Reihe beigetragen. Viele Kommentare und Besprechungen waren lobend. Trotzdem ist es angebracht, die Frage nach dem Sinn und Zweck der «Fortschritte» zu stellen und zu überprüfen.

Nach wie vor ist es unser Ziel, neueste Forschungsergebnisse in Form von Übersichten darzustellen und dem Leser auf diese Weise zu ermöglichen, sich verhältnismäßig rasch und mühelos über bestimmte aktuelle Richtungen der Arzneimittelforschung zu informieren. Es wird ihm somit die Möglichkeit gegeben, sich im komplexen und sich rasant entwickelnden Fachgebiet auf dem laufenden zu halten und den Kontakt zur aktuellen Forschung aufrechtzuerhalten.

Die Übersichten der «Fortschritte» bieten dem Spezialisten eine wertvolle Quelle der Originalliteratur dar, erlauben ihm nützliche Vergleichsmöglichkeiten, und sie können u. a. seine eigene Forschung befruchten. Für alle Leser der «Fortschritte» stellt die Reihe mit ihren ausführlichen Verzeichnissen eine nützliche Quelle von enzyklopädischem Wissen dar, so daß das gesamte Werk auch als Nachschlagewerk dienen kann.

Zum Gedeihen der Reihe haben die Autoren maßgebend beigetragen; ihnen allen sei hier gedankt. Dank gebührt auch dem Birkhäuser Verlag, insbesondere Frau L. Koechlin und den Herren H.-P. Thür und A. Gomm.

Basel, April 1994   Dr. E. JUCKER

Progress in Drug Research, Vol. 42
Edited by Ernst Jucker
© 1994 Birkhäuser Verlag Basel (Switzerland)

Moral challenges in the organisation and management of drug research

By Michael J. Parnham

Parnham Advisory Services, Von-Guericke-Allee 4, D-53125 Bonn, Germany

1   Introduction

The organisation of drug research has become a burgeoning field for business consultants in recent years who have found a gold mine in investigating, advising on and writing reports on the optimal orga-nisational structure for a company. These activities, however, are predominantly occupied with the "how" of organisation. How can the most profitable structure be established? How can the employees best be motivated? How can costs be kept to a minimum?

Within an ethical context it is also essential to consider "why" a particular structure or course of action is desirable. This fact has been described and emphasised by Graner [1] who draws attention to the need in scientific investigation and decision-making not just to "fol-low the rules", but also to call into question the moral principles behind our actions.

Since the major aims of the pharmaceutical industry are to develop new drugs and to make money in the process, the organisation of research is generally strictly "goal-orientated", as in most other branches of industry. However, it must always be borne in mind that while the product and the profit gained are inanimate, the means to achieve the goals involve people, both to decide on and to implement the work. The importance of the underlying ethical validity of the organisational structure and decision process with regard to the people involved in drug research will be emphasised here. In addition, the type of product developed by the pharmaceutical industry de-mands that decisions with regard to drug research and development cannot be taken purely on the basis of economic considerations, but must take into account the potential application of the product in medical practice, i. e. by thinking people. In other words, organisation within the drug industry is essentially a balancing of economically profitable solutions against solutions which are motivating for the people involved, while ensuring that the drugs being developed meet the requirements of a critical market exhibiting increasingly demand-ing expectations with regard to efficacy, safety and price. In such a climate, reflection on decisions taken is essential. This is basically the prerogative of research managers, but needs to be understood by all those involved in drug research.

1.1   The basic problem

Unfortunately, the practical reality is that little opportunity is available to the research manager to consider the ethics of decisions taken. Those who choose and are chosen to become responsible for research organisation are generally those who want to further their personal careers, while their employers are often far more concerned with profit than the morality of the means used to achieve it. The result is that decisions taken are frequently those which are most beneficial to the career of the individual involved (taken often out of fear of losing personal standing within the company, to enhance personal power base, revenge etc.) and/or provide short-term financial benefit for the company. These attitudes are encouraged by the rewarding of employees who follow cost-saving, turnover-enhancing and profit-bringing policies, irrespective of their long-term social and economic effects [2]. This chapter considers some of the approaches taken within the pharmaceutical industry towards the organisation of drug research and the challenges to more ethical approaches arising out of these structures.

1.2   Types of organisational structures

Peters and Waterman [3] define five different types of company organisational structures which can be detected in US business:
I) Functional organisation, with strict divisions according to principle tasks and functions.
II) Business organisation, divided according to research or market indication.
III) Matrix structure, in which complex interactions between various groups are established in an attempt to meet the requirement for multiple competence and expertise.
IV) "Adhocratie", in which the structure regularly readjusts to requirements.
V) Organisation according to the mission of the company.
As far as the pharmaceutical industry is concerned the first three structures are those most commonly encountered.

2   Functional organisation and manager stress

The classical structure is the functional organisation, upon which
many research-based pharmaceutical companies have been built.
Under this system, clearly defined units are formed with their respective heads and an extensive hierarchy exists, as shown in Fig. 1. In
most cases, decision-making occurs vertically. In a small company this
has the advantage that everyone knows his place and to whom he/she
must go for a decision; also the immediate superior usually has a
compatible background and training. In a large company, horizontal
contacts between departments and divisions are likely to suffer, unless
a specific mechanism (such as project management) is built into the
functional organisation to deal with interdisciplinary contacts. If
decision making is not delegated to such groups, the problem may
arise that a busy top manager may need to take decisions on matters
he or she is not fully informed about.

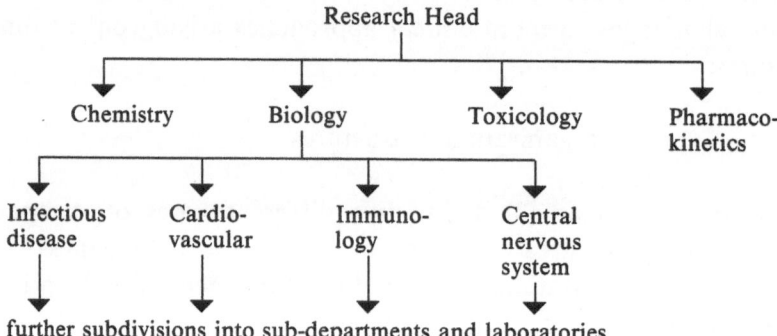

Fig. 1
The functional line organisation of a pharmaceutical research division, as exemplified
by Biology Research.

2.1   Pressures on managers

The pressures facing managers within a functional organisation are
similar in most companies, irrespective of the industry. Here I shall
discuss how these affect some of the situations which arise within
pharmaceutical research. As long as the relevant superior is good at
making decisions, functional organisation can work on a small scale.
The area of responsibility is generally clear and provided that not too
many projects are being pursued at the same time competence, at least

theoretically, can be maintained. However, this type of system is very dependent on the personalities and capabilities of the managers at each hierarchical level. The individual is held personally responsible for his/her own area and the quality of its research and is expected to be able to answer questions on every detail of the department's activities as well as the implications of the research data in association with those of other departments. For instance under the structure shown in figure 2, the head of Biology will be expected to present the results of experiments from any of the four research field represented in his or her department and to discuss the implication of these results for further chemical synthesis, toxicological and pharmacokinetic investigations.

He or she will also have to provide detailed advice to colleagues in the other departments on the approach they should take in following up his/her recommendations. Conversely, he or she will need to be able to interpret the relevance of chemical structural changes and toxicological and pharmacokinetic data on a compound for further biological testing on specific experimental test systems for each area within a particular field of responsibility. The wide range of detailed knowledge required for such a position demands that such a structure can only be successful when the different areas of expertise (e. g. immunology, cardiovascular etc.) are restricted to a small number. In this case, the responsible person is able to maintain a reasonably detailed knowledge of his subject(s) by reading the scientific literature, attending scientific congresses and discussing with colleagues. He/she is able to stay on top of the job and retain integrity and competence as well as feeling capable of fulfilling the relevant responsibilities towards his/her employer. As soon as the field of responsibility becomes too large or diverse, this one person can no longer maintain detailed knowledge of all areas. Stress results!

A number of possibilities remain open. The obvious and most sensible approach is to delegate, thereby not only spreading responsibility, but also training subordinates to make their own decisions. Trust is an essential factor in delegation, not only in that the department head must select capable and trustworthy colleagues, but also in that the scientist who takes the responsibility for his/her own ideas and actions is motivated by being shown trust. As a factor in building an efficient team, trust which is based on a general attitude and not affected by the occasional mistake, in my opinion is far more important than intellectual excellence. There are, of course, degrees of delegation, depending on the capabilities of both the manager and the subordinates and I shall come to some of the problems a little later on.

Another possibility is that the department head doesn't delegate directly but through concentrating on specific areas of interest, such as budgetary matters, external contacts or personal scientific interests, leaves whole areas uncoordinated. The scientist whose field is of no interest to the boss will either take matters into his or her own hands, carrying out investigations and building up contacts without any managerial control or will feel neglected, lose interest and probably look for another job. Neither results are right, on the one hand leaving a subordinate without direction will inevitably produce friction and loss of team spirit, while on the other hand, losing good scientists who have not been integrated is bad for the team and will leave the victim feeling bitter.

All scientists have their hobby horses. I have come across research managers who were very good politicians and highly capable at hammering out legal agreements who should have delegated decisions on specific research projects to those who knew more about the material. Then there are other managers so keen on keeping up to date with the latest results from the lab that strategic decisions concerning the whole research group are only cursorily planned. More delegation and trust would have helped, but at least they didn't all try to do everything.

This is the worst scenario, when the department head tries to keep abreast of all developments personally. These people feel guilty for not knowing everything they need to know and are likely to be asked and try to work longer hours. They feel – rightly – obligated towards their employer, but to the extent that they feel unable to take any holiday. Anxiety is continually present because they are always waiting for that awkward question in the important strategy meeting which they know they won't be able to answer for lack of knowledge. A vicious circle starts because in an attempt to remember everything the manager starts forgetting details and the now painful stress-gastritis impairs ability to concentrate. The person becomes aggressive in meetings in an attempt to preempt searching questions and starts putting pressure on subordinates to produce the needed results. These people may become more withdrawn, not allowing themselves to be drawn into discussions they feel inadequate to cope with. For a company to force a valuable employee into such a position, without making attempts to relieve or relax the workload, is morally wrong, because the individual is made secondary to the organisational structure and quite simply this is a destructive waste of creative potential. The manager is expected to provide and demands from him or herself expert informed suggestions and decisions without acknowledging natural human limitations. Achievement is demanded without accepting the limits of possibility.

I well remember a similar situation in which my superior was responsible, in a vertical hierarchy, for 60 people working on hypertension, atherosclerosis, inflammation, immunology and toxicology. It wasn't long before his working hours were so long that his family life was suffering and he finally decided to put his family first and left the company. I was asked to take over temporarily and although I requested successfully that the responsibility in the department should be delegated in part, 10 months of keeping up with all those different areas, dealing with personnel problems, as well as carrying responsibility for external collaborative projects took its toll of my gastric mucosa!

2.2   Stress and productivity

Overloading in a vertical hierarchy can also be counterproductive since the level of scientific expertise at points of decision has a tendency to become diluted and inadequate. Some people seem to thrive under conditions of high activity, their minds being sharpened by the challenge of constant decision making. Others have a remarkable capacity to store and process facts and are a real asset in a multi-disciplinary research meeting. Yet others have an uncanny knack of getting straight to the core of a problem despite its confusing and complex nature (a frequent challenge to modern drug research). One such person is Sir John Vane, for many years Director of Research and Development at Wellcome Research Laboratories. Before his move to industry, I spent a year as an undergraduate project student in his department. The department was full of staff, postgraduate students and several visiting scientists crammed into little labs and working till all hours at exciting projects. Vane's advice was frequently sought and he made a point of keeping abreast of the experimental work. I had the impression that his sixth sense would tell him when a mistake was being made, since he often entered the lab just as something was going wrong. Whether it was a malfunctioning pen recorder, a blocked tube or an incorrectly drawn figure, John seemed to be able to put his finger on it immediately.

Top jobs require exceptional people and the ability to sort out the wood from the trees under crowded circumstances is a valuable commodity in a research environment. Unfortunately, the Peter Principle – everyone rises to their highest level of incompetence – can be seen at work in drug research, just as it can in any other hierarchical structure. The higher the level of incompetence, the more pronounced the lack of scientific expertise becomes. Insufficient detailed knowledge is brought to bear on the overloaded situation and the input of creativity, thought and involvement inevitably decreases. Consequently, the decisions likely to be taken under such conditions will often be ill-considered, materially deficient and possibly irrelevant, because the relevant discussion material is not available. With such constraints, the mind usually concentrates itself on the immediate; how can I obtain the quickest solution, what is the most obvious next step or even what can I do to get myself out of this mess and pass on the buck to someone else? The path to the next immediate goal, for many people in such a situation, completely outweighs a reflective consideration of the morality or outworking of the decision.

An inevitable result of the dilution of creativity and detailed knowledge at laboratory level is a reliance in the drug discovery process on simple screening systems. While a certain degree of routine screening is essential to be able to find a suitable candidate compound under a rational, mechanistic approach to testing, most of the better companies have developed automatic systems to deal with screening. In addition, biotechnology and some basic research provide a broad front for the search for a new drug. Generally speaking the sheer quantity of compounds tested cannot make up for the role of intelligence and creativity in making the chemical and mechanistic selections. Ideas are the life blood of research, and can best be achieved when the researcher works in a stimulating environment. This is created by the better companies through a mix of basic research and screening. Boring routine dulls the mind and has a destructive influence on the motivation of the researcher, who needs (in addition to a certain amount of routine) the opportunity to develop new ideas.

Companies must learn to recognise that achievement has its limits. Success can not always be measured in terms of short-term benefit. A company which encourages its employees to limit excessive overtime and make more time for family and relaxation, will in the long-term undoubtedly create conditions under which new ideas can be born more easily. Laziness is certainly not to be encouraged, but physical fitness, mental alertness and a clear conscience are assets to an employee which cannot be measured either in hours or dollars. In the long-term, a healthy employee given time to think and consider the decisions he takes at work will prove far more productive than when he is continually under pressure to meet short-term deadlines. This is of particular importance in drug research in which products take many years to develop and are heavily dependent on good ideas. Managers must be encouraged to take morally acceptable and not just financially beneficial decisions. Why not reward a manager who has the civil courage to take an ethical decision which may have negative economic results in the short term [2]? Safety at work is a prime example. Investment in laboratory safety measures may require initial unwanted expenditure, but the long-term benefits to employees' morale and on litigation costs saved will be considerable.

2.3   Effects on subordinates and the role of delegation

In a vertical, functional hierarchy the members of a particular department are very much dependent upon their departmental head for all matters related to their employment, including the implementation of their experimental results, environmental safety and comfort as well as personal matters. This is one of the clear disadvantages of the functional or discipline organisation, since there is a communication bottle neck; the possibility of horizontal interdisciplinary communication and decision-making is reduced, since the head of department must be informed about everything and be allowed to take final decisions on all these varying matters. If the lab head is under pressure, time available to motivate and encourage subordinates becomes very limited and tensions build up. These may not only disturb the willingness of subordinates to approach the manager and his willingness or capacity to deal with the needs of his staff, but also results in tensions and difficulties between the staff because the boss is not available to mediate.

Some years ago I was working with a group of technicians with whom I had very good contact, professionally and socially. When the promotion to acting head of department arose, which I have described above, in which I had too little time for too many tasks, these technicians were the first to suffer. I didn't have the time to discuss results, assist with malfunctioning apparatus or plan the Christmas party. The next few months were very hard as the antipathy grew – it was like walking into a steaming sauna to come to work. Fortunately, time was a good healer and the staff adjusted to the new situation but with a different, cooler attitude.

A partial solution to the problems of overloaded managers is delegation. Most people who have taken a couple of steps up the promotion ladder are very conscious of their need to succeed in order to sustain the upward movement of their professional career. This frequently engenders a feeling that one must try to become almost indispensable to attract the attention of senior management. This is thought to be possible by ensuring that no stone is left unturned and every detail of the department's activities must be intimately known and checked upon by the manager himself. (Such managers become workaholics, devoting all their time to work and can be absolutely devastated when a change in company policy deprives them of their sole source of satisfaction). The opposite approach – leaving a group to its own devices – can succeed with a good team. Apart from the danger of generating too many individualists, management by helicopter can result: a sudden arrival blowing up a lot of dust, followed by an abrupt departure, leaving everyone a little confused. Learning to delegate both tasks and responsibilities not only brings a sense of balance into the manager's work, but also gives the subordinate a degree of responsibility and a realization that he/she is wanted and appreciated. Those who have been crushed too often by dictatorial, critical and pedantic superiors are unlikely to develop into future managers themselves.

Teamwork is the basis of successful drug discovery and development. Few individual academic scientists working in isolation are now able to make significant therapeutic breakthroughs and the consistent, continual interaction between chemists, biologists, pharmacists and clinicians is crucial. Some may play less obvious roles, but all are important cogs in the machinery [4].

Each individual needs to know that they have worth in themselves, that they have expertise to offer to the team which contributes to its effectivity. A manager must recognise that he/she does not know everything, can not hope to and – most important – is not expected to. Failure to acknowledge, accept and incorporate into the team the knowledge and ideas which differ from those of the manager himself, is morally wrong and exceptionally arrogant.

2.4   Communication and the need for shared decisions

The vertical, functional organisation thus requires very careful consideration of the employees involved. The decision bottlenecks demand that sufficient opportunity exists for subordinates not directly involved in the decision-making process to air their ideas, views and suggestions, for the good progress of the research projects and for the motivation and well-being of the people involved. Not only this, but the "decision-makers" must maintain a good communication net, to compensate for the relative lack of interdisciplinary interactions under this system [5]. Unfortunately, functional organisation and a pronounced hierachy tend to reinforce personal ambition and "empire-building". Ultimately, the manager is responsible for ensuring the efficient, cost-effective and speedy development of company projects. A manager in a strict hierarchical system, under pressure from management and solely responsible for subordinates, is however running a considerable risk of taking decisions according to personal ambition and interest rather than for the interest of the company's projects and programmes. "A burden shared is a burden halved" is an often quoted proverb, which is very applicable in this situation. How many managers can remember situations in which they would have been able to make a better decision if they had felt able to share the responsibility with someone from another area or discipline who could have provided an alternative way of looking at the situation? In this respect, drug research strategies can benefit considerably from regular contacts with academic researchers. Most companies have university consultants who advise them from time-to-time on particular research programmes or projects. Whether the advice given is accepted is of course a different matter. Closer collaboration in the development of a particular project can be even more fruitful. I experienced this as manager of an international project in which two university research groups were involved at an early stage of research.

This meant that the academic researchers were not just being asked for advice, they were integrated into the research programme. Consequently, they had a personal interest in the fate of the project and promoted interest in the project among other external researchers, as well as making active contributions to the research project itself.

In all contacts between industry and universities, though, each side must ensure that no conflicts of interest arise which will either open the company to accusations of malpractice or the academic to lack of objectivity [6].

A possible approach that can be applied to internal communication within research divisions is, at the same time, a way of making the most of older scientists who are no longer able to generate new research ideas [7]. Often these people are pushed into a dusty corner, retired early or even fired. Many of them have been in the company for years and are well acquainted with the company culture. This wealth of experience can be put to good use by creating liaison officers whose major task is a to act as an interface between different departments and between research and other divisions, such as sales and marketing.

2.5   Responsibility to company versus responsibility to individuals

Power has a tendency to corrupt. Any manager, and particularly one in a strong hierarchical position, is under a moral obligation to carefully balance the interests of his individual subordinates, the interests of the company and the progression of its projects against his own personal ambitions and short-term interests in order to be able to take ethically sound decisions [6].

In this situation, it is, nevertheless, not always possible to determine which decision is morally correct, even when one takes the time to decide upon the morality of the issue (which is unfortunately not a frequent occurence). Sometimes one is confronted with a decision which is a true moral dilemma [8]. One case in point was when the research division of the company I was working for was told that 30% of the research personnel would have to be reduced by retirement, transfer or if necessary firing. I was told that two of my subordinates would have to go and this produced a series of disturbed nights' sleep as I turned the problem over in my mind. On the face of it, this seemed an unfair situation, since all of my staff were good workers and didn't deserve to be treated in this way. However, I also had an obligation to the company which paid my salary to face economic facts. The decision expected of me was not illegal but I felt I had to deal with my staff individually to come to an ethically acceptable solution. As it turned out, the most logical and reasonable solution, for each individual concerned, was to select for transfer those who were allergic to animal hair and thus limited in the experiments they could perform with biological samples. Although the separation was painful, the new tasks for the transferred staff subsequently proved to be satisfying and fulfilling. Principles are important, but one must also have the courage to act upon them in practice, particularly when this acutely works to one's own disadvantage.

Such morally challenging decisions are most frequent at the top of the hierarchical ladder, where pressure of time is the most intense. The most logical and ethically acceptable solution is to seek to maintain openness and transparency in all transactions and agreements and where necessary to put everything down in writing which can be assessed by objective observers.

2.6   Short-term planning

It has always seemed to be a rather hazardous approach to provide managing directors and chief executive officers with 3 or 4 year contracts in the pharmaceutical industry, as is often practised. When one considers that drug development can take anything up to 10–12 years, how can one possibly expect the top manager to implement effective policies in 3–4 years which are not going to be overturned by his successor? The temptation for the company director to take short-term decisions to secure his own position, rather than furthering the company's future prospects must be very great! Why not reward a successful director with a longer contract and avoid hasty firing on the basis of acute difficulties? The now traditional US management approach of high-stress, short-term performance with a hire-and-fire attitude is ultimately totally counterproductive since it degrades the human being to little more than a robot and bears little relationship to the long-term nature of pharmaceutical development and production. This same fact was born out very clearly, with regard to the electronics industry, in an interview with Akio Morita, the chairman of the highly successful Sony company [9]. Certainly, development of a new video recorder requires far less time than that of a new drug, yet Sony always plans at least 10 years in advance. In Morita's view, US industry has begun to suffer because of short-term management, concern about quarterly finance reports and rapid firing of top managers, together with insufficient investment in research. But an alternative is hardly conceivable if top management as well as middle management is not given the opportunity to put long-term plans into action.

The classic example of short-term planning is to develop "me-too" drugs. This involves a minimum of investment into research on new chemical entities for the sake of a rapid development process and a quick return on investment once the compound reaches the market. Therapeutic advantage is not seen as a goal in itself but as a means to deflect some of the competitors profits to the company's own product. Drastic changes in reimbursement by various governments over recent years, however, have made it increasingly less financially attractive for companies to develop such "me-too" drugs. The costs of research and development, particularly with the increased burden of the safety testing now demanded by regulatory authorities, mean that only compounds with an obviously advantageous mechanism of action or tolerability are economically viable projects.

2.7   Organisation by therapeutic indication

Organisation according to business is to some extent a variation of the functional organisation. Within pharmaceutical research this generally means division of research activities according to therapeutic indication. Within this scheme, the departments of infectious diseases, cardiovascular diseases, immunology and central nervous system disorders in figure 1 become major research divisions, each with their own chemists, biologists, clinicians, chemists, analysts etc, working together to develop drugs for a particular disease area (Fig. 2). The major advantage of this system is that it brings together people from differing disciplines and thereby enhances the collaborative nature of the organisation [10]. Each manager within the still pronounced hierarchy has, however, a more clearly circumscribed area of responsibility and is, theoretically, more likely to be able to make informed decisions, since his/her training and experience can be brought to bear more precisely upon problem-solving. The increased tendency toward collaboration also facilitates "burden-sharing" so that more team decisions can be taken.

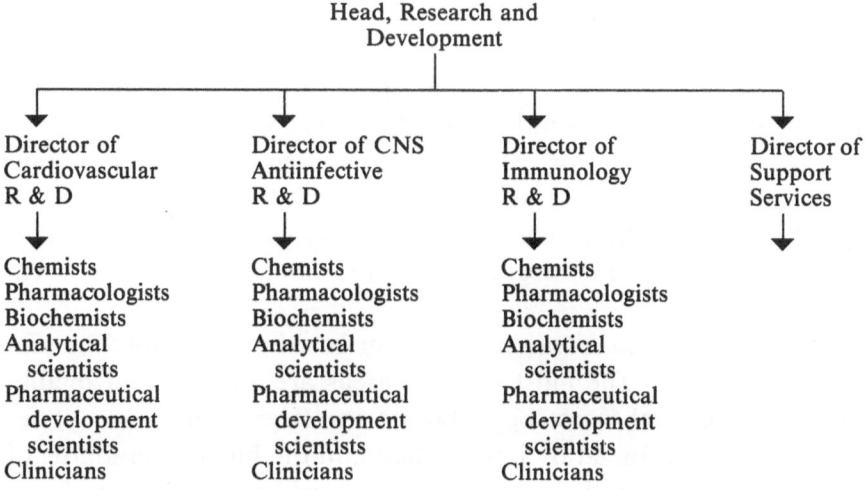

Fig. 2
Therapeutically based organisation of research and development activities in a drug company.

2.8   Inflexibility of indication-orientated organisation

A disadvantage of this system is a greater degree of inflexibility, since only projects which are clearly related to the relevant therapeutic indication are likely to be undertaken. An excellent example of the sort of problem which might arise is provided by receptor antagonists of platelet activating factor (PAF) [11]. This ether phospholipid mediator was first discovered as a product of basophils released during immediate hypersensitivity (allergic) reactions. It was subsequently found to be a potent stimulator of platelet aggregation (and thus thought to be involved in thrombosis) and to cause hypotension. Consequently, the majority of pharmaceutical companies in the 1980's set up research groups looking for PAF receptor antagonists as possible anti-thrombotic compounds or PAF agonists as potential anti-hypertensive compounds. In most companies, these activities were confined to the cardiovascular research programme. Then came the discovery that PAF is a potential mediator of airway hyperreactivity in asthma and that PAF antagonists may be effective anti-asthma drugs [12]. At one company, asthma research was being performed as part of the inflammation programme while PAF antagonists were still under the control of the cardiovascular programme. The result was research on anti-asthmatic PAF antagonists being carried out by cardiovascular specialists – not an optimal organisation! (PAF antagonists were subsequently not very successful in clinical trials in asthma and are currently under consideration for septic shock; i. e. back to a cardiovascular indication.) Such a situation can give rise to dissatisfaction among the researchers concerned and is not guaranteed to motivate experts who are familar with the topic they are not given! While continual reorganisation is also counter-productive to research progress, some degree of organisational flexibility is essential.

Certain areas of the research effort can best be maintained in centralized divisions. The most obvious areas are analysis and quality control and central toxicology laboratories. Every company is under an obligation, enforced by law, to maintain the highest standards of quality and safety in their products, which will be administered to a variety of patients in different countries living under widely disparate conditions. Central analytical laboratories ensure that all products developed by a single company are assessed under the same conditions and by identical criteria and are not subject to national, economic or indication-dependent differences. The same is true also for toxicological investigations, which provide an added incentive to centralization. The time and costs involved in toxicity testing are so great these days that it does not make economic sense to have more than one centre for toxicology within a company. In fact, many medium-sized companies have dispensed with toxicology laboratories altogether and now rely on experienced contract research institutes. Particularly in Europe, where intensive efforts are being made to achieve homogeneity in the research and development of drugs, toxicological and analytical investigators need to be well-informed of the latest regulatory changes in order to continue to meet legal requirements and thereby avoid unnecessary delays and expense arising from additional studies at the registration stage.

Like the functional organisation structure, organisation according to therapeutic indication is effective and encourages collaboration as long as the individual therapeutic divisions do not become too large. Under these conditions the decision-makers at each level are once again confronted with too many differing problems and too little detailed information at their fingertips, with the ensuing stress, decreasing competence and ethical problems discussed above.

3 Matrix organisation and problems of responsibility

Most large companies have sought to overcome the problems of increasing size in a strongly hierarchical organisation by introducing matrix organisation. This system involves the inclusion as a complement to the vertical, line management, of a horizontal organisation with project management and co-ordination. In the pharmaceutical industry this means that when a drug reaches the stage at which a clear but limited biological profile is available it is assigned to a project team and its leader who reports to a project co-ordinator who also reports to the research and development director. Many of the ethical problems faced under this organisation system, including manager stress and lack of motivation and time, are similar to those faced under the functional organisation structure. However, with the matrix organisation, problems of diffuse responsibility and conflict-of-interest become particularly noticeable.

3.1 Project leader

The project leader is usually appointed by the research and development director on the basis of his/her personality, leadership quality and motivation for the project. For this reason it is usual to select someone who has a personal interest in the compound in question and a desire to push the project. For instance, I was involved in the initial pharmacological studies on an anti-inflammatory compound and had a personal interest in its development. I subsequently became project leader and rapidly found that it was not just important to coordinate effectively the various activities required, but found that I was pinning my own professional career to this compound. A project leader is viewed as the project champion and is encouraged to view the task as a privilege and honour rather than a burden [13]. It is common practice to start a project with a scientist as leader and then to change to a clinician during phase II trials, while the first project leader remains on the team. Many companies now use professional project managers who are responsible for several projects within a distinct project management department and are thus likely to be somewhat more objective about individual projects. They are also likely to have more time for the project than „amateur" project leaders who also have line management functions in addition [13]. Team members are appointed according to expertise and usually include a pharmacologist, chemist, pharmaceutical chemist, analyst, clinician and someone from regulatory affairs. A big advantage of this system is that its flexibility and cooperative nature gives the project team members greater visibility within the company and thereby greater opportunities for career advancement and clear individual motivation.

3.2   Project responsibility

The task of the project team is to co-ordinate the various stages of the development of the drug, to anticipate problems and find their solutions. The advantage of this system over the traditional line management is that it minimizes the number of people involved in the decision-making process while markedly enhancing collaborative teamwork; it is more flexible, because the small project team can rapidly adjust to changes, but it has the disadvantage that the project leader is still dependent on the „good will" of managers in the vertical hierarchy for the performance of tasks which compete with those for other projects. In the final analysis, the success of this organizational structure is very much dependent on the project leader. In this respect, the pressure of responsibility lies with an individual as with functional organisation, but with a clear distinction: the project leader is not solely responsible for the performance of the various tasks associated with the project. For example, the head of pharmacology will be responsible for the quality and speed of animal experiments with the compound, while the head of pharmacokinetics will be responsible for data on absorption of the drug. The project leader, however, will be held responsible by the management for ensuring that everything possible is done to perform each stage of project development within the right department and by the right people at the time planned.

3.3   Conflict-of-interest: line managers vs. project leader

The ethical problems most prominent in matrix organisation are conflict-of-interest issues [6] and nebulous responsibility. The matrix functions by a balance being maintained between hierarchical responsibilities and project responsibilities. I have already commented that the strict hierarchical system is subject to interference from personal ambition and interests. The project leader and the combined project team now offer a challenge to this personal sphere of influence. The line manager is further challenged to maintain priorities which put the company's above personal interests in permitting additional capacity to be taken up within his/her department by project activities or by relinquishing a member of staff as a project leader. Since the line manager is not personally responsible for the project, he/she must be prepared, if necessary, to set aside personal short-term intentions in order to accommodate the project plans. This becomes a particular problem when the project is one which the line manager does not particularly support or approve of. Several times, as project leader, I gained the impression that a line-manager was "stonewalling" my attempts to have an experimental study carried out in his department because he did not believe that the compound had a chance of being developed successfully. Excuses about priorities, lack of capacity or doubts about the value of the planned studies then become effective arguments to stall the project. A common practice is for the line manager to "hide" behind the decision of a strategy committee chairman or research director who has, at some stage, expressed doubts about some aspect of the compound. In such situations the project leader is very much dependent on the moral objectivity of the line manager and his ability to view the planned studies independently of his own personal preference or career. The line manager, as with experts in all disciplines, must overcome narrow-minded vanity; no-one has the whole truth and consideration of others in such a situation – perhaps to one's own detriment – becomes a moral imperative to the success of the project.

3.4   Conflict-of-interest: project leader as line manager

A further conflict of interest arises for the project leader when he/she has a line function in addition to the project-related task. In my experience a successful project tends to take time and energy away from the line management task, with resulting problems among subordinates! On the other hand a project in its early stages or a project which is not running too smoothly can often suffer because the project leader ist spending too much time on routine administration.

In both instances the "tyranny of the urgent" plays an important role – the person involved starts to find he is acting more like a fire-fighter, trying to extinguish conflagrations rather than trying to anticipate where the next fire might break out. In such situations one is presented with a considerable moral dilemma. Do I ensure that the project is pursued with all due speed and attention? Do I invest the time and energy my subordinates require to keep them motivated? Do I concentrate on line managerial activities, administration and meeting? This is a frequent managerial problem [3]. I believe the answer lies in facing up to reality rather than trying to achieve perfection in every area – this is simply humanly impossible! Everyone makes mistakes. I found that trying to live up to my own idealised standards and those I assumed were expected of me from my employer only resulted in stress, poor health and lack of time for my family. This is neither helpful for professional activities nor is it sensible. I found very helpful a clear mental acceptance of the fact that, while seeking to maintain the highest standards of excellence, mistakes would be inevitable and no-one can be expected, by worrying, to avoid making mistakes. Such an attitude is not only healthy but liberating since one is not continually under self-accusation, a very destructive process. It also leads to a more objective analysis of priorities which helps to solve conflicts-of-interests.

3.5   Nebulous responsibility

The other ethical problem with matrix organisation is nebulous responsibility. I have already stated that the project leader is dependent upon line managers for approval of activities in their areas of responsibility. This means that while the project leader is held responsible by senior management for the progress of the project, he/she has no hierarchical authority to enforce project activities. As I said, this situation is coloured to a considerable degree by the moral principles of the line managers. In addition, the project manager may report to various superiors: to his/her line superior for individual department activities, to the project co-ordinator for project activities and to various strategic committees responsible for overseeing and planning projects and programmes. For me this meant continual presentations at meetings, repeating the same things several times for different people. Unless communication between the various superiors is good, the inevitable result is either that no-one is sure who is responsible for what, or that no-one is prepared to take responsibility, but everyone passes the buck. Alternatively, one strong-willed senior manager can ride roughshod over everyone else who ducks his own responsibilities. Ultimately, this leads to frustration for the project leader and damage to the project. In such a matrix system, everyone (or at least the majority) must be prepared to shoulder responsibility in an objective manner, otherwise the whole structure becomes so nebulous that all that is ever done is to talk and procrastinate. Nobody can then point the finger, because no-one has stood up to be pointed at! Everybody is talking to everyone else in an attempt to obtain an informed consensus but no progress is achieved. The organisation balloons, becomes bureaucratic, non-creative and tends towards anarchy [3]. The solution is to keep the organisation in small groups and to encourage decision-makers to have the courage to stand behind their own decisions.

4   Centralisation and the balance of power

A major concern among upper management in all companies is to ensure that decisions are passed down the line rapidly, with maximal effect and minimal waste. In a strict functional organisation, this involves passing down decisions from the top and their implementation by middle and lower management. Two major obstacles have to be overcome: one is to ensure that the decisions are actually implemented in the efficient manner desired (i. e. suitable communication down the hierarchical pyramid) and the second is whether the decisions taken at the top have any relevance to the actual situation at grass roots level (i. e. communication back up the pyramid). In some companies decisions continually come from the top without feedback from lower levels, while in others information is collected from below, but the decisions are not properly communicated back downwards [5]. This is a common complaint among French companies in which decisions are often "allowed to happen" – employees only learning about them once they have become a "fait accompli".

4.1   Geographical flexibility

Centralisation of decision-making has the clear advantage that a relatively small group of experienced top managers are able to maintain an overview of all the company's activities and are thus best able to balance resources and power amongst the various functional groups [14]. However, how can one be sure that the decisions taken by such a small group of people are optimal, since it is humanly impossible for the few top managers to be aware of the different ramifications of local issues or the particular problems in a specific area of the pharmaceutical business, such as basic research? For instance, a centralized organisation based, say, in the United Kingdom cannot possibly be intimately informed about the daily challenges facing the daughter company in, say, India, so that a certain degree of devolving of responsibility must be allowed to maintain the flexibility needed in meeting local demands.

4.2   Functional flexibility

Centralisation not only affects geographical flexibility, it also affects functional flexibility; in other words, the flexibility of specific areas of expertise within the company is restricted. This is particularly true for research. Should one concentrate all research on one centre or distribute activities among several research centres in different geographical locations? Should strategic decisions be taken only by the central organisation or delegated? Is top management capable of making detailed decisions on research or should such responsibility be delegated to those with the necessary expertise? In answering these questions, I am not concerned here so much with the facts or outworking of such organisational structures as with the rights and wrongs of the issues. However, analysis of a variety of highly succesfull US companies has shown that centralisation is not a recipe for success, but rather division into semi-autonomous groups, where individual concerns are emphasised, results in much greater productivity [3].

4.3   Management qualifications

Why should this be so? For a start, top managers tend, for obvious reasons, to be trained in finance rather than in science. It is very difficult to pursuade someone trained to think in economic and market-orientated terms that an analysis of the market for a particular type of drug is not the only method to determine a strategy for new drug development. From bitter experience, I can vouch for the fact that the sound scientific argument that research on a new mechanism might open an as yet unknown drug market, but that this possible market size is difficult to estimate on the basis of known drugs, cuts little or no ice with a market-orientated top manager. I wonder though how they explain the decision to develop the histamine H2-receptor blocker cimetidine and later ranitidine as anti-ulcer drugs when only antacids were known to be effective at the time? In fact, when the search for inhibitors of histamine-stimulated gastric acid secretion was started by Smith, Kline and French in 1964, only one type of receptor for histamine (H1) had been described and gastrin, rather than histamine was regarded as the major hormone controlling gastric acid secretion [15, 16]. In other words, there was absolutely no proven basis for the assumption that just because histamine stimulated acid secretion in the rat, inhibition of histamine action in man would be therapeutically effective, particularly since the predominant opinion was that if any improvement over antacids were to be achieved, gastrin inhibitors would be the most promising candidates. The research management at SKF would seem to have been either open to new ideas and/or they had considerable faith in the capabilities of their own scientists. Alternatively, Sir James Black was so tenacious that he was able to maintain his convictions in the face of failures such as burimamide and metiamide, due to lack of oral activity and agranulocytosis, respectively. Whichever was true, any support from upper management would have been very motivating for the researchers involved.

To be successful in new drug development, upper management in the pharmaceutical industry either must have some understanding of the nature of research, devolve decisions in their area or both. It is surely of no coincidence that Roy Vagelos, the chief executive officer of Merck and Co., the most successful of all drug companies and "America's Most Admired Company", is medically qualified and thus able to understand the challenges and problems facing researchers [17]. Top managers are often recruited from successful companies in other branches of industry or from management consultancies. These people may have no idea about research or how to manage a laboratory. A common and ethically dubious result is that research expertise is acquired by taking over other companies rather than developing in-house research potential.

From an ethical standpoint, it is undoubtedly unjust to penalise an economist-manager for failing to encourage the development of new, profitable drugs when the individual concerned neither has the training nor the experience to understand the long-term, mechanistic attitudes and scientific processes involved in drug research. However, without this knowledge, should he ever have been given such a responsible position? It is folly for a pharmaceutical company to develop a good drug and then sit on its laurels and expect that simply through effective sales techniques and cost management its profits will be sustained. Sooner or later the competition heats up and the euphoria turns to depression. The moral responsibility for the avoidance of such situations lies both with the top managers themselves and with those who appoint them. Just because someone has been able to turn around the fortunes of a car- or soap-manufacturing concern, this is no guarantee of his ability to do so in such a specialised area as drug research. On the other hand, such an appointment might be successful if the manager avoids the ivory tower of his/her plush executive office or jet and listens to the ideas and attitudes of subordinates who have far more specialised knowledge of the problems involved. As I have said before, no-one has a monopoly on the truth and a willingness to learn from others is a far greater guarantee of success that the bull-headed, arrogant determination to demonstrate one's personal prowess at dealing with the problems singlehanded. In fact, a drug stocks analyst recently suggested that the "ego and arrogance" of many senior pharmaceutical executives has made a major contribution to the poor public standing of the industry in the US [18].

4.4   Concentration of personal power

Unfortunately, many top managers are more interested in developing their own personal power base than encouraging initiative and responsibility in their subordinates. Centralisation encourages this concentration of power and does not facilitate delegation. The result is that middle management, while understanding the problems better, are not consulted in the decision-making process and become frustrated as they see good projects destroyed or abandoned for lack of management understanding. Inevitably, the company suffers for lack of innovative products. Short-sightedness, for instance, can lead to the abondonment of a programme because upper management fails to understand that a drug being developed on the basis of a new particular mechanism may not only be therapeutically effective for the initial, primary indication, but is likely to be shown, empirically, to be effective for other therapeutic indications. Once a project has been abondoned, though, it is pointless to cry over spilt milk as no-one can know whether the project would have been successful or not. Fortunately, several examples exist, other than that of James Black, of individual scientists who were able to push through a successful drug in the face of opposition from above.

A rebound effect of such personalized concentration of power is that, whether they realise it or not, upper management can not be certain that the decisions they take are fully carried out at lower management levels because of lack of confidence in the top managers. Particularly in research, where the style of work is less routine and less formalized there is a tendency to rebel against ill-considered management decisions. I have heard it said by a research manager "Go to a meeting to agree about what the upper management is telling you and then go off and do what you consider to be right. Just keep them happy and they won't bother you". In this same company, the chief executive officer called together a meeting of his upper management to find out where the ten greatest problems lay within the company. Over 40% considered personnel management the major problem, which caught him completely off-guard. He hadn't expected the answer because he had become divorced from grass-roots opinions. The result in many cases is that the most creative and energetic of researchers leave, inducing a vicious circle of inconsiderate management, loss of interest and creative potential and thereby poor corporate sales and image.

4.5   Decentralization and the individual

One of the advantages of decentralization of research organisation is that an overloaded, cumbersome, central bureaucracy and service centre is less likely and that it "allows the collaborators to become more autonomic and responsible in the organisation of the everyday life of their research and increases their performance" [19]. Ideas, which I have said are the lifeblood of research, can be most easily tested, because they are better unterstood by those taking the decisions to implement them. Once again, the individual is placed at "stage-centre" and is not just an unnamed cog to be used or dispensed with at the whim of a manager either too "power-hungry" or too "stress-distressed" to appreciate the results of his or her decisions.

4.6   "Small is beautiful"

It is a basic tenet of business that successful companies will grow. However, it is not necessarily true that big companies are successful. The spate of takeovers in the late 1980's and early 1990's is a testament to this fact. Peters and Waterman [3], in their analysis of successful US businesses emphasise that large, successful companies have recognised the importance of dividing into small functional units. This is not only applicable for successful production and sales but also for research. Admittedly, a small research centre which is too diversified in its activities will inevitably be inefficient, with competence thinly spread, attended by chronic understaffing and only superficial experimental investigations being possible, reliance on external institutes being very strong. On the other hand, an excessively large research centre becomes bureaucratic, logistics being cumbersome and decisions being taken very slowly [19]. Project delays become inevitable because it proves impossible either to bring together everyone needed to take a decision or to place, say, a required toxicological study because the available laboratory space is occupied by experiments being run on other projects.

Quite apart from the fact that the development of drugs will inevitably become slower, a giant research centre raises specific ethical questions. Firstly, unless communication is good, depersonalization of the individual employee can arise. Strategic decisions may be taken by senior research managers who are never seen by the ordinary laboratory personnel and whose decisions are inevitably divorced from the day-to-day routine and challenges at the laboratory bench. The laboratory personnel and managers may feel unimportant, their ideas and suggestions unheard and they become distrustful towards superiors and identify less with the company itself. Individual motivation suffers because flexibility and the chances of changing a research approach through the energies and ideas of a single scientist are low. In the worst scenario, the employee finds the lowest common denominator which justifies his appearance at work each day and becomes unwilling to adjust or respond to any extra demands made on his time and capabilities. Because of the large size of the research centre, it is almost always possible to find someone else to perform the required task or, more likely, to find a bureaucratic excuse why the job has not been carried out! It is often the demotivated, disinterested scientist whose initiative and creativity has been crushed by an excessive, suffocating research bureaucracy that has given pharmaceutical industrial research a poor reputation amongst academic colleagues and the media.

The other ethically questionable aspect of a large research centre is that the huge amounts of money being poured into research by the company may not be used efficiently. There is inevitably duplication of effort and of equipment because it is not possible for anyone to have a wide enough overview to decide whether duplication is justifiable or not. Research groups may be running inefficiently with demotivated and poorly qualified staff, but those who know about this are not likely to draw attention to the deficiencies in their departments, while those who are in a position to deal with the wasteful budget administration are too distanced from the situation to know anything about it. The research budget expands and ultimately cuts have to be made. It is then often the highly creative but high risk research groups which are axed while the unobtrusive, inefficient sluggards remain to eat up further budgets!

Smaller research groups are more intimate, encourage cooperation, because most people know each other and whom to ask for advice, permit individuals to make their voices and ideas heard (if they so wish!) and discourage "hangers-on" because they are more easily noticed. Greater flexibility is also ensured, because the whole group can respond to changes and greater contact is possible between managers and staff – though not always, depending on the personalities involved.

5   Conclusions

It is a relatively straightforward (if time-consuming) task to analyse the different approaches taken to the organisation of research in the pharmaceutical industry and describe the theory behind them [10]. Unfortunately, in practice, the picture is always more complicated. As a general rule, the most ethical approach is to build an organizational structure which does not place the unnecessary pressure of an unwieldy size and excessive numbers of decisions on its managers, thereby reducing stress and the tendency towards acquisition of personal power empires and which distributes the load of responsibility more widely. Nevertheless, the success of such an organisation depends on the willingness to take responsibility and to co-operate, where the principle of "give-and-take" is utilised at all levels of the company and where the knowledge and capabilities of colleagues are respected and taken into account.

Any one individual is incapable of taking alone all the decisions with which he or she is confronted. A willingness to accept fallibility both in oneself and in colleagues and subordinates, together with the ability to forgive when toes are trodden upon and to be sufficiently humble to ask for advice when needed are essential attributes for a healthy working atmosphere and a successful team.

This implies that researchers and their managers must take time not just to consider *what* needs to be done, but *why* they should take a particular course of action. "No man is an island", the poet John Donne declared and a readiness to serve others has characterised most great leaders. Scientists are no exception and function most effectively when they recognize that their superiors are doing their best to provide conditions conducive to good research. A well-qualified scientist is no guarantee of good research. Provide clear goals and the means to reach them, but don't forget that the scientist needs to accept the reasons behind the goals and to approve of the means to achieve them in order to be motivated. A scientist or manager who finds it difficult to accept that a course of action is right will inevitably drag his or her feet on the issue. Perhaps this may eventually mean a change in employment, but that is better than a disillusioned colleague.

Even acceptance of such principles is not always sufficient. Knowing what to do is one thing, the readiness to act upon these ethical principles – even when short-term personal and economic benefits are not visible – is another.

Acknowledgements

I am very grateful to Dr. Bert Spilker and Dr. Erich Graf for their critical comments on the draft manuscript.

References

1 J. L. Graner: Lancet *II*, 150 (1989).
2 K. M. Leisinger: Management Wissen *1*, 100–103 (1990)
3 T. J. Peters and R. H. Waterman Jr: In Search of Excellence, Harper & Row, New York 1982.
4 J. F. Cavalla: Trends Pharmacol. Sci. *1*, 225–227 (1980).
5 B. Spilker: Drug News Perspect. *5*, 236–246 (1992).
6 B. Spilker: Drug News Perspect. *5*, 561–571 (1992).
7 M.J. Parnham: Drug News Perspect. *6*, 123–128 (1993).
8 P. Vardy: Business Morality, Marshall Pickering, London, 1989, pp 58–74.
9 M. Funk and T. Terzani: Der Spiegel *48*, 154–164 (1989).
10 B. Spilker: Multinational Drug Companies. Issues in Drug Discovery and Development, Raven Press, New York, 1989, pp 213–215.
11 M. Koltai, D. Hosford, G. Guinot, A. Esanu and P. Braquet: Drugs *42*, 174–204 (1991).
12 M. Pretolani, P. Ferrer-Lopez and B. B. Vargaftig: Biochem. Pharmacol. *38*, 1373–1384 (1989).
13 Ref. 10, pp 255–267.
14 Ref. 10, pp 119–134.
15 M. Ennis and W. Lorenz: in: Haemodynamics, Hormones and Inflammation. Discoveries in Pharmacology, ed. M. J. Parnham, J. Bruinvels, Elsevier, Amsterdam, *2*, 623–645 (1984).
16 J. Black. Science 245, 486–493 (1989).
17 G. Bock: TIME Magazine, pp 30–31. February 22, 1988.
18 Anon: SCRIP No. 1806, p 13, March 26, 1993.
19 G. Bartholini: in: Decision Making in Drug Research. ed., F. Gross, Raven Press, New York, 1983, pp 123–139.

Progress in Drug Research, Vol. 42
Edited by Ernst Jucker
© 1994 Birkhäuser Verlag Basel (Switzerland)

Luteinizing hormone regulators: Luteinizing hormone releasing hormone analogs, estrogens, opiates, and estrogen-opiate hybrids

By Vera M. Kolb

Department of Chemistry, University of Wisconsin-Parkside, Kenosha, Wisconsin 53141, USA

1   Introduction

This chapter deals with certain aspects of luteinizing hormone (LH) regulation. LH is a large glycoprotein which is secreted from the anterior pituitary [1]. The mechanism of action of LH is very complex. LH is a part of a hormonal cascade [2]. Luteinizing hormone releasing hormone (LHRH), also known as gonadotropin releasing hormone (GnRH), a decapeptide produced in the hypothalamus, controls release of LH and follicle stimulating hormone (FSH) from pituitary to general circulation. LH and FSH are known as gonadotropins, since they act on gonads of both sexes. In the gonads they regulate gamete maturation and the production of sex hormones. For example, in males LH stimulates testosterone synthesis and secretion from testes. In females it acts on corpus luteum of ovary to increase production and release of progesterone. LH triggers ovulation. FSH promotes spermatogenesis in testes and production of estradiol in ovaries.

LH regulation is extremely complex. The entire hormonal cascade is regulated via feedback loops [2]. In addition, endogenous opioid peptides (EOP) are involved in LH regulation, via their inhibitory effect on LHRH [3].

Design of drugs to regulate LH as a part of the hormonal cascade is a great challenge. The purpose of this chapter is to describe the influence on LH level of selected synthetic drugs or potential drugs. They are non-endogenous analogs of LHRH, opiates, estrogens, and opiate-estrogen hybrids. Some of these compounds are in the clinical phase of testing as LH regulators, while some may still be in the in vitro stage of investigation. However, we shall term them all as drugs.

2   Background literature

In this section we provide some key references, reviews in particular, on the general topic of this chapter. In the subsequent sections we give references which are more specific and more narrow in their scope. Regulation of LHRH and thus LH with opiates has been subject of numerous reviews [3–15], which have, however, different emphasis. Jaffe et al. [4] emphasized that LHRH release is regulated by a complex interaction of opioids, steroids, catecholamines and other neurotransmitters. Vobis and Gruen [5] review the role of endogenous opiates on gonadotropin secretion as it pertains to farm animals. Genazzani and Petraglia [3] emphasize opioid control of LH secretion in children, women during the ovarian cycle, and postmenopausal women. Negro-Vilar et al. [7] review the regulation of LH by LHRH in the absence of gonadal steroids, and by opiates under conditions of vanishing gonadal steroid input. Kalra and Kalra [8] discuss regulation of LHRH with endogenous opioids, gonadal steroids, and catecholamines. Malven [10] reviewed endogenous opioid inhibition of LH release which is reversible by action of opiate antagonist naloxone, and discussed mechanisms and receptor subtypes for this inhibition. Cicero reviewed the effects of opiate agonist morphine and antagonist naloxone on LH [12] and the role of opiate mediated LH control in the development of narcotic tolerance and dependence [13]. The estrogen-opiate-LH connection in the context of this chapter is examined in the brain. Thus, references related to the estrogen and opiate receptors in the brain are relevant.

Steroid receptors in the central nervous system are reviewed by Freeman and Breedlove [16]. Molecular mechanisms of action of steroid hormones are reviewed by O'Malley et al. [17]. Muldoon and Watson address steroid hormone receptor functionality in the brain and anterior pituitary [18]. Bettini et al. [19] established the structural identity among the estrogen receptor (ER) mRNA expressed in the hypocampus, hypothalamus, and uterus. The greatest density of ER mRNA neurons is in hypothalamus, as shown by an in situ hybridization study by Simerly et al. [20].

Opioid receptors and their endogenous and non-endogenous ligands are reviewed by Pleuvry [21]. Enkephalins, endorphins, and dynorphins are endogenous peptides. They are derived from prohormones proenkephalin, pro-opiomelancortin, and prodynorphin, respectively. These prohormones are coded by mRNAs derived from three separate genes. Beta-endorphin and [Met]enkephalin bind to mu receptors (not selectively), [Leu]enkephalin is selective for delta receptors, while dynorphins interact preferentially with kappa receptors. The existence or specificity of epsilon and sigma opioid receptors, and mu1, mu2, kappa1 and kappa2 opioid receptor subtypes is controversial. Unnatural ligands exist which are specific agonists or antagonists to various opioid receptor subtypes, such as DADLE (delta agonist), ICI 174864 (delta antagonist), norbinaltrophimine (kappa antagonist), etc.

More about these will be said in the subsequent sections of this chapter. Mu and delta receptors are capable of interconverting. The activation of one receptor changes the affinity of the other. While both mu and delta receptors appear to be coupled to potassium channels, kappa receptors are coupled with calcium channels. Mu opioid receptors are distributed widely. In the brain, they are most dense in the areas associated with pain regulation. Delta receptors are distributed less widely than mu. Kappa receptors are found mainly in the areas associated with pain perception, and also water and food intake. Opiate-estrogen connection is established at the receptor level. A series of estrogenic steroids has been found to specifically bind to opiate receptors in the brain by LaBella et al. [22]. Vertes et al. [23] studied naloxone and estradiol binding in the rat estrogen sensitive tissues, uterus and hypothalamus. Specific naloxone binding was found in both tissues. The densities of naloxone binding sites in hypothalamus are decreased by treatment with estrogen or estrogen plus progesterone [24]. While the receptor density of the mu opioid receptors in hypothalamus is decreased by estradiol plus progesterone, the affinity constant of the receptor for a mu ligand is not changed [25].

3   LHRH agonists and antagonists as LH regulators

LHRH is released by the hypothalamus. It reaches pituitary via a portal system. In the pituitary it stimulates the release of LH.
As opposed to LH, which is a very large glycoprotein, LHRH is a decapeptide. Thus, LHRH is more amenable to drug design than LH. Chemical features and structure-activity relationships of LHRH have been reviewed by Conn et al. [26] and Karten and Rivier [27]. Conn et al. [26] also address in depth all the aspects of LHRH receptor structure and function and the molecular mechanism of LHRH action on pituitary.
The primary structure of LHRH is pyro-Glu-His-Trp-Ser-Tyr-Gly-Leu-Arg-Pro-Gly-NH2. The cyclic conformation in which the two termini interact appears to be both the most stable and biologically active [28].
The drug design efforts were directed toward synthesis of LHRH analogs stable against enzymatic degradation, super agonists, and antagonists.

The two LHRH termini are crucial for the binding to the receptor. The enzymatic termination of LHRH action occurs by cleavage of the peptide bond adjacent to the sixth residue. When the latter is substituted with a D-amino acid containing bulky, hydrophobic groups, enzymatic stability is achieved. Since a beta-turn in the molecule characterizes the biologically active conformation, substituents which stabilize this turn enhance the activity [26].

A very interesting feature of LHRH agonist action is a rather dramatic difference in acute vs chronic administration. In the former administration the agonists induce the synthesis and release of LH, as expected. The chronic administration, however, leads to suppression of LH due to the receptor down-regulation [29]. This further translates to a decrease of the levels of sex steroids, a property exploited for therapeutic purposes [26, 29]. A problem arises in the treatment with LHRH agonists, since the desired gonadotropin suppression is accompanied by their initial surge. Thus, the need arises for LHRH antagonists, which should be devoid of these problems, since they would suppress gonadotropins all the way from the beginning throughout the treatment.

In contrast to successful development of LHRH agonist drugs, such as buserelin, leuprolide, and nafarelin [26], the LHRH antagonist drugs development lags behind. This is due in part to the side effect to release histamine [29].

Very creative and interesting examples of design of LHRH antagonists are given in references 29–31. De et al. [31] worked on a series of non-peptide competitors for the pituitary LHRH receptor. The lead compound was the antifungal drug ketoconazole, which exhibits weak but competitive binding affinity to LHRH receptor. Structure-activity relationship of the ketoconazole series was established. Structure-activity relationship in the peptide series of LHRH antagonists is still being explored [26, 29, 30]. Antagonistic action is generally promoted by substitution of D-amino acids at positions 1, 2, 3 [26] and 10 [29]. Conversion of LHRH agonists to antagonists was effected by specific N-methyl substitution in the peptide backbone; this was established by a systematic substitution of each peptide bond in leuprolide, deslorelin, and nafarelin by N-methyl [30]. This work also contributed to the understanding of bioactive conformation of LHRH analogs, which was shown not to be a simple type II' beta turn as postulated earlier. This was demonstrated by surprisingly high receptor affinities of several agonists and antagonists strategically methylated at the positions in which the N-methyl group would interfere with the beta turn. The extension of methylation study on antagonists was equally fruitful. The N-methylation of residue 5 (Tyr) in a series of LHRH antagonists yielded potent, water-soluble compounds [29]. These effects were ascribed to the peptide conformation which favors the bioactive conformation, and interacts better with the aqueous environment. It was also found that the beta turn of the antagonists differs from that of the agonists.

In summary of this section, the results on non-endogenous LHRH agonists and antagonists show that it is possible to design drugs to regulate LH by modifying another part of the hormonal cascade, in this case LHRH.

4   Estrogens as LH regulators

Regulation of LH via endogenous estrogens is very complicated. The negative feedback of estradiol involves different mechanisms for the central (brain) and peripheral (pituitary) systems [32]. Estrogens mediate regulation of LHRH system primarily via estrogen receptive interneurons; most LHRH neurons are not directly estrogen responsive [33].

The overall sequence of events involves interaction of estrogens with their receptors in the brain. These receptors are nuclear and cytoplasmic. This was shown by staining in the brain cell nuclei and cytoplasm in an immunocytochemical study using three antibodies directed against different epitopes on the estrogen receptor protein [34]. The neural estrogen receptors undergo different conformational changes when bound to estrogen agonists and antagonists. This was suggested by Etgen and Robisch [35] who found that the nuclear estrogen receptors from brain were extracted more easily by both ionic agents and DNA intercalators following injection of estrogen antagonist tamoxifen than of estradiol. The relationship between estrogens and their brain receptors is not static, since circulating estrogens suppress the biosynthesis of the estrogen receptors by reducing the levels of estrogen receptor mRNA [36].

In this section we discuss the effects of selected non-endogenous estrogens [37–39] and estrogen derivatives which carry a chemical attachment which enhances brain delivery [40–43].

Most steroids do not have any problems reaching the brain, due to their lipophilicity which enables them to pass the blood-brain barrier (BBB). Estrogens would be useful drugs for decreasing the LH levels if their brain-peripheral equilibrium maximizes the brain concentration and minimizes the peripheral concentration which is responsible for unwanted side effects [42]. Another approach would be to try to minimize the peripheral side effects by using weak estrogens or partial estrogen agonists/antagonists while hopefully achieving sufficient brain effect on LH.

RU 16117 is an orally active weak estrogen which is a partial estrogen the LH response to LHRH. Low doses which block ovulation by 100% have no effect on vaginal cornification. This indicates a greater sensitivity at the hypothalamus/pituitary than on the periphery. In postmenopausal women RU 16117 decreased LH levels and alleviated hot flushes symptoms.

A series of methylestrogens [39] have been found to bind to cytoplasmic estrogen receptors in hypothalamic, pituitary and uterine tissues of the ovariectomized rat. The capacity of these compounds to translocate in vivo estrogen receptors into the cell nuclei of pituitary and uterine tissues varied according to dosage in both tissues: higher dosage yielded higher potency. Perhaps some manipulation of the dosage levels could transform these compounds into useful LH regulators.

A very successful and creative work on redox-based chemical delivery system for estrogens [40–42] led to novel LH regulators. A dihydronicotinate conjugate of an estrogen is made first. This conjugate undergoes in vivo enzyme-catalyzed oxidation to give a nicotinate salt, which is quickly eliminated from the systemic circulation but is trapped in the brain since it cannot easily cross the BBB. The nicotinate salt is slowly hydrolized in the brain and releases estrogens. As a net result, the estrogen is delivered to the brain, while its peripheral action is minimized. This unique chemical delivery system was applied also to other drugs [42, 43], notably progesterone [43]. A series of estrogens derivatized with the chemical delivery moiety was evaluated for its effects on LH [40, 41]. It was found that these compounds suppressed LH levels over a long period of time, which testifies for a prolonged release of estrogen in the brain. No significant peripheral estrogenic effects were observed. Thus, these drugs appear to be potentially very useful as LH regulators.

Anti-estrogens stimulate LHRH secretion from hypothalamus by interfering with the negative feedback of estradiol. This property has lead to their well-known use in ovulation induction; clomiphene citrate is a drug clinically used for this purpose. Its action, however, does not seem to be mediated by EOP [38].

5   Opiates as LH regulators

Effects of opiates which bind specifically to mu, delta, and kappa opioid receptors on the secretion of LH have been studied extensively. Leadem and Yagenova [44] found that the mu agonist DAGO suppressed the LH secretion in ovariectomized rats. DPDPE, a delta agonist, and U 50488 H, a kappa agonist, also suppressed LH but only at high doses. Pfeiffer et al. [45] also found that DAGO suppresses LH, but found no significant effects of DTE12, a delta agonist, and MRZ, a kappa agonist, at equivalent doses. In another study Pfeiffer et al. [46] found that MR 2034, a kappa agonist, suppressed LH levels, while another kappa agonist, MRZ 2549, had no effect on the LH levels. Pretreatment with beta-FNA, a highly selective mu antagonist, blocked the action of mu agonists morphine and DAGO as well as MR 2034. It appears that mu receptors are involved predominantly in LH secretion. Weaker effects of delta agonists could be related to relatively small number of delta receptors in the hypothalamus.

The effects of opiate antagonists on LH secretion also indicate predominant role of mu receptors. Panerai et al. [47] found that naloxone, a predominantly mu antagonist, and MR 1452, a kappa antagonist, affect LH concentrations, while a delta antagonist, ICI 154129 does not. However, Wiesner et al. [48] found that ICI 154129 blocked the suppressive effect of beta endorphine on LH levels. The mu antagonists naloxazone and beta-FNA had no effect. This study indicated mediation of LH release by delta receptors. Dyer et al. [49] compared the action of MR 2266, a primarily mu and kappa antagonist, and naloxone on estrogen-stimulated LH surges in ovariectomized rats. These surges can be inhibited by opiates and potentiated by blocking the opiates. At higher doses naloxone increased the size of LH surge while MR 2266 did not.

However, at small doses the reverse was true. It seems that at the present time the role of the delta and kappa receptors needs to be considered in LH regulation, because of the sometimes contradictory data on these receptors.

Influence of opiate antagonist naltrexone on LH was studied thoroughly. It was found that the receptors which mediate the acute effects of naltrexone on LH secretion are central and stereoselective [50]. This was established by using both enantiomers of naltrexone, dextro and levo, and quaternized naltrexone. Levo enantiomer of naltrexone elevated the LH levels in very small doses, while the dextro isomer was largely inactive. The combined results prove the stereoselectivity of the receptors involved. A lipophobic quaternized naltrexone derivative evoked no LH responses upon an intravenous injection, but increased the LH levels upon intracerebroventricular injection, indicating the central action. Other opiate antagonists were studied, for example WIN 44441-3 [51] and nalmefene [52, 53]. Quaternized nalmefene, which does not cross the BBB, was also studied to elucidate the site of the opioid influence on secretion of LH from the anterior pituitary [54]. The quaternized nalmefene was ineffective in blocking morphine-induced antinociceptive responses, but was effective in blocking morphine-induced LH suppression. The latter result indicated mediation by receptors located outside the BBB. Novel opiate antagonists, 14 beta substituted morphines and morphinans, led to orally active LH stimulators [55, 56].

Cicero et al. studied various aspects of the control of LH secretion by opiates in the male rats. Out of a long and very significant series of papers we just quote a selected few [57–60]. Naloxone has been shown not to reverse the inhibitory effect of morphine on LH secretion in the prepubescent rats, in contrast to full reversal of his effect in adult animals [57]. This naloxone-irreversible effect of morphine was specific to LH, since naloxone successfully antagonized other effects of morphine, such as other neuroendocrine effects and its analgesic activity. These results indicate the complex involvement of EOP system in sexual maturation. Opiate antagonists do not increase LH levels in the prepubescent rat, but with the onset of puberty they become effective [58]. Difference has been found in the young and adult animal sensitivity to action of mu, kappa, and delta agonists and antagonists on LH. For example, kappa antagonists are not active in young animals, but increase LH in adults [58]. In the male rats naloxone and naltrexone increase LH levels, but not via a testosterone-dependent mechanism [59]. Narcotic antagonists do not displace testosterone from its receptors, and vice versa [60].

In summary of this section, a myriad of opiate agonists and antagonists exists which acts at different opioid receptors and affect LH levels differently. The experimental results of different research groups are sometimes difficult to compare, due to different animal models used, different stages of hormonal cycle, or different doses and mode of administration. However, the biggest problem may be the unwanted side effects of opioids. The answer to a successful opiate drug for LH regulation is perhaps a very specific mix of opioid receptor subtype affinities, coupled with relatively low activity, to avoid acute perturbations of other EOP functions.

6   Estrogen-opiate hybrids as LH regulators

Steroid-opiate hybrids were synthesized in which the steroid moiety is androstene dione, pregnenolone or estrone, and the opiate moiety is oxymorphone, an opiate agonist, or opiate antagonists naloxone or naltrexone [61–63]. The chemical linkage between the steroid and opiate moiety is the azine, which comprises of $C=N$-$N=C$ unit. While the azine moiety allows flexibility around the N-N single bond, it also imposes geometric restrictions due to the existence of four possible isomers, syn-syn, anti-anti, anti-syn, and syn-anti [64]. Stereochemistry of steroid-opiate hybrids has been determined by C-13 NMR [64] and X-ray crystallographic technique [61]. The interaction of these hybrids with the opiate receptors was measured [62, 63] and molecular modeling of their receptor binding sites was performed [65]. In this chapter we concentrate on naltrexone-estrone azine, EH-NX. The name EH-NX denotes the mode of preparation of this compound; i.e., from estrone hydrazone, EH, and naltrexone, NX [64]. EH is a hydrazine with an anti configuration. EH-NX is assigned an anti-anti configuration [61].

Naloxone analog of EH-NX, EH-NAL, was initially prepared and was studied extensively. Obviously, EH-NX and EH-NAL are very closely related and many of their effects are almost the same.

EH-NX and EH-NAL are opiate antagonists which cause a prolonged blockade of mu receptors in vitro. The long-lasting effect is probably due to the bulky steroid moiety which causes "locking" of the drug to the receptor [63]. EH-NAL shows selectivity towards delta receptors. Its affinity for the mu receptor is 10 times less as compared to naloxone, but its affinity for the delta receptor is 7 times larger. When tested against DALE, a delta agonist, EH-NAL is 9 times more potent than naloxone. EH-NAL is 22 times less potent than naloxone at the mu receptor, tested against normorphine, a mu agonist. EH-NX is assumed to have similar delta selectivity as EH-NAL. EH-NX is a pure opiate antagonist in vivo, as shown in the mouse tail-flick test [66]. It was found that EH-NX reduces body weights among rats [67] which could imply its central estrogenic activity [68].

EH-NX effects on LH secretion were studied [69–71]. The effects of EH-NX on pituitary LH secretion in ovariectomized (OVX) rats are different than those caused by either of its components, EH and NX, or their combination, and were not obvious [70]. EH-NX was found to behave as an estrogen and not like an opiate antagonist. No stim-ulatory effect on LH secretion was observed with EH-NX in estra-diol-3-benzoate (EB) primed OVX rats. Inhibition of LH secretion and uterine proliferation were observed in rats treated chronically with EH-NX. Both central and peripheral effects appear to be the result of estrogenic activity of EH-NX. However, EH-NX has an interesting pharmacological profile; the data suggest a faster transport and/or binding of EH-NX to the estrogen receptors in the hypothalamus and/or the pituitary, as compared to EB and EH. The NX component of the hybrid is likely a cause of a faster brain intake of EH-NX. The suppression of LH levels occurs within 20 minutes, time more charac-teristic for opiate brain effects than those of estrogens; the latter is typically 40–60 minutes.

EH-NX has also been shown to have estrogenic activity at the level of the pituitary gland [71]. The EH-NX effect starts more rapidly than that of EB or EH. Again, faster uptake and/or transport of EH-NX as compared to that for EB and EH is observed.

EH-NX thus inhibits LH secretion both by a direct effect on the pituitary and indirectly via inhibition of LHRH secretion at the hypothalamic level. The negative pituitary effect is partially blocked by NX, suggesting the involvement of the EOP.

In summary, EH-NX is a hybrid drug in which the estrogenic moiety exerts a predominant effect on LH secretion. The NX part of the molecule appears to act as a carrier to the brain, leading to a fast action of this drug.

Modification of the estrogenic moiety of EH-NX to diminish the estrogenic activity may reverse the estrogen-opiate character of

EH-NX. Such a drug may cause stimulation of LH in hypoestrogenic conditions, without the addition of gonadal steroids.

7   Perspective

Progress has been made in understanding the mechanism of LH secretion within the hormonal cascade and a broader system which includes EOP. Numerous potential drugs exist. However, most of them are still in the in vitro basic research stage. Some LHRH analogs are developed as drugs for human use. This particular class of compounds yields the most promising results at the present time.

References

1   A. Korolkovas: "Essentials of Medicinal Chemistry", Second Ed., Wiley-Interscience, New York, 1988, pp. 1005–1009.
2   G. Litwack: "Biochemistry of Hormones. I. Peptide Hormones", in: T. M. Devlin, Ed., "Biochemistry with Clinical Correlation", Third Ed., Wiley-Liss, New York, 1992, pp. 848–858, 876–881.
3   A. R. Genazzani and F. Petraglia: J. Steroid Biochem., 33, 751–755 (1989).
4   R. B. Jaffe, S. Plosker, L. Marshall, and M. C. Martin: Am. J. Obstet. Gynecol., 163, 1727–1731 (1990).
5   V. Vobis and E. Gruen: Montsh. Veterinaermed., 45, 844–848 (1990).
6   A. N. Brooks, G. E. Lamming, and N. B. Haynes: Res. Vet. Sci., 41, 285–299 (1986).
7   A. Negro-Vilar, M. D. Culler, and C. Masotto: J. Steroid Biochem., 25, 741–747 (1986).
8   S. P. Kalra and P. S. Kalra: "Hypothalamic microenvironment controlling LHRH secretion", in: K. W. Kerns, A. Aakvaag, and V. Hansson, Eds.: "Regul. Target Cell Responsiveness", Vol. 2, Plenum, New York, 1984, pp. 127–155.
9   S. P. Kalra and C. A. Leadem: "Control of luteinizing hormone secretion by endogenous opioid peptides", in: G. Delitala, M. Motta, and M. Serio, Eds.: "Opioid Modulation Endocr. Funct.", Raven, New York, 1984, pp. 171–184.
10   P. V. Malven: Domest. Anim. Endocrinol., 3, 135–144 (1986).
11   A. Loviselli, S. Balzano, E. Atzeni, E. Lai, A. M. G. Farci, P. Farci, and A. Balestrieri: Rass. Med. Sarda, 88, 447–456 (1985).
12   T. J. Cicero: NIDA Res. Monogr., 55, 14–23 (1985).
13   T. J. Cicero: NIDA Res. Monogr., 54, 184–208 (1984).
14   R. J. Bicknell: J. Endocrinol., 107, 437–446 (1985).
15   E. DelPozo: Recent Adv. Clin. Biochem., 3, 177–193 (1985).
16   L. M. Freeman and S. M. Breedlove: Methods in Neurosciences, 11, 1–15 (1993).
17   B. W. O'Malley, S. Y. Tsai, M. Bagchi, N. L. Weigel, W. T. Schrader, and M.-J. Tsai: Recent Progress in Hormone Res., 47, 1–26 (1991).
18   T. G. Muldoon and G. H. Watson: "Steroid hormone receptor functionality in the brain and anterior pituitary", in: I. Cummings, Ed., "Endocrinol. Proc. Int. Congr. Endocrinol., 6th", Elsevier, Amsterdam, 1980, pp. 106–109.

19 E. Bettini, G. Pollio, S. Santagati, and A. Maggi: Neuroendocrinology, 56, 502–508 (1992).
20 R. B. Simerly, C. Chang, M. Muramatsu, and L. W. Swanson: J. Comp. Neurol., 294, 76–95 (1990).
21 B. J. Pleuvry: Br. J. Anaesth., 66, 370–380 (1991), and the references cited therein.
22 F. S. LaBella, R.-S. S. Kim, and J. Templeton: Life Sci., 23, 1797–1804 (1978).
23 M. Vertes, Z. Pamer, and J. Garai: J. Steroid Biochem., 24, 235–238 (1986).
24 N. G. Weiland and P. M. Wise: Endocrinology, 126, 804–808 (1990).
25 R. Maggi, P. Limonta, D. Dondi, and F. Piva: Pharmacol. Res., 91–92 (1989).
26 P. M. Conn, W. R. Huckle, W. V. Andrews, and C. A. McArdle: Recent Progress in Hormone Res., 43, 29–68 (1987), and the references cited therein.
27. M. J. Karten and J. E. Rivier: Endocr. Rev., 7, 44–46 (1986).
28 F. A. Momany: J. Amer. Chem. Soc., 98, 2990–2995 (1976).
29 F. Haviv, T. D. Fitzpatrick, C. J. Nichols, R. E. Swenson, N. A. Mort, E. N. Bush, G. Diaz, A. T. Nguyen, M. R. Holst, V. A. Cybulski, J. A. Leal, G. Bammert, N. S. Rhutasel, P. W. Dodge, E. S. Johnson, J. B. Cannon, J. Knittle, and J. Greer: J. Med. Chem., 36, 928–933 (1993), and the references cited therein.
30 F. Haviv, T. D. Fitzpatrick, R. E. Swenson, C. J. Nichols, N. A. Mort, E. N. Bush, G. Diaz, G. Bammert, A. Nguyen, N. S. Rhutasel, H. N. Nellans, D. J. Hoffman, E. S. Johnson, and J. Greer: J. Med. Chem., 36, 363–369 (1993), and the references cited therein.
31 B. De, J. J. Plattner, E. N. Bush, H.-S. Jae, G. Diaz, E. S. Johnson, and T. J. Perun: J. Med. Chem., 32, 2036–2038 (1989).
32 C. A. Johnston, M. Tesone, and A. Negro-Vilar: Braz. J. Med. Biol. Res., 18, 125–130 (1985).
33 R. E. Watson, Jr., M. C. Langub, Jr., and J. W. Landis: J. Neuroendocrinol., 4, 311–317 (1992).
34 J. D. Blaustein: Endocrinology, 131, 1336–1342 (1992).
35 A. M. Etgen and D. M. Robisch: Brain Res., 452, 1–10 (1988).
36 R. B. Simerly and B. J. Young: Mol. Endocrinol., 5, 424–432 (1991).
37 J. P. Raynaud, G. Azadian-Boulanger, M. M. Bouton, M. C. Colin, N. Faure, L. Fernand-Proul, J. P. Gautray, J. M. Husson, A. Jolivet, P. Kelly, F. Labrie, T. Ojasso and G. Précigoux: J. Steroid Biochem., 20, 981–993 (1984).
38 S. J. Judd, J. Alderman, J. Bowden, and L. Michailov: Fertil. Steril., 47, 574–578 (1987).
39 J. Kirchhoff, X. Wang, R. Ghraf, P. Ball, and R. Knuppen: Brain Res., 294, 354–358 (1984).
40 M. E. Brewster, K. S. Estes, and N. Bodor: J. Med. Chem., 31, 244–249 (1988).
41 W. R. Anderson, J. W. Simpkins, M. E. Brewster, and N. Bodor: Life Sci., 42, 1493–1502 (1988).
42 N. Bodor: "Novel site-specific chemical drug delivery system", in: E. Mutschler and E. Winterfeldt, Ed., "Trends in Medicinal Chemistry", VCH, New York, 1987, pp. 195–210.
43 M. E. Brewster, N. Deyrup, K. Czako, and N. Bodor: J. Med. Chem., 33, 2063–2065 (1990).
44 C. A. Leadem and S. V. Yagenova: Neuroendocrinology, 45, 109–117 (1987).
45 D. G. Pfeiffer, A. Pfeiffer, Y. Shimohigashi, G. R. Merriam, and D. L. Loriaux: Peptides, 4, 647–649 (1983).
46 D. G. Pfeiffer, A. Pfeiffer, O. F. X. Almeida, and A. Herz: J. Endocrinol., 114, 469–476 (1987).

47 A. E. Panerai, F. Petraglia, P. Sacerdote, and A. R. Genazzani: Endocrinology, 117, 1096–1099 (1985).
48 J. B. Wiesner, J. I. Koenig, L. Krulich, and P. L. Moss: Endocrinology, 116, 475–477 (1985).
49 R. G. Dyer, S. Mansfield, and A. D. P. Dean: Neurosci. Lett., 49, 111–115 (1984).
50 M. S. Blank, D. R. Mann, D. T. Daugherty, T. Dwayne, R. Sridiran, and J. R. Murphy: Life. Sci., 39, 1493–1499 (1986).
51 C. S. Whisnant and R. L. Goodman: Biol. Reprod., 39, 1032–1038 (1988).
52 P. Limonta, C. W. Bardin, E. F. Hahn, and R. B. Thau: Steroids, 46, 955–965 (1985).
53 D. A. Van Vugt, M. Y. Webb, and R. L. Reid: Neuroendocrinology, 49, 275–280 (1989).
54 J. W. Simpkins, D. Swager, and W. J. Millard: Neuroendocrinology, 54, 384–390 (1991).
55 L. Revesz, R. A. Siegel, H. H. Buescher, M. Marko, R. Maurer, and H. Meigel: Helv. Chim. Acta, 73, 326–336 (1990).
56 R. A. Siegel and L. Revesz: J. Pharmacol. Exp. Ther., 249, 265–270 (1989).
57 T. J. Cicero, B. Nock, and L. O'Connor: J. Pharmacol. Exp. Ther., 264, 47–53 (1993), and the references cited therein.
58 T. J. Cicero, E. R. Meyer, B. T. Miller, and R. D. Bell: J. Pharmacol. Exp. Ther., 246, 14–20 (1988), and the references cited therein.
59 T. J. Cicero, C. E. Wilcox, R. D. Bell, and E. R. Meyer: J. Pharmacol. Exp. Ther., 212, 573–578 (1980).
60 T. J. Cicero, R. D. Bell, E. R. Meyer, and C. E. Wilcox: "Narcotic antagonists increase serum luteinizing hormone levels by a nontestosterone-dependent mechanism", in E. L. Way, Ed.: "Endog. Exog. Opiate Agonists Antagonists", Pergamon, Elmsford, New York, 1980, pp. 421–424.
61 V. M. Kolb, D. H. Hua, and W. L. Duax: J. Org. Chem., 52, 3003–3010 (1987), and the references cited therein.
62 A. Koman, V. M. Kolb, and L. Terenius: Pharmaceutical Res., 4, 147–149 (1987), and the references cited therein.
63 A. Koman, V. M. Kolb, and L. Terenius: Pharmaceutical Res., 3, 56–60 (1986).
64 V. M. Kolb and D. H. Hua: J. Org. Chem., 49, 3824–3828 (1984).
65 V. M. Kolb and J. P. Snyder: NIDA Res. Monogr., 75, 41–44 (1986).
66 M. D. Aceto, E. R. Bowman, L. S. Harris, and E. L. May: NIDA Res. Monogr., 90, 468–515 (1989).
67 V. M. Kolb: "Prospects for Developing More Specific Opioid Antagonists", in L. D. Reid, Ed.: "Opioids, Bulimia and Alcohol Abuse and Alcoholism", Springer Verlag, New York and Berlin, 1990, pp. 281–288.
68 V. M. Kolb: "Opiate receptors: Search for new drugs", Progress in Drug Res., 36, 49–70 (1991).
69 M. C. Armeanu: "Opioid Antagonists and Gonadotropin Secretion", PhD Dissertation, Vrije University, Amsterdam, The Netherlands, 1991, ISBN 90-900-4608-9.
70 M. C. Armeanu, J. A. M. J. van Dieten, V. M. Kolb, J. Schoemaker, and J. de Koning: Life Sci., 50, 913–921 (1992).
71 M. C. Armeanu, J. A. M. J. van Dieten, V. M. Kolb, J. Schoemaker, and J. de Koning: Life Sci., 52, 1311–1318 (1993).

Progress in Drug Research, Vol. 42
Edited by Ernst Jucker
© 1994 Birkhäuser Verlag Basel (Switzerland)

53

Natural products as anticancer agents

By Shradha Sinha and Sudha Jain

Medical Chemistry Division, Central Drug Research Institute, Lucknow 226 001, India, and Department of Chemistry Lucknow University, Lucknow 226 007, India

1   Introduction

Cancer is perhaps one of the most active anti-human factor operating in the world today, and efforts are being made all over the scientific world to prevent and eradicate it. All possible avenues are being tapped; from the most obvious to the least probable sources are under study.

It may appear a little ridiculous when we turn to the world of vegetation for the cure of this dreaded monster. But our ancient lore has many instances where incurable and inexplicable diseases were cured by the use of such drugs (in India the famous Hindu religious book Ramayan describes that when Lakshman faints, Hanuman is despatched to fetch the plant for his cure).

New agents with chemotherapeutic value in the fight against cancer is obviously a medical problem of high importance to modern man. But the development of new drugs in the cancer field is a difficult task given that anticancer agents must be lethal to, or incapacitate tumor cells, but they should not do excessive damage to normal cells. At present the state of knowledge in cancer biology and in medical chemistry does not warrant the designing of new classes of molecules which may be effective antitumor agents. Despite the great progress made in cancer biology, molecular pharmacology, pharmacokinetics, medical chemistry and allied fields, the knowledge sought after, is still elusive and may defy our past for many years to come. Theoretical researchers and the empiricists are at variance with each other. It is only to be hoped that in due course these differences will disappear.

Since the concept of chemotherapeutic treatment of malignant diseases had come to the forefront during the last decades, plant principles and their derivatives have been intensively investigated by several western scientists as new antitumor inhibitors.

The chemical structures of substances in plants are varied, and as such, the usefulness in the discovery of new drugs would be limited. It leads to the conclusion that compounds produced biologically tend to have biological activity.

In the present treatise we present a concise review of the plant products used as anticancer agents with antitumor activity of vinca alkaloids and taxol described in detail.

2 Acronychia

Acronycine was first isolated in 1948 by Hughes and coworkers from the bark [1, 2]. Two possible structures [I] and [II] were established for acronycine [3–5]. Degradative evidence and physical properties suggested that [I] was the correct structure [6]. Proof of the angular structure for acronycine was done through X-ray crystallography [7].

Svoboda *et al.* [8] reported the antitumor activity of acronycine and found its significant inhibitory activity in 12 of the 17 tumor systems tested including leukemias, sarcomas, carcinomas und melanoma lines in mice. Sullivan and coworkers [9] studied the mammalian metabolism of acronycine and found that predominant metabolites were produced by hydroxylation of ring and or side chain. Belts *et al.* [10] and Brannan *et al.* [11] showed that the same major metabolite 9-hydroxyacronycine that was produced in mammals was also made by microorganisms. Schneider *et al.* [12] reported the synthesis of sixteen analogs of acronycine and found that none of these were superior to the parent compound.

Acronycine showed no activity in most of the murine tumor systems including the B-16 melanoma, L-121-leukemia, P-388 leukemia, Lewis lung carcinoma and Walker 256 carcinosarcoma but was active in LP-1 plasma-cell and Ridgeway osteogenic sarcoma.

3 Brucea

B. antidysenterica Mill is a simaroubaceous tree which is used in Ethiopia for the treatment of cancer. Alcoholic extract of the plant showed significant inhibitory activity *in vitro* against cells derived from cancer of the nasopharynx and two standard animal tumor systems. Three new bitter principles bruceantin [III], bruceantinol [IV] and bruceantarin [V] were isolated. III (KBED50 4.9×10^{-3} (μg/ml) and IV (ED50 2.2×10^{-3} μg/ml) showed potent antileukemic activity at microgram/kilogram dose levels and over a wide dosage range. In contrast **V** $(3.7 \times 10^{-2}$ $\mu g/ml)$ and bruceine B **[VI]** (ED50 2.8×10^{-1} $\mu g/ml)$ showed diminished antileukemic activity [13, 14].

B. javanica (L.) Merr

Oleic acid isolated from the fruits of *B. javanica* at a dose of 0.2 and 2.0 mg/ml *in vitro* inoculated with mouse Ehrlich ascites cells, inhibited the incorporation of ^3H thymidine in the DNA 56.8 and 66.7%, respectively [15]. This inhibition lasted for ›4 hours. Bruceene **[VII]** was found to be active against KB cells *in vitro* [16].

VII

Bruceoside A **[X]** and B **[XXIII]** exhibited antileukemic activity by inhibiting the growth of Walker carcinoma cells and Ehrlich ascites carcinoma cells [17]. Some of the related bruceolides such as **V** showed only moderate activity. **III** was active at 1 mg/kg/day against P-388 lymphocytic leukemia (T/C 197) and at 2 mg/kg/day against B 16 melanoma (T/C 178) in mice. **III**, bruceine D **[VIII]**, E **[IX]** and bruceoside A **[X]** significantly inhibited P-388 lymphocytic leukemic cell RNA and protein syntheses in cell culture [18]. However DNA synthesis inhibition seemed to correlate more directly with the antineoplastic activity of these compounds in the *in vivo* P-388 survival system. In *in vitro* tests brusatol **[XII]** marginally inhibited 10-day P-388 lymphocytic leukemia, DNA polymerase, RNA polymerase, thymidylate synthetase, dihydrofolate reductase, phosphoribosyl pyrophosphate aminotransferase and cathepsin protease activities. Purine synthesis was inhibited drastically by **XII** *in vivo*. Histone phosphorylation and ribonucleotide reductase activity were also inhibited marginally by **XII** while bruceine A [**XI**] is highly toxic to TLC-5 and lymphoma cells [19]. Lee *et al.* [20] reported that **VIII** inhibited the growth of Walker 256 carcinosarcoma.

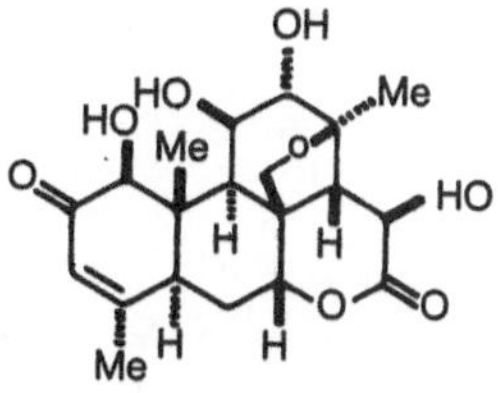

VIII

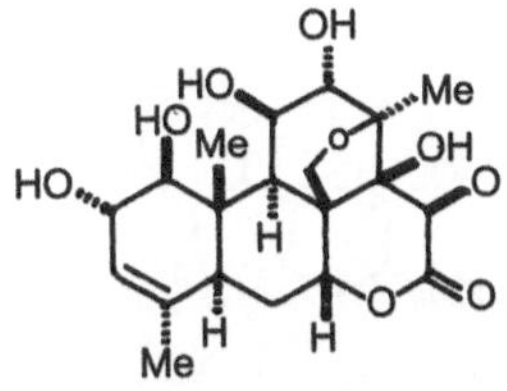

IX

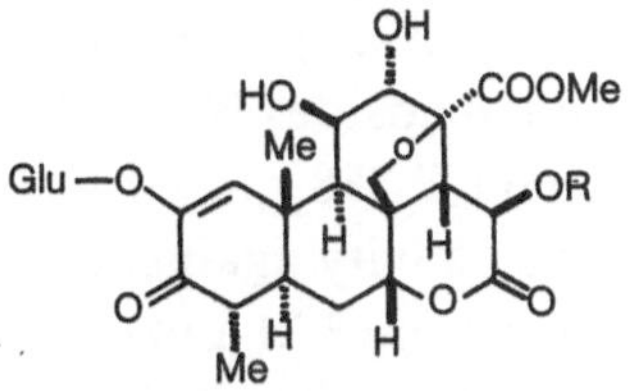

X   R= CO—

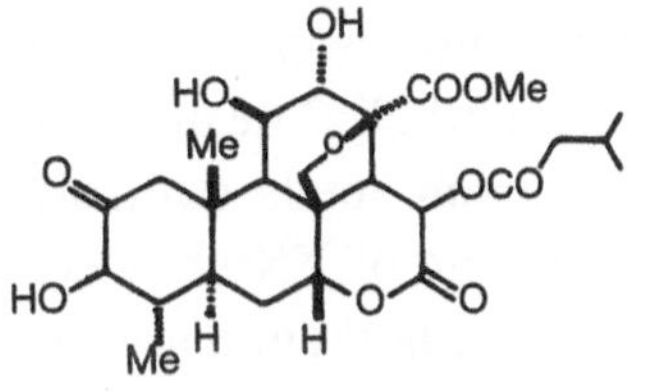

XI

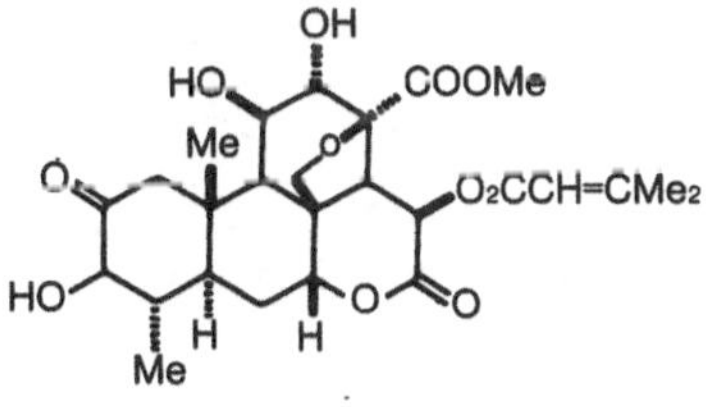

XII   R=H
XXIII R=Glu

Roots and fruit extracts inhibited the uptake of ^{3}H-labelled thymidine into TLX-5 mouse lymphoma cells [21]. The most potent cytotoxic fractions of extracts contained bruceolides. ID50 of **XI** was 0.031 μg/ml, whereas the most active bruceolide **III** had an ID50 value of 0.003 μg/ml.

XII showed potent antileukemic activity in P-388 leukemia (T/C 158 at 0.125 mg/kg/day, i.p. dose) [22–25], but **XII** showed weak antitumor activity against sarcoma-180 in mice [26]. Cleomiscosin **[XIII]** isolated from *B. javanica* and other plants is also active in the *in vitro* P-388 lymphocytic leukemia (ED50 = 0.8 μg/ml) [10] and **[XIII]** is not active *in vitro* KB system. Handa *et al.* reported ED50 values for **XIII** in the *in vitro* P-388 and KB test system as 2.8 μg/ml and 4.9 μg/ml, respectively [27].

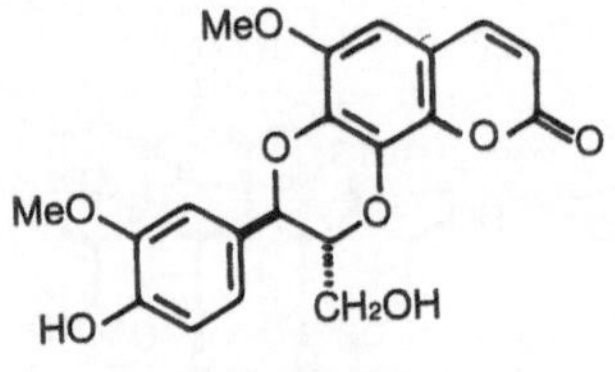

XIII

Yandanziosides A **[XIV]**, C **[XV]**, F **[XVI]** and G **[XVII]** were isolated from seeds and showed antitumor activity [28]. Yandanziosides K **[XVIII]**, I and L were also reported to be active against leukemic P-388 cells in mice [29]. The aglycone of Yandanziosides N **[XIX]** and O **[XX]** isolated from seeds controlled leukemia P-388 growth in mice [30]. The aglycone of **XX** showed antitumor activity against murine P-388 lymphocytic leukemia and its ILS values were 37.1 and 47.2% at 2 and 4 mg/kg/day dose levels respectively [31]. Yandanzioside P **[XXI]** also showed antileukemic activity [32].

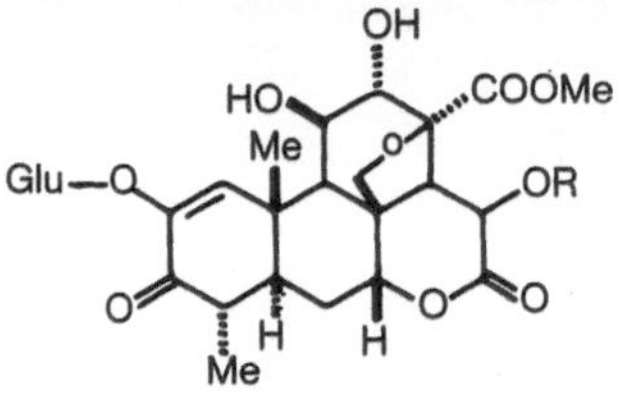

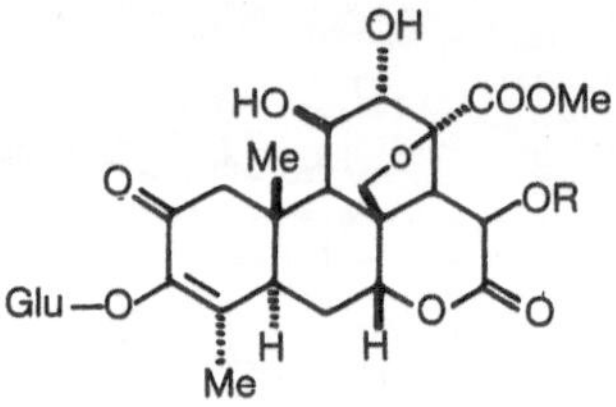

XIV	R=3,4-dimethyl-4-hydroxy-2-pentenoyl
XV	R=3,4-Diemthyl-4-acetoxt-2-pentenoyl
XVI	R=2-Methylbutanoyl
XVII	R=R=OAc

| XVIII | R=Acetic acid residue |
| XXI | R=CCCH=CMeCHMe₂ |

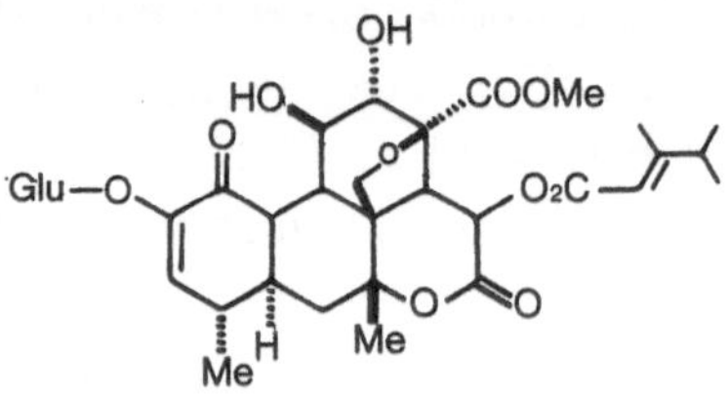

XIX

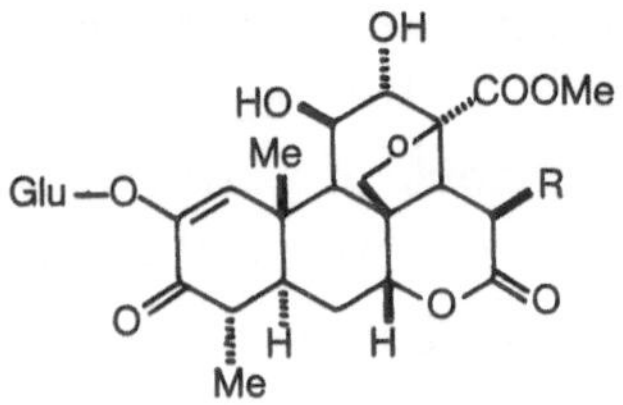

XX   R= O₂C─ ... ─OAc

Fukamiya *et al.* [33] reported the isolation of bruceoside C [**XXII**] KB (ED50 ‹0.1 μg/ml, A-549 (ED50 0.44 μg/ml) HCT-8 (ED50 451 μg/ml), RPMI (ED50 ‹0.1 μg/ml), TE-671 (ED50 0.29 μg/ml) as well as murine lymphocytic leukemia P-388 tumor cells (ED50 5.11 μg/ml).

XXII R= CO

4   Catharanthus

C. roseus (formerly *Vinca rosea* Linn.)

Extracts of *Catharanthus roseus* were used as early as 1653 for hemostasis and for treating gingivitis and diabetes [34]. It was ›300 years later that the leukopenic and antitumor activities of such extracts were noted. Indeed, it was the reported hypoglycaemic activity of extracts which led to the first detailed studies of their biological effects. Later on, their hypoglycaemic activity turned out to be of miniscale importance compared to their cytotoxic properties. These studies demonstrated that the extract has myelosuppressive activity and could induce peripheral leukopenia; this component was then isolated and termed as vincaleukoblastine [**XXIV**], now termed as vinblastine, simultaneously at two different places [35, 36]. Later on, another alkaloid with antileukemic properties, named leurocristine and now known as vincirstine [**XXV**] was isolated [37]. Since then over 90 alkaloids have been isolated from *C. roseus* and because of the complexity of alkaloid mixture it required the most advanced isolation and structure determination techniques. The interest in the broad spectrum of antitumor activity of these compounds has resulted in numerous achievements in the pharmaceutical, clinical, pharmacologic and therapeutic sciences. Both the alkaloids **XXIV** and **XXV** are present in *C. roseus* to approximately 0.00025 and 0.0003 %. **XXV** has the lowest level of any medicinally useful alkaloid produced on a commercial basis.

XXIV has also been obtained from *C. ovalis* [38], *C. longifolius* [39] and *C. trichophyllus* [40]. Several procedures have been reported for the large-scale separation of **XXIV** and **XXV** [41–47]. The structure elucidation of **XXIV** has been reviewed [48]. An extensive ^{1}H and ^{13}C NMR study on **XXIV** [49–52] established chair conformation of the piperidine ring in the velkanamine moiety. The absolute configuration of the stereocenters (chirality centers) of **XXIV** was determined by the X-ray crystal structure of vincristine methiodide [53, 54], as the relationship between **XXIV** and **XXV** has already been established. The absolute stereochemistry at C-18 in **XXIV** and related derivatives was also established by ORD and CD spectroscopy [55, 56]. The structure of **XXV** has been reviewed extensively. **XXV** possesses an indole nucleus (the catharanthine portion) and a dihydroindole nucleus (the vindoline portion). Both **XXIV** and **XXV** are structurally identical except for the substitution attached to the nitrogen of the vindoline nucleus where **XXV** possesses a formyl group and **XXIV** has a methyl group. The most interesting point here is that although these are structurally similar, they are dramatically different in their antitumor activity and clinical toxicities [44, 57].

	R^1	R^2	R^3	R^4	R^5
XXIV	Me	OMe	Ac	⌇	OH
XXV	CHO	OMe	Ac	⌇	OH
XXVI	Me	OMe	H	⌇	OH
XXVII	H	OMe	Ac	⌇	OH
XXXI	Me	OMe	Ac	OH	Et
XXXVI	Me	NH$_2$	H	⌇	OH
XXXIX	CHO	OMe	Ac	H	Et
XLI	Me	NHCHR'(COOR")	H	⌇	OH

(R', R" = Different amino acids)

Deacetylvinblastine [XXVI] (formerly named desacetylvincaleuko-
blastine) was isolated as a minor alkaloid [58]. The 4-deacetylvinblas-
tine amides are quite active antitumor agents [59] and the tubulin
binding activity of several of these agents has been described. De-
methylvinblastine [XXVII] (formerly named N-desmethylvincaleuko-
blastine and N-deformyl-vincristine) isolated as a minor alkaloid is
now converted in the crude alkaloidal mixture into more active base
XXV [60, 61]. Catharanthamine [XXVIII] isolated from the post-
leurocristine fraction [62] was found to be cytotoxic in the KB test *in
vitro* with significant activity in the P-388 lymphocytic leukemia test.
The structure of pleurosine [XXIX] isolated by Svoboda *et al.* [63] was
confirmed by high resolution ^{1}H- and ^{13}C-NMR spectroscopic data [64]
as leurosine N'b-oxide [65]. It was highly cytotoxic in KB test system
(ED50 0.019 μg/ml) *in vitro*. It also showed activity in two *in vivo*
systems. Exceptional activity was observed in the B16 melanoma test.
In a parallel test, XXIV showed test control (T/C) 309% at 0.5 mg/kg
with five survivors, XXIX showed good dose response in the dose
range 2.5–10.0 μg/kg, at the highest dose, T/C values in excess of
300% with five cures in one instance and four cures in another. It is
one of the most active compounds in the B16 test system isolated so
far.

XXVIII

5'-Oxoleurosine [XXX] and leurosidine N'b-oxide [XXXI] were cytotoxic in the KB test *in vitro* [65, 66]. Leurocolombine [XXXII] isolated
later with an additional hydroxyl group compared to XXIV exhibited
antimitotic activity and marginal antitumor activity against the Ridgeway osteogenic sarcoma (27% inhibition at 15 mg/kg) [67]. Roseadine
[XXXIII] was isolated by the bioassay-guided fractionation of *C. roseus* using the P-388 lymphocytic leukemia and Eagle's carcinoma of

the nasopharynx (KB) systems. It was active in the P-388 test showing
T/C 176% at 2 mg/kg [51].

XXIX	R = HNb'oxide	XXXII
XXX	R = O	
XXXV	R = H,H	

Serpentine [**XXXIV**] showing antitumor activity in mice infected with
mammary cancer MS 301 was isolated from *C. roseus* and also from
the leaf organ cultures of the plant [68, 69].

XXXIII

Confirmed antitumor activity was also found in indolindoline alkaloid leurosine [**XXXV**] (isomeric with **XXIV**). The highest activity was
against the P-1534 acute lymphocytic leukemia in DBA/z mice [70].
The base was also isolated from *C. ovalis, C. longifolius, C. lanceus*
and *C. pusillus* along with *C. roseus*.

XXXIV

A number of synthetic analogs of **XXIV** and **XXV** have been prepared and evaluated for biological activity, but very few have advanced beyond initial clinical trials; although these molecules have served as biochemical probes in several areas of biology, especially in those of microtubule assembly and drug resistance. But only **XXIV** and **XXV** remain the bisindole alkaloids approved for cancer treatment in the United States. A third vinca alkaloid analog vindesine [**XXXVI**] (desacetylvinblastine carboxyamide) a synthetic derivative and human metabolite of **XXIV**, was combined with **XXIV** and **XXV** for clinical trials in Europe. Then vinleurosine and vinrosidine were also found to possess antitumor activity but due to their exceptional toxicities, the clinical trials were abandoned [39]. Recently, two more semisynthetic derivatives of **XXIV**, specifically vinorelbine (Navelbine) [**XXXVII**] and vinzolidine [**XXXVIII**] are the subject of ongoing research and appear to be exciting for several reasons. The most important factor is that both **XXXVII** and **XXXVIII** are oral preparations, contrary to all other vinca alkaloids (administered by parenteral routes). Relevant aspects of vinzolidine's clinical pharmacology and early phase I/II trials have been reported [72, 73].

A number of reviews and monographs have been published describing the isolation, identification, synthesis and pharmacology of vinca alkaloids [71, 74–76].

Compounds **XXXVI** and **XXXVIII** represent structural modifications of the lower portion (vindoline) of the "dimeric" molecule at position 3. **XXXVI** was obtained by replacing the carbomethoxy function of **XXIV** by a carboxamide. Although compounds **XXIV**, **XXV** and **XXXVI** are closely related structurally, the profiles of biological activity are quite different; e. g. **XXIV** treatment is much less likely to result in neurotoxicity than treatment with **XXV**. **XXIV** produces much more perturbation of bone marrow function than does **XXV**. On the other hand **XXV** is more effective than **XXIV** in the treatment of acute leukemia in children.

XXXVII   XXXVIII

Biological evaluation and application:

A quite large number of papers, reviews and monographs have appeared describing the pharmacology and medicinal properties of vinca alkaloids [34, 35, 74, 76]. We have described concisely the mechanism of action, resistance, pharmacology (biochemical, cellular and preclinical) preclinical toxicology followed by clinical pharmacology and toxicology of major vinca alkaloids **XXIV, XXV, XXXVI** and **XXXVII.**

C. roseus alkaloids induce cytotoxicity by direct interactions with tubulin. The mechanism of action thus involves (a) entry into the cell by competing for transport of amino acids into the cell and (b) interference with cellular metabolic functions as inhibition of purine biosynthesis, RNA, DNA and protein synthesis, disruption of lipid metabolism, inhibition of glycolysis, alterations in the release of antidiuretic hormone, inhibition of release of histamine by mast cells and enhanced release of epinephrine and disruption in the integrity of the cell membrane and membrane functioning [71, 77]. Microtubules are the most strategic subcellular targets of anticancer chemotherapeutics and are ubiquitous to all cells. These are responsible for maintaining the cell shape, mitosis, meiosis, secretion, intracellular transport and axonal transport. Vinca alkaloids bind to a site on tubulin that is distinctly different from the binding sites of colchicine, podophyllotoxin and taxol, thus exerting antimicrotubules effect [78, 79], and this binding leads to disruption of microtubules. Further binding to tubulin prevents the polymerizations of these subunits into microtubules; instead the subunits form highly ordered paracrystalline arrays of tubulin termed as "paracrystals" [80] containing one mole of bound drug per mole of tubulin [81]. The overall effect of these processes includes the blockage of the polymerization of tubulin into microtubules, thus leading to the inhibition of vital cellular processes and cell death. Because the aggregation of tubulin units into microtubules is required not only for the formation of the mitotic spindle but also for the transport of materials in nerves. An excellent correlation between drug concentration required to produce inhibition of cell colony formation and those required to dissolve mitotic spindle was observed. The effects of **XXIV** on the mitotic spindle occur very rapidly and can be observed within 30 sec. Mitotic arrest is the principal cytotoxic effect of vinca alkaloids but it is also assumed that the lethal effects of these agents may be attributable in part to effects on other phases of the cell cycle [82].

XXIV, XXV and other structurally related analogs inhibit microtubule polymerization by 50% at concentration of $0.1–1\,\mu M$. Vinepidine [**XXXIX**] was twice as potent as **XXIV** as an inhibitor of steady-state tubulin addition but nearly 10-fold less potent than **XXIV** as an inhibitor of cell growth [83]. Apparently **XXIV** and not **XXV,** is lethal for Hela cells in the G1 phase (gap before DNA synthesis) of the cell cycle [84].

A review was published describing the mechanisms other than interaction with tubulin that may play a role in the biological actions of **XXIV** and related compounds; it says that "the mechanism(s) responsible for the cytotoxic and antitumor activities of vinca [sic] alkaloids is not clear". A synthetic photoaffinite labelled derivative of **XXIV** was used to identify alkaloid binding sites in P-388 murine leukemia cells [85].

A review describing the cellular pharmacological aspects of resistance to **XXIV** and related compounds has been published by Beck *et al.* [86]. The important cellular characteristics frequently associated with resistance to **XXIV** include cross-resistance not only to structurally related compounds such as **XXV** and **XXXVI** but also to other basic, naturally occurring compounds. Resistance to **XXIV** and representative anthracyclins (e. g. doxorubicin) may involve reduced abilities of resistant cells accumulate these cytotoxic drugs and the expression of a moderately sized surface glycoprotein, the so-called P-glycoprotein. The expression of this glycoprotein is a hallmark of the multiple drug resistance (MDR) phenotype. Those cells which exhibited high levels (several hundred fold) of resistance to **XXIV, XXV** and **XXXVI** have an extremely limited capacity to accumulate radiolabelled **XXIV** [86]. A substantial number of unrelated compounds including calcium channel antagonists [87], phenothiazines and other "calmodulin antagonists" [88, 89], antiarrhythmic agents such as quinidine and amiodarone [90], cephalosporins [91] and cyclosporin A, have been demonstrated to reverse drug resistance related to MDR phenotype. Treatment of cells resistant to **XXV** and adriamycin (doxorubicin) with the calcium entry blocker verapamil increases the susceptibility of the cells to the antitumor drugs. This phenomenon is related to either calcium channel antagonism or immuno-modulation since inactive isomers are considerably more active in reversing this type of resistance [92, 93]. Resistance to **XXIV** and other drugs can be produced in mammalian cells by transfer of specific gene sequences that code for P-glycoprotein [94].

XXV is a component of chemotherapeutic regimens used in the management of Rhabdomyosarcomas (common soft tissue sarcomas in children). Some cross-resistance to the alkylating nitrogen mustard derivative L-phenylalanine mustard (L-PAM) was exhibited by Rhabdomyosarcoma xenografts resistant to **XXV** which is of potential clinical pertinence in view of the relatively low degree of activity of L-PAM in pediatric patients unresponsive to drug regimens including **XXV** [95]. During a study of **XXV** resistance in Chinese hamster ovary cells, it was observed that cells resistant to **XXV** are also resistant to **XXIV** and **XXXVI** [96].

Compound **XXIV** enhances the accumulation of folate antagonist methotrexate in murine leukemia cells [96] and both **XXIV** and **XXV** in human leukemia cells [97]. It has been suggested that the effect of **XXV** on methotrexate efflux may be related to alterations of cell membrane electrical activity that appear to occur when cells are treated with **XXV**.

Although vinca alkaloids have broad clinical use, still not much data are available about their pharmacology in humans as compared to other antineoplastic agents. This is because of a lack of a sensitive assay capable of measuring the minute plasma concentration which results from the wide distribution of mg doses of these bases. The earlier studies conducted on animals and humans used radiolabelled vinca alkaloids, with further separation of parent drug and metabolites by high-pressure liquid chromatography (HPLC) [98–100]. With the advent of sensitive radioimmunoassay (RIA) and enzyme-linked immunosorbent assay (ELISA) methods it is now possible to detect picomolar concentrations [101–104].

Earlier it was shown that both **XXIV** and **XXV** share the ability to produce marked prolongations of life span in mice bearing intraperitoneally inoculated leukemic cells and at relatively low doses (<1 mg/kg/day for 10 days) could prolong the life span of leukemic animals by 100% and more [105]. The base **XXV** was particularly effective in treating mice with P-1534 leukemia and could achieve "cures" in leukemic mice. It was observed that P-1534 leukemia which was sensitive to both **XXIV** and **XXV** developed resistance afterwards [106]. **XXIV** was inactive against the Ridgeway osteogenic sarcoma in mice but **XXV** strongly inhibited the growth of this tumor (0.15–0.2 mg/kg/day) and **XXXVI** inhibited this tumor by 90–100% when administered intraperitoneally (0.3–0.4 mg/kg/day for 8 days) [107].

Compound **XXIV** and related substances had no significant activity when administered to mice inoculated with L-1210 leukemia cells. Compounds **XXIV** and **XXXVI** prolonged the life of mice with P-388 by 200–300% while mice with L-1210 leukemia showed little or no prolongation of life. All three bases **XXIV, XXV** and **XXXVI** are active against the murine B16 melanoma *in vivo* with many long-term survivors [107]. Selectivity exists in the relation of **XXV** in tumor tissue and normal tissue of mice [108].

The activities of **XXIV** analog in experimental tumors have been reported but none was superior to **XXXVI**. One dimer of **XXXVI** bisvindesine [**XL**] has shown comparable antitumor activity to **XXXVI** but the difference is in its ability to inhibit the growth of P-388 leukemia resistant to **XXXVI** and **XXIV** [109].

The amino acid derivative [**XLI**] of **XXIV** also showed good activity against P-388 leukemia; some treated mice survived for 60 days after inoculation of tumor cells (average survival time for control mice was 10 days) [110].

CONHCH₂CH₂-S-S-CH₂CH₂NHCO

XL

As mentioned previously with respect to verapamil, there are drugs that have little or no antitumor activity alone but are capable of restoring sensitivity to **XXIV** or **XXV** in resistant tumor cell populations, a phenomenon known as "synergization"; e. g. the acridone derivative quinacrine in combination with **XXV** increases the life span of mice inoculated with P-388 leukemia [111].

Pharmacokinetic studies with tritiated **XXV** in rats and dogs demonstrated the elimination from the blood of both species in a biexponential manner. Uniform distribution of radioactivity did occur in tissues like liver, kidney, lung and small intestine by i. v. injection of tritiated **XXV**. From 1 to 6 hrs after drug administration, the activity was lower in brain than other tissues but no marked difference was observed at a later time. Base **XXV** and its metabolites are excreted in urine and feces [112]. **XXV** rapidly concentrates in the bile with an initial bile: plasma concentration ratio of 100 : 1 declining to 20 : 1 at 72 hrs post injection [113]. Studies both in man and animals demonstrated the production of at least 6 to 11 metabolites [114–118]. Not all of the metabolites have been characterized. The major metabolite in dog has been identified as 4-deacetyl vincristine [114]. 4-Deacetyl vincristine and N-deformyl vincristine were isolated from human bile [115–116]. From the *in vitro* incubation of **XXV**, 4'-deoxy-3'-hydroxy-**XXV** and 3',4'-epoxy vincristine N-oxide were isolated from dog's bile and tentatively characterized [117]. In tumor tissue sensitive to **XXV** but not to **XXIV**, the elimination of **XXV** is monophasic with very little of the drug leaving the tissue over a period of 72 hrs, the elimination of **XXIV** is biphasic in these tissues.

This toxicological studies for **XXIV** and **XXV** provided LD50 values for **XXIV** of 17 mg/kg following single i. v. injection to mice with **XXV** approximately 10-fold less, the toxicity for **XXIV** and **XXV** was higher if administered intraperitoneally [105]. The reported LD50 for **XXVI** in mice is approximately half that of **XXIV** [106].

In the rats treated with **XXIV** the depression of white blood cell count (leucopenia) was reversible and dose related and the death of animals in these cases was due to an overwhelming bacterial infection secondary to the leukopenia. A summary of the major toxicological observations after the administration of **XXIV** or **XXV** has been given by Johnson *et al.* [105]. **XXIV** is lethal in dogs (0.05 mg/kg, i. v., 5 times in one week) and monkeys (1 mg/kg 5 times weekly).

Monkeys treated with **XXV** had degenerative changes in liver and kidney. **XXXVI** produced leukopenia and reduced spermatogenesis in rats without altering neural function at doses 0.1–0.3 mg/kg weekly [119]. The LD50 for **XXXVI** in mice is 6.3 mg/kg and for **XL** 6.9 mg/kg [109].

No accepted experimental model is available for peripheral neurotoxicity produced by **XXV** in humans although it is suggested that chronic treatment of rabbits with **XXV** might serve as a useful model for neurotoxicity [120].

The paracrystal formation of the cells in neuronal tissue of a softwater snail upon treatment with **XXIV** or **XXV** was proposed as a model for the neurotoxic effects of vinca alkaloids and analogs [121]. **XXV** was found to be 10-fold more active as an inducer of paracrystal formation than **XXIV**. Further it was observed by Johnson *et al.* [105] that the toxicity of high doses of **XXV** could be counterbalanced in mice with folinic acid which lowered the mortality to 25% from that of 90%. If folic acid was substituted for folinic acid, no similar protection was observed; however, reports are also available which indicate that the protection can be achieved by comparable treatment with isotonic saline solution [122].

The important breakthrough in cancer chemotherapy happened in the 1960s with the recognition of **XXV** as the most active agent in acute lymphocytic leukemia. Today, acute lymphocytic leukemia in children and adults is treated with **XXV** as a component regimens. The combination includes use of corticosteroid-analog prednisone and anthracyclin daunorubicin, cytosine arabinoside, 6-thioguanine and 5-azacytidine [123]. The same combination (with prednisone) is also used to treat acute lymphoblastic crisis of chronic mylogenous leukemia [124] and Philadelphia chromosome positive childhood acute lymphocytic leukemia [125]. Compound **XXV** is not generally used in most conventional treatment regimens although it is incorporated in several induction and post remission therapies for adult acute non-lymphocytic leukemia [126, 127]. On the other hand, **XXIV** has been shown to be only modestly active in acute lymphocytic leukemia and is at present playing no role in the therapy of acute leukemias. **XXIV** has been demonstrated to be the most active agent producing complete and overall responses in 33% and 65% of patients respectively. However its action is of limited duration if given alone. For the treatment of Hodgkin's disease **XXIV** is used in combination with doxorubicin, procarbazine and bleomycin although it was used in the first successful and most popular regimen for Hodgkin's disease. This is due to a relative lack of myelosuppressive properties. The substitution of **XXIV** for **XXV** in combination with nitrogen mustard, procarbazine, and prednisone (MOPP) regimens, including others, has resulted in less neurotoxicity [128–130].

Compound **XXV** is an important component of multiagent chemotherapy regimens used in the palliative treatment of indolent lymphomas and in both the palliative and curative treatment of aggressive lymphomas [131–133]. The complete responses were achieved with cyclophosphamide, **XXV** and prednisone in about 70% of the patients [134]. Some other more aggressive regimens are also available [135, 136], but the survival of untreated and/or palliated patients is quite long; still, the **XXV**-based regimens (**XXV**, cyclophosphamide and prednisone) is commonly used in both first line and salvage therapies [137] as compared to **XXIV**. However, the combination chemotherapy regimens containing **XXIV** are clearly active and may be useful in first-line and salvage therapies [138]. **XXV** is also used as a component in other lymphomas and pediatric tumors such as Wilnis tumor and embryonal Rhabdosarcoma.

For treatment of non-small cell lung cancer a regimen has also included compound **XXXVI** with cisplatin but it also produces substantial toxicity including neurotoxicity [139]. The administration route for both **XXIV** and **XXV** is i. v. reflecting the relatively poor bioavailability in preclinical studies of the drugs indicated. Although vinzolidine (analog of **XXIV**) showed some antitumor activity *via* oral route, it was discontinued due to unpredictable toxicities [140].

Although **XXV** is active in plasma cell dyscrasias and incorporated into several treatment schemes, no clear indication is available that addition of **XXV** to conventional combinations of alkylating agents and prednisone results in improved therapy. The regimen consisting of **XXV**, doxorubicin and dexamethasone is particularly useful in myeloma complicated by renal failure [141]. Compound **XXIV** is used as an integral component of both curative and palliative treatment regimens for several advanced cerological malignancies, particularly germ cell carcinoma, transitional cell carcinoma of the urothelial tract and renal cell carcinoma. Several **XXIV** based regimens have been developed for the treatment of gonadal and extragonadal germ cell malignancies [142].

The combination of **XXIV** with cisplatin (a platinum complex) and the heterocyclic glycopeptide antibiotic bleomycin is suitable for the treatment of metastatic testicular cancer [143]. Good results are obtained with a regimen of **XXIV** and biological agents such as recombinant interferon alpha [144].

Similarly, **XXV** is used in combination for the treatment of small cell carcinoma of pulmonary or extrapulmonary sites, and a very high response rate has been recently reported by Murray *et al.* [145] with **XXV**, cyclophosphamide, doxorubicin and etoposide.

Both **XXIV** and **XXV** are active in metastatic breast cancer as single agents and are frequently used in combination regimens. In the case of **XXV** severe neurotoxic events were observed in early phase-II single agent trials [146]. Compound **XXIV** is incorporated into secondary and tertiary regimens [147].

XXV in combination regimens is frequently used in the treatment of many pediatric solid tumors [148] and has also been shown to be active in several non-malignant hematologic disorders. In case of refractory auto-immune thrombocytopenia [149], thrombotic thrombocytopenia purpurea [150], lymphomatoid granulomatosis [151] and hemolytic uremic syndrome, infusion of **XXV** or **XXV**-loaded platelets was effective.

XXIV is active alone and in drug combinations in Kaposi's sarcoma associated with the acquired immunodeficiency syndrome [152]. It is also active in gestational trophoblastic disease [153], metastatic non-small cell lung cancer [154] and adjuvant programs [155]. Anti-neoplastic activity has also been observed with **XXIV** alone or in regimens in gastric [156], vaginal [157] carcinomas, the terminal phase of chronic myelogenous leukemia [158] and malignant histocytosis [159]. Like **XXV**, **XXIV** is also used in patients with refractory idiopathic thrombocytopenic purpura [128].

Without significant toxicity, modulation of resistance has been observed with tamoxifen and cyclosporin A [160–163]. A triexponential elimination pattern has been revealed for both **XXIV** and **XXV** by clinical pharmacokinetic studies. As discussed earlier nowadays pharmacokinetic studies are being done using radioimmunoassay rather than the administration of a radiolabelled drug that also measures structurally related drug metabolites if data are cautiously interpreted. Half-lives after administration of **XXIV** to patients were estimated as 4 min, 1.6 hrs and 25 hrs, suggesting the rapid distribution of the drug to most tissues, relatively rapid clearance and a subsequent slow terminal elimination process. Compound **XXV** was also found to have similar distribution and initial clearance phase with half-lives of 4 min and 2.3 hrs, respectively. However **XXV** has a three to four times longer terminal elimination phase than that estimated for **XXIV**, and the slow elimination of **XXV** from susceptible neuronal tissue is perhaps one of the causes of neurotoxicity commonly observed with **XXV** but not with **XXIV** [163].

Both **XXIV** and **XXV** are mainly eliminated by hepatic metabolism and bile excretion in human [164]. **XXIV**, **XXV** and **XLI** have an extremely high volume of distribution, the mean value for **XXIV** is approximately 2000 lts (estimated for 70 kg individual) and those for **XXV** and **XXXVI** are approximately 600 lts [163]. These high estimates for the apparent volume of distribution suggest that extensive binding to various tissues is a prominent feature of the pharmacokinetics of these drugs.

It is recommended to reduce the dose of both **XXIV** and **XXV** in patients with liver disease. The dose for **XXV** conventionally administered i. v. to adults is 1.4 mg/m^2 with a total dose not exceeding 2 mg for a given administration, whereas the initial dose of **XXIV** for adults is 3.7 mg/m^2, with a typical dose later increasing to the 5.5–7.4 mg/m^2 range administered weekly [163].

Both **XXIV** and **XXV** have different profiles of toxicities during treatment of patients with malignant diseases. Patients treated with **XXIV** start developing leukopenia 5–10 days after completion of a treatment cycle that lasts for 1–2 weeks. Patients having undergone radiotherapy or taken some other drugs toxic to bone marrow may show enhanced thrombocytopenia after **XXIV**. The other effects are stomatitis (mouth sores) and gastrointestinal dysfunction including nausea, vomiting and constipation. Alopecia (hair loss) is a reversible effect commonly observed in patients receiving **XXIV** and **XXV**. With a number of basic natural products (including **XXV** and **XXVI**), **XXIV** shares the capacity for producing severe local tissue damage if the agent leaks from the site of administration (extravasation) or if excessively high concentrations are given to vascular tissue.

Contrary to **XXIV**, the dose-limiting toxicity for **XXV** is usually leukopenia [165]. The major manifestations of neurotoxicity are loss of the Achilles tandon reflex, paresthesias, loss of muscle strength (e. g. in foot and wrist) and ataxia. **XXV** is a potent tissue irritant and may produce a syndrome of inappropriate secretion of antidiuretic hormone. Some manifestations of neurotoxicity, e. g. seizures, are considered to be due to electrolyte disturbances associated with the relative excess of the antidiuretic hormone [165].

Several reports are available on the incidents of **XXV** overdosage, some of which involved inadvertent administration of the intravenous formulation into the central nervous system by the intrathecal route. The overdosage toxicities are initially vomiting and diarrhea with subsequent constipation and paralytic illness, mental confusion and hallucination also persisted for 2–3 weeks. Toxicity episode was larger in patient who received folinic acid as compared to others who did not. It was finally concluded that "apart from animal experimentation no reason exists for recommending this procedure [folinic acid rescue] as a treatment for vincristine overdose" [69].

Compound **XXXVI** has the same toxicological profile as that of **XXIV** and **XXV** and the effects observed with **XXXVI** are bone marrow depression, alopecia, and peripheral neurotoxicity.

We now come to the only semisynthetic analogue of vinblastine – Navelbine [**XXXVII**] (vinorelbine ditartrate; 5'-noranhydrovinblastine) used clinically [166]. It was synthesized from catharanthine and vindoline isolated from *C. roseus* plant. Compound **XXXVII** has structural peculiarities which can partly or entirely explain its distinct pharmacological profile. It contains an eight-membered ring instead of the nine-membered ring common in **XXIV** or related compounds. Nb' of vinblastine type compounds must be 'free' (protonated?) to exhibit antitumor activity. Whatever may be the exact mode of interaction with tubulin it is quite probable that after their recognition by tubulin (hydrophobic interactions) further interaction comes into play and protonation of Nb' of the upper part of vinblastine-type compounds by an amino acid of tubulin is possible whereas in vinblastine-type compounds, there is no further consequence of this protonation. In **XXXVII**, protonation of Nb' of the 'gramine portion', of that alkaloid instead of the 'tryptamine portion' in the equivalent vinblastine-type compounds can be followed by a fragmentation reaction thus offering the possibility of nucleophilic addition of a suitable group of tubulin onto the newly formed conjugated imminium indolic ion [**XLIa** and **XLIb**]

XLIa   XLIb

This results in the formation of a "reversible covalent bond" which plays an important role in the control of the fate of the tubulin, microtubules, spindles etc. Preclinical studies have shown that although **XXXVII** is cytotoxic like other vinca alkaloids by inhibiting microtubule assembly, it is more specific in preferentially affecting the microtubules of the mitotic spindle [167–168]. At a lower concentration (2.0 μM) in intact tectal plate microtubules from mouse embryos, **XXIV, XXV** and **XXXVII** inhibit mitotic microtubule formation and induce cell cycle blockade in metaphase [167], but at higher concentrations (25 μM) **XXXVII** is the only agent which induces blockade in prophase. Compound **XXV** depolymerizes axonal microtubules at 5 μM concentrations whereas **XXIV** and **XXXVII** do not induce this effect below 30 μM and 40 μM respectively, suggesting that **XXIV** and **XXXVII** may have a reduced potential for causing neurotoxicity (167–169). **XXXVII** is also active in murine tumor models P-388, L-1210 leukemias and M-5076 reticulosarcoma, B16 melanoma, producing high T/C ratios and many cures [170], active against several human tumor xenografts including non-small cell lung cancer, small cell lung, gastric and breast carcinomas and also in ovarian cancer [170].

For investigational purposes **XXXVII** is available only in the United States. It also demonstrated activity against advanced breast and non-small cell lung carcinomas in Europe. However broad phase-II trials have not yet been performed. High response rate was observed when **XXXVII** was given in combination with either doxorubicin or 5-fluorouracil, in untreated patients with advanced breast cancer [171]. The major toxicity of both regimens was reversible neutropenia [172]. The pharmacokinetic behavior of **XXXVII** is similar to that of other vinca alkaloids in rats, monkeys and humans. Both 2 and 3 compartment models were used to describe the drug disposition in plasma [173, 175]. Within the first hour an extensive decay of initial concentration is observed which is followed by a slow elimination phase. Consequently navelbine's plasma clearance is quite high, its steady-state volume of distribution is large with a long elimination half-life (20–49 hrs) [173, 174]. Tissue distribution studies in several animal species have shown a high **XXXVII** level in several tissues (tissue/plasma ratios of 20 to 80), except brain [143], and the distribution is more intense compared to other vinca alkaloids. The principal route of excretion for 3H-**XXXVII** in both animals and humans is in the fecus (70–80%) while in urine only 20–30% of total eliminated radioactivity was observed [176].

The liver is the principal site of drug disposition excreting large quantities of both **XXXVII** and metabolites [176]. The structures of all metabolites have not been established; however, a comparative study with standards shows that 2 metabolites are eluted with a retention time similar to deacetyl navelbine and an N-oxy derivative [177] from urine while no metabolites have been detected in serum [174].

The major toxicities of **XXXVII** are hematologic neuralgic and gastrointestinal. Leukopenia is the most common adverse effect of **XXXVII** and has been dose limiting. Anemia and thrombocytopenia are rare but asymptomatic thrombocytosis is fairly common [178].

The common neurotoxic manifestations of **XXXVII** are constipation (gastrointestinal toxicity) and cumulative loss of deep tendon reflexes. Tumor pain and jaw pain has also been reported in some patients [179].

5   Cephalotaxus

It is a genus of yew-like coniferous trees and shrubs consisting of many species. The genus is a source of a unique group of alkaloids, the prototype of which is cephalotaxine. The antitumor activity in Cephalotaxus was first detected in an aqueous extract of seeds against sarcoma 180 tumor.

Powell *et al.* [180] reported the isolation of first active principle harringtonine [**XLII**] form *C. harringtonia* var. *drupacea* and the structures of [**XLII**], homoharringtonine [**XLIII**] and isoharringtonine [**XLIV**] were reported later on by the same authors [181].

XLII, XLIII and deoxyharringtonine [**XLV**] showed greatest activity at 1–2 mg/kg, **XLII** being the most active. In the same system the alkaloid **XLV** has the greatest activity at 7.5 mg/kg. Alkaloid fractions were highly effective in treatment of several types of leukemia in man [182]. Against L-1210 lymphotic leukemia the alkaloids **XLII, XLIII** and **XLIV** showed only marginal activity [183].

XLII	R = (Me)$_2$C-(CH$_2$)$_2$-C-CH$_2$CO$_2$Me
XLIII	R = (Me)$_2$-C-(CH$_2$)$_3$-C-CH$_2$CO$_2$Me

XLIV   R = (Me)$_2$-CH-(CH$_2$)$_2$-C-CH(OH)CO$_2$Me

XLV   R = (Me)$_2$CH-(CH$_2$)$_2$-C-CH$_2$CO$_2$Me

The esters of cephalotaxine [**XLVI**] and substituted malic and tartaric acids exhibited significant activity against P-388 lymphocytic leukemia over a wide range of dosage [185, 186]. **XLVI** and acetylcephalotoxine [**XLVII**] are both inactive in the P-388 leukemia system. Partially synthetic pseudo-deoxyharringtonine showed only marginal activity at 40 mg/kg [184].

The three esters of cephalotaxine [**XLVIII-L**] and rearranged esters [**LI**] are also inactive, although **XLIX** does show marginal activity at 135 mg/kg [187].

XLVIII	R = CO-C(OH)-CH$_2$Me
XLIX	R = CO-C-CH$_2$CH$_2$CHMe$_2$
	CHCOOMe

L   R = CO-CH-CH$_2$CH$_2$CHMe$_2$
     CH$_2$COOMe

XLVI   R = OH
XLVII   R = Me

LI

$$R = -C(OH)-CH_2CH_2CHMe_2$$
$$\quad\ \ \ CH_2COOMe$$

XLII and **XLIII** were both found to be orally effective against i. p. implanted P-388 leukemia, although the activity was reduced by 20–40% and the doses were approximately double of those that were optimum for i. p. treatment. Against the s. c. implanted B16 melanoma, there was little tumor inhibition at nontoxic doses upon oral treatment, whereas i. p. treatment showed 60–90% tumor inhibition [188]. Intraperitoneal injection of **XLII** and **XLIII** into mice inoculated with L-1210 leukemia produced apoplosis in leukemic cells. DNA synthesis was severely inhibited.

XLIII caused swelling of nuclear membrane, endoplasmic reticulum, and mitochondria as well as formation of membrane vacuoles, expansion of perinuclear space and a type of small membrane-bound organelle [189].

XLIII showed significant antitumor activity against sarcomas, breast tumors and ovarian and endometrial carcinomas in human tumor clongenic assays, while **XLII** was only active against ovarian and endometrial cancers, but using 1-hr exposure there was no significant difference between the two drugs [190]. **XLIII** was tested against surgical explants of human tumors in a 6-day *in vivo* subrenal capsule assay in nude mice, 16% response rate observed. This was similar to adriamycin, but lower than other clinically useful agents such as cytoxan and 5-fluoruracil. It showed the most activity against lung, ovarian and cervical tumors and least against breast and colorectal tumors [191].

XLIII was metabolized in dogs to one major and two minor metabolites. Biliary excretion of tritium level was 14% in 5 hrs, but only 2% as parent drug. In 72 hrs 40% of labelled drug was excreted in urine and 43% of the excreted drug was **XLIII**, indicating that metabolism is extensive [192]. **XLII** showed additive activity with dexmethasone or cytosine arabinoside *in vitro* but combinations with 5-fluorouracil, adriamycin, acivicin or L-asparaginase were at least partially antagonistic [193].

XLIII in phase I study caused a severe but reversible hypotension 6–16 hrs after bolus injection of 5 mg/m². This could be alleviated by giving the drug as a constant infusion. Examination of this phenomenon in rats showed that delayed hypotension was clearly associated with changes in the electrocardiogram [194].

Yan *et al.* [195] showed that **XLII** *in vitro* was stronger on the proliferation human leukemic progenitors than on hematopoietic progenitors. It may be useful in bone marrow transplant in treatment of leukemia. Liu *et al.* [196, 197] reported that a drug containing **XLII** and **XLIII**, anethole, oleanolic acid and ginsenoside is effective in the treatment of nonlymphatic leukemia without cardiotoxicity and damage to hematopoietic organs. The LD50 of the drug in mice was 1005 mg/kg body wt whereas that of a drug containing only **XLII** (2.5 mg) and **XLIII** (1.25 mg) was 4.01 mg/kg body wt.

Wilsonine [**LII**] isolated from *C. sinensis* had a weak antileukemic activity in mice [198]. Geran *et al.* [199] reported that cephalomannine [**XII**] isolated from *C. manii* showed potent anticancer activity in KB cell culture and in lymphocytic leukemia P-388 in mice. **LIII** shows potent inhibition of PS leukemia in mice. The antileukemic ED50 of **XII** against lymphocytic leukemia cells of strain P-388 implanted in mice was 3.5 x 1.0–3 μg/ml [200–201].

LII

LIII

R' = OC(O)CH(OH)CHPhNHCOC(= CHMe)Me

Mikolajczak *et al.* reported the structure-activity relationship in cephalotaxus alkaloids. The inactivity of **XLVI** indicates that an ester function at C-6 is necessary for activity. Furthermore, the inactivity or substantially reduced activity of esters **XLVII**, pseudodeoxyharringtonine and **XLVIII-LI** suggests a high degree of structural specificity in the acyl moiety. An alpha-hydroxy group and a hindered tertiary carbonyl group in the acyl portion are required for activity. However, some variations in the acyl side chain are allowed. Insertion of an additional methylene group in the terminal portion of the side chain has little effect on activity (**XLII** and **XLIV**). Removal of a hydroxy group from the side chain causes a 50% reduction in activity. Shifting of an ester function from C-6 to C-8 results in an inactive molecule.

6   Ellipticine

The ellipticines are very promising because they not only show a broad spectrum of activity (i. p. implanted tumor and tumors implanted at other sites) but are also effective by a variety of routes (i. p., i. v. and oral) [202–204]. The first report of the isolation of ellipticine from *Ochrosia elliptica* and *O. sandwichensis* appeared in 1959 [205]. Later on, the base was isolated from other *Ochrosia* spp., *Bleekeria vitiensis* [206, 207] and some other plants including *Strychnos dinklegi* Gelg. (Loganiaceae) [208–210].

In 1967 came the first report of antitumor activity of ellipticine [**LIV**] and 9-methoxyellipticine [**LV**] [211] and subsequently the activity of 9-hydroxyellipticine [**LVI**] [212, 213] and the quaternary compounds were reported [214]. The L-1210 leukemia model was used in most of the *in vivo* studies although some other mouse and rat systems have also been used [215]. Among the bases evaluated, **LIV** [216], **LV**, **LVI** and 2-methyl-9-hydroxyellipticine acetate [**LVII**] [217] have been shown to be the highly active compounds on various experimental tumors and leukemias. **LV** has at the moment the broadest spectrum of

	R¹	R²	R³	R⁴	R⁵	R⁶	X
LIV	H	Me	H	–	Me	H	–
LV	OMe	Me	H	–	Me	H	–
LVI	OH	Me	H	–	Me	H	–
LVII	OH	Me	H	Me	Me	H	OAc
LIX	H	H	Me	O⁻	Me	H	–
LXI	H	H	Me	–	Me	H	–
LXIII	-OCOEt	Me	H	–	Me	–	–
LXVII	H	Me	H	–	-CH₂OCONHMe	H	–
LXVIII	OH	Me	H	(CH₂)₂NHEt₂	Me	H	2Cl⁻
LXX	OMe	Me	NH(CH₂)₃NHEt₂	–	Me	H	–
LXXI	NH₂	Me	H	–	Me	H	–
LXXII	Cl	Me	H	–	Me	Cl	–
LXXVI	H	Me	H	Me	Me	H	–

antitumor activity [76] and is also active against leukemia and solid
tumor (not responsive to *Catharanthus roseus* alkaloids).

LV has also been isolated through bio-activity directed fractionation
of the ammoniacal benzene extract of the bark of *O. maculata* Jacq.
[204]. The ethanolic extract of the bark of *O. maculata* Jacq. showed
moderate activity against adenocarcinoma 755 [218] while the extracts
of *O. moorei* F. Muell and *Excavatia coccinea* (Tejs & Bin) Mgf. were
active against sarcoma 180, adenocarcinoma 755, and the L-1210 lymphocytic leukemia [219]. *Aspidosperma* alkaloids when evaluated
against the Walker 256 carcinosarcoma system demonstrated the
higher activity of uleine [LVIII] and olivacine 2-oxide [LIX] when
compared with guatambuine [LX] or olivasine [LXI], while the synthetic carbazole [LXII] derived from [LVIII] was found to be most
active.

LVIII   LX

LXII

An ellipticine drug has been combined with the appropriate carrier
molecule to deliver it to specific biological targets. Of the various
ellipticine-estradiol receptor conjugates synthesized, only leurocolombine [LXIII] had good activity against L-1210 mouse leukemia system
in vitro (IC50 0.5 μM; ellipticine IC50 0.85 μM; elliptinium [LVII],
IC50 0.08 μM), the IC50 refers to the inhibitory concentration that
reduces by 50% the growth rate of the cells after 24 or 48 hrs of drug
exposure, providing a good indication of the efficacy of drugs against
human cancer [220]. LXIII also showed activity against the human
breast cancer cell line MCF-7 [221]. The ellipticine enkephalin conjugates [LXV] exhibited *in vitro* binding properties to both DNA and
opioid receptors in NG 108-15 mouse tumor cells [222].

A-LV low density lipoprotein (LDL) complex was found to be 10 times
more active than [LV] against L-1210 and P-388 leukemia *in vitro*. The

activity depends on the **LDL**-high affinity receptor since **LDL** itself reduces antitumor activity [223].

LXV

Alberici *et al.* [224] synthesized various elliptinium [**LVII**] mono-clonal antibody conjugates (by oxidizing **LVII** with HRP/H_2O_2 in presence of mono-clonal antibody), and one Fab AF01-5 was found to be at least 100 times more cytotoxic *in vitro* against human hepatocarcinoma cell lines than **LVII**.

Upon encapsulation of [**LVII**] within phospholipid vesicles, Sauterau *et al.* [225] showed that the drug as such is less cytotoxic against L-1210 cells *in vitro* and *in vivo* than when it is free. However, the entrapped drug has higher antitumor activity than the free form if the onset of leukemia is delayed in mice [225]. Ali-osman *et al.* [226] showed that [**LVII**] is able to cross the blood-brain barrier in rats and is cytotoxic *in vitro* against three human glioma cell lines (SE 126, SF 375, SF 407).

Alworth and Slaga [227], while studying the effects of various agents including **LIV** on the initiation of skin tumors in mice by polycyclic aromatic hydrocarbons (PAH), showed that **LIV** can either stimulate or inhibit skin tumorigenesis depending on the dose of **LIV** and the nature of the PAH. The mechanism involves binding to microsomal membranes and strong inhibition of aryl hydrocarbon hydroxylase (AHH) activity. Ditercalinium [**LXVI**] and **LVII** when studied as agents against small cell lung cancer in bone marrow *in vitro*; it was found that the former has high activity against NCI-H449 and NCI-N417 human cells (IC50 1.2 x 10-3 and 10-2 μM, respectively) [228].

LXVI

Of the modified ellipticine derivatives developed [229, 230], ellipticine glycosides [**LXIV**] were found to possess antitumor activity. Ellipticine carbamate [**LXVII**] ("RPI-6") also has excellent antitumor activity [231] (1000 times higher than doxorubicin) against two human small-cell lung cancer lines (NCI H69c, N417) and two human non-small cell lung cancer lines (H460, H385).

LXIV

In addition to these three new elipticine derivatives, datelliptium [**LXVIII**] [232], pazellipticine (PZE or BD-40) [**LXIX**] [233] and BD-84 [**LXX**] [234] were evaluated; of these **LXVIII** and **LXX** showed better *in vivo* activity than **LVII** towards P-388, L-1210, B-16 colon 38 and M-5076 reticulosarcoma while **LXIX** has excellent *in vitro* activity against L-1210 cells.

LXIX $R^1 = H$, $R^2 = NH(CH_2)_3NHEt_2$, $X = 2Cl^-$
LXXIII $R^1 = Me$, $R^2 = H$, $X = 2Cl^-$

Mechanism of action – Although the mechanism of action of ellipticines *in vivo* has been studied in detail, and the results are supported experimentally, they are rarely confirmed. The DNAs were the biological targets of this type of molecules. Several reviews appeared in the literature discussing the mechanism of action of ellipticines [210, 215, 218, 235–237]. The other important cellular targets are metabolic activation of an ellipticine to a quinone imine or related species of high electrophilicity, DNA intercalation (not only binding) and topoisomerase II.

It has been shown that both **LIV** and **LV** caused inhibition of DNA, RNA and protein syntheses [238] with a strong inhibitory effect on DNA polymerase and RNA polymerase [239]. Any compound believed to be an antitumor agent acting on DNA must penetrate the cell, then cross the cytoplasm and enter the nucleus before being able to interfere with the DNA structures in the nucleus (unprotected by their usual chromatin). While crossing the cytoplasm, these agents can well encounter other nucleic acid structures e. g. RNAs, which are important in transferring genetic information, protein synthesis and in other basic biological processes (cofactors, ATP, GTP etc.). That these reactions could occur *in vivo*, was suggested by the high reactivity of ribonucleosides or ribonucleotides with 9-hydroxyellipticine derivatives under oxidative conditions leading to the formation of regiospecific and stereoselective ketal linkages between 2'- and 3'-hydroxyl groups of the ribose moiety of these compounds and the 10-position of ellipticine derivatives. The order of reactivity for hydroxyellipticine for the naturally occuring ribonucleosides used in this reaction is A, G, T [or U], C is A›G›››T(U)›C. The decreasing reactivity in going from purines to pyrimidines is probably due to a better affinity (recognition) of adenine and guanine for the pyrido-carbazole moiety of ellipticine as evidenced by NMR techniques [239].

The intercalation effects on DNA are manifested by DNA breaks of both the single-strand and double-strand types. It has been observed [240] that **LIV** produces a large number of protein associated single-strand breaks, and it was assumed that the breaks could be caused by nicking of DNA by intracellular enzymes to reduce the torsional strain resulting from intercalation. **LIV, LVI**, 9-aminoellipticine [**LXXI**] and 2-methyl-9-hydroxyellipticinium caused DNA breaks at concentrations corresponding to their order of cytotoxicity. Further it has been shown that strand breaks caused by **LIV** were not (after wash out) reversible while those caused by 2-methyl-9-hydroxyelliptinium were almost completely reversible [241, 242] thus suggesting that **LIV** itself has other molecular targets or is retained in the cell in a depot bound to cellular components. Later on it was suggested [243] that the reported strand breakage of DNA is not necessarily the primary cause of cytotoxicity of **LIV** and 9-hydroxyellipticine; other factors such as the interaction with phospholipid monolayers, the formation of free radicals and quinone imines and the interaction with cytochrome P-450 could all be important as the effects are demonstrated at same concentration. When the interaction of ellipticine derivatives with phospholipids in artificial or natural membranes was studied [243, 244] it was observed that compounds without a polar group in position 9 ([LIV] and [LV]) bind strongly to acidic lipids, while LVI and LXXI do not. It is also proposed that this type of binding could effect:

(i)   Pharmacokinetics by a depot effect,

(ii) Interaction with enzymes at the microsomal membrane and,

(iii) Direct cell killing through membrane permeability changes.

LV was found to penetrate deeper into the membrane lipid layers than LXXI or LVI [245].

The inhibition of AHH activity by LIV, LVI and 9-fluoroellipticine is quite marked, and it is suggested that binding to heme iron (through pyridinic nitrogen at position 4) in cytochrome P-450 may be involved [246, 247]. AHH inhibition was seen, both using human liver microsomes and rat liver microsomal preparations [248]. Structure-activity relationship (SAR) study of AHH activity inhibition [246] showed that LIV, LVI and 9-fluoroellipticine are the most promising compounds, whereas 7-hydroxyellipticine, 7,9-dichloroellipticine [LXXII] and 9-azaellipticine [LXXIII] derivatives are less effective. From these studies Lesca [246] derived the idea that it may be possible to develop an ellipticine that is a fairly pure AHH inhibitor and is devoid of antitumor (DNA binding) effects. This type of compound could be used successfully to treat accidental exposure to metabolically activated carcinogens or drug substances.

Ross [235] has summarized the importance of topoisomerase II as a potential target for anticancer drugs. Since the activity of topoisomerase II is thought to be higher in malignant cells as compared to normal cells (improved selectivity), topoisomerase II was pursued as a drug target. The topoisomerase II bonds to the 5'-phosphate on adjacent DNA strands four base apart to form an enzyme-DNA complex during cleavage and rejoining of DNA strands (catenation, decatenation, relaxation, unknotting). It is the interaction between this complex and many drugs, e. g. LIV, that results in the stabilization of the complex and the formation of a "clearable complex" leading to the cleavage of double-stranded DNA. The cells which are resistant to 9-hydroxyellipticine have fewer DNA double-strand breaks than normal cells, suggesting the role of breaks in the antitumor activity of topoisomerase II inhibitors [249, 250]. A good correlation has been observed between antitumor activity and topoisomerase II inhibitory activity in vitro for 9-hydroxyellipticine, elliptinium, 9-aminoellipticine and 9-fluoroellipticine [251].

Alternatively, **LIV** and its derivatives can act by their quinone imines **LXXIV** and **LXXV,** and it has been hypothesized that the quinone imine is involved in the observed covalent binding *in vivo* to DNA in L-1210 cells exposed to elliptinium [259]. The binding of **LIV** derivatives to DNA destroys kinoplastic DNA and base pairing ability, thus denaturing DNA [210]. The strong activity of 9-hydroxyellipticine, an easily accessible metabolite of **LIV,** suggests that **LIV** has to be metabolized to this compound before being active. In the patients who are kept on barbiturates, this metabolization is enhanced, since they are known to be potent cytochrome P-450 inducers.

LXXIV   R = H
LXXV   R = Me

Since it was found that most of the effective anticancer drugs are mutagenic in the Ames test, several reports appeared describing the mutagenicity of **LIV** and derivatives [253–256]. It is observed that all of the unchanged compounds evaluated (ellipticine and its 9-hydroxy-, 9-methoxy-, 9-bromo-, and 9-amino-derivatives) were mutagenic, whereas the quaternized derivatives, 2-methyl-9-hydroxyellipticinium and 2-methylellipticinium [**LXXVI**] were not mutagenic either with or without microsomal activation. Later on Pinto *et al.* [257] reported these charged ellipticines as potent inducers of mitochondrial mutations in *Saccharomyces cerevisiae,* indicating that significant differences in response exist between prokaryotic and eukaryotic organisms and that multiple types of assay systems are indicated for proper evaluation.

Paoletti *et al.* [258, 259] concluded that to be active *in vivo,* a compound in the ellipticine series must have either a hydrogen at C-9, which is readily oxidizable to a 9-hydroxy group or a 9-hydroxy group or derivatized 9-hydroxy group. The **LVI** was terminated in clinical trials because of the solubility problems [217].

9-methoxyellipticine lactate was the first candidate for clinical trials of ellipticine derivative in 1971 [269] on 34 patients with acute lymphoblastic leukemia (ALL), acute myeloblastic leukemia (AML), or

Hodgkin's disease. Out of 15 cases of AML, complete remission in 3 was observed and no responses in ALL or Hodgkin's disease. The phase I and Phase II clinical trials [261–263] with 2-methyl-9-hydroxy-ellipticinium acetate showed positive responses in thyroid and renal cancer, soft tissue sarcomas and in bone metastases from advanced breast cancer.

LVII given to patients i. v. (100 μg/ml in a 5% dextrose solution for 1–2 hrs), responded well in metastatic soft tissue sarcoma [264] and breast cancer [265]. When LVII was in combination with mitomycin, vinblastine, and/or etoposide it showed potent activity and was well tolerated by advanced breast cancer patients [266]. Elliptinium was also useful in metastatic renal cell carcinoma [267].

The toxicities observed are: severe inhibition of salivary secretion, oral infections, loss of appetite, loss of sensation of the tongue, rarely renal shutdown and hemolytic reactions related to high antibody level.

These results suggested a promising future for ellipticines. The development of various "second generation" ellipticine analogs of azaellipticines, the bispyridocarbazoles, ellipticine glycosides and carbamates opens a new era to keep the ellipticine as antitumor agents in the spot light of cancer chemotherapy with a bright future.

7   Erythrophleum

Several cytotoxic alkaloids in the cassamine series [268, 269], and the amide alkaloids [270] were not cytotoxic. 3a-acetoxynorerythrosuamine [LXVIIa] isolated from bark exhibited an ED50 of 0.0003 μg/ml in the KB assay a thousand times more active than its parent alcohol norerythrosuamine [LXVIIIa].

LXVIIa R = COMe, R^1 = COOCH$_2$CH$_2$NHMe
LXVIIIa R = H, R^1 = COOCH$_2$CH$_2$NHMe

Cassaine was inactive against the B16 melanoma, L-1210 leukemia, Lewis lung, P-388 leukemia, P-1534 leukemia, sarcoma 180, P-1798 lymphosarcoma and Walker 256 carcinosarcoma tumor systems *in vivo,* but is active against KB cells in culture (ED50 = 0.8–1.0 µg/ml). Cytotoxicity towards KB cells has also been commonly observed with digitalis-type cardenolides as well as bufodienolides, both of which are likewise inactive *in vivo* indicating that there is no selective activity against tumor cells, but rather a general cytotoxic effect. It would, therefore, seem evident that the Erythrophleum alkaloids are unlikely to be useful as antitumor agents [271].

8   Maytansinoids

Maytansine [**LXIXa**] and the related maytansine esters are potent antileukemic agents isolated from *Maytenus ovatus, M. buchananii* and *Colubrina texensis* [272–275]. A review of the chemistry and pharmacology of maytansine has appeared [276], and a quantitative microbiological assay for µg/ml concentration of maytansine has been developed using *Penicillium avellaneum* [277].

Putterlickia verrucosa is the richest source of **LXIXa** yet found (12 mg/kg) [278]. Maytansinol [**LXXa**] and maytanacine [**LXXIa**] were also isolated from this plant. **LXIXa** is a highly active inhibitor of cell division. At 6×10-8 M **LXIXa** irreversibly inhibited cell division in the eggs of sea urchins and clams. **LXIXa** and **XXV** showed comparable inhibition of the *in vitro* polymerization but **XXVa** showed lower inhibitory action in the division of marine eggs [279–280]. **LXIXa** is also a potent inhibitor of murine sarcoma virus in mice [281]. Injection of **LXIXa** (50 µg/kg/day, i. p.) for 5–10 days after one-day inoculation of various tumors in mice inhibited the growth of mouse sarcoma, Lewis lung cancer and brain tumor 22 by 42.8 to 31.8 and 32% respectively, and injection of maytanprin [**LXXIIa**] inhibited growth of these tumors by 23.8, 28.0 and 15.8% respectively. **LXIXa** at 25–50 µg/kg prolonged survival time of mice with leukemia P-388 and L-121 by 104–133 and 71.3–166% respectively. **LXXIIa** treatment prolonged the survival time of P-388, L-121 and L-615 leukemic mice by 138.0, 63.4 and 41.6% respectively. **LXIXa** at 25 µg/kg also prolonged the survival time of mice with hepatoma and Ehrlich ascites tumor by 250.0 and 26.4% and **LXXIIa** at the same dose prolonged the survival time by 202.8 and 263.9% respectively [282].

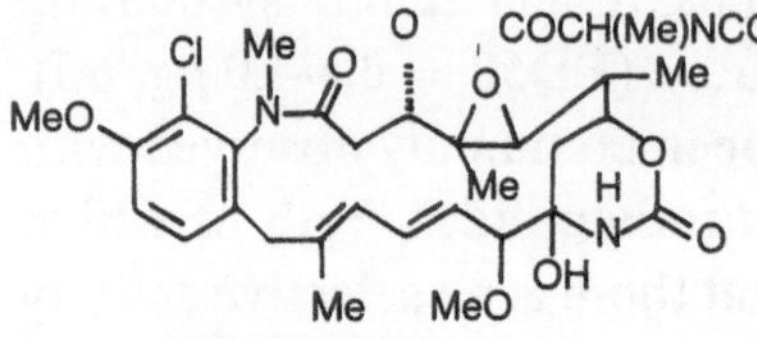

LXIXa R=Me
LXXIIa R=Et

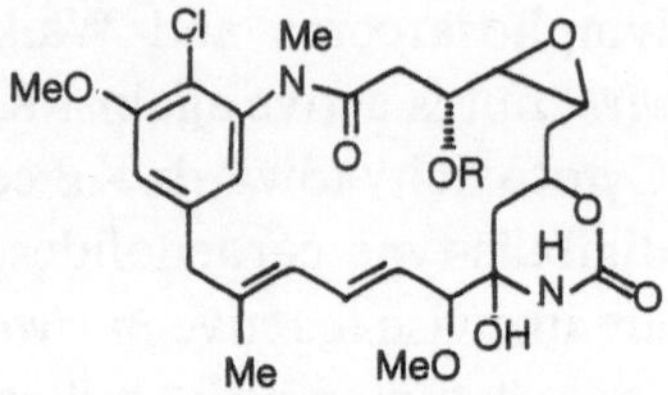

LXXa R=H
LXXIaR=COMe

Nozaki *et al.* reported that the tritepenes 3-oxofriedelan-29-oic acid, 3-oxofriedelan-28-oic acid and 28, 29-dihydroxyfriedelan-3-one isolated from *M. diversifolia* showed cytotoxicity against the A-549 lung carcinoma cells with ED50 values of 0.21, 1.18 and 0.64 μg/ml respectively [283].

Kuo *et al.* reported [284] that methanolic extract of stem and branches of *M. emerginata* was found to display significant *in vitro* cytotoxicity against KB cell culture and *in vivo* antitumor activity against P-388 lymphocytic leukemia. Emarginatine A [**LXXIIIa**] and emarginatine B [**LXXIVa**] were isolated from *Maytenus emerginata* [285]. **LXXIVa** was found to be active against KB cells with ID50 of 4.0 μg/ml. In comparison, **LXXIVa** was found to be much more active against the same cell line with ED50 of 0.4 μg/ml. Evidently the placement of benzoate group at C-9 position potentiates the cytotoxicity.

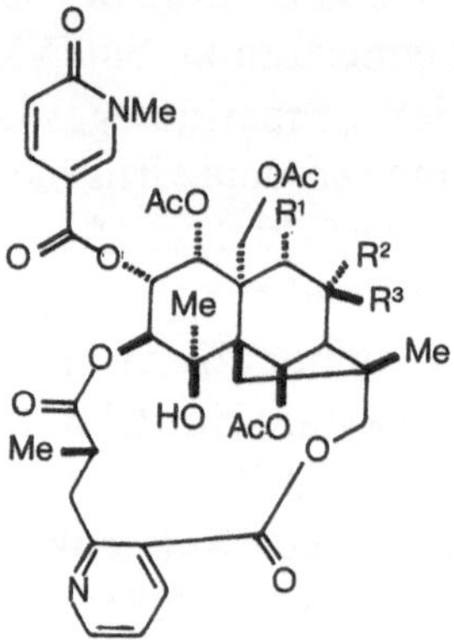

LXIIIa R¹=R²=OAc, R³=H
LXXIVa R¹=OCO—⟨phenyl⟩, R²=H, R³=OAc

9   Panax

Ginsenoside Rgl [**LXXVa**] (50 mg/kg/7 days) showed 52% tumor inhibition in mice infected with sarcoma 180 [286]. Its effectiveness was demonstrated against stomach cancer in human and in mice bearing sarcoma 180 [287]. Yuki *et al.* [288] reported the antitumor mechanism of ginsenoside Rh2 and the role of gene C-myc in cell proliferation in cultured B16 melanoma Meth-A and HL-60 cell lines. Results showed that ginsenoside Rh2 does not act on expression of C-mye directly. Notoginsinoside R1 [**LXXVIa**] affected synthesis of DNA and RNA while it induced differentiation of HL-60 cell. At 48 hrs the incorporate inhibition was 26.32% with [3H] Tdr and 18.57% with [3H]-VR and at 72 hrs the inhibition was 17.46 and 21.76% respectively [289].

LXXVa R = Glu
LXXVIa R = Glu (2–1)Xyl

Ether extract of Korean ginseng roots was toxic to mice and inhibited sarcoma 180 and adenocarcinoma 755 roughly in proportion to weight loss of hosts. Its ethanol extract also significantly inhibited growth of sarcoma 180 [290]. Panaxytriol [**LXXVII**] isolated from Panax ginseng roots significantly prevented the decrease in glutathione peroxidase activity and ornithine decarboxylase induction caused by croton oil. In addition it significantly inhibited croton oil induced edema in mice and afforded protection by delaying the subsequent development of skin tumors [291].

Matsunga *et al.* [292] showed the *in vitro* effect of **LXXVII** on the cell growth *in vitro*. The concentrations of **LXXVII** required to give 50% growth inhibition (ED50) were 0.8, 1.7, 2.2, 2.3, 10.7 and 11.7 µg/ml against MK-1, B16, L-929, SW 620, HeLa and K-562 cells. However **LXXVII** did not inhibit the growth of human fibroblasts MRC-5 cells by 50% even at concentration of over 40 µg/ml. Mitsuo *et al.* [293] reported that cell growth inhibition of **LXXVII** seemed to be tumor specific. Its action was more dose dependent than time dependent. **LXXVII** (40 mg/kg, i. m.) produced tumor growth inhibition in mice.

$CH_2=CH-CH(OH)-C\equiv C-CH_2-CH(OH)-CH(OH)-(CH_2)_6-Me$

LXXVII

Kim *et al.* [294] studied the tumoricidal activity of murine macrophase against K-562 tumor cells in the presence of lipopolysaccharide (LPS) and ginseng saponin. The tumoricidal activity was increased more by LPS plus ginseng total saponin (44% in 24 hrs) than by LPS alone (22% in 24 hrs). In the case of diol saponin the tumoricidal activity was increased as much as 35% at concentration of 10-3 to 10-7%. Triol saponin slightly increased the tumoricidal activity, more than LPS alone treatment, at each concentration. When total diol and triol saponins were added to K-562 tumor cells in various concentrations without macrophase it was found that saponins had no tumoricidal effects. This result suggests that ginseng saponin increases the tumoricidal activity against K-562 tumor cells through the tumoricidal activity of macrophase.

10   Podophyllum

Podophyllin is a resin isolated from the dried roots and rhizomes of *P. peltatum* (American species) and *P. emodi* (Indian species). Both species are herbaceous perennials. *P. peltatum* is indigenous to the US and Canada and is usually called the "May apple" or "American mandrake" [295]. *P. emodi* resembles *P. peltatum* and grows in the enterior ranges of the Himalaya mountains from Sikkim to Hazara. Natives have long been familiar with the cathartic properties of the aqueous extract of roots.

Kaplan *et al.* [296] reported that the topical application of podophyllin in oil was effective in the treatment of condyloma acuminata. This was soon followed by a report of King and Sullivan [297] demonstrating that podophyllin caused pronounced cytologic changes in normal human and rabbit skin. Miller *et al.* [298] reported the podophyllin treatment of condyloma acuminata without side effects. Sullivan *et al.* [299] also reported that podophyllin caused mitotic arrest during metaphase.

Heyenga *et al.* [300] reported the isolation of tumor inhibitory lignans podophyllotoxin **[LXXVIII]** 4'-demethyl-podophyllotoxin **[LXXIX]** and podophyllotoxin 4-O-glucoside **[LXXX]** from callus culture of seedlings.

The lignans potentially useful as anticancer agents have now been chemically modified to produce the clinically useful drug **[IV]** and teniposide **[LXXXII]**. **LXXXI** is of particular value in the treatment of

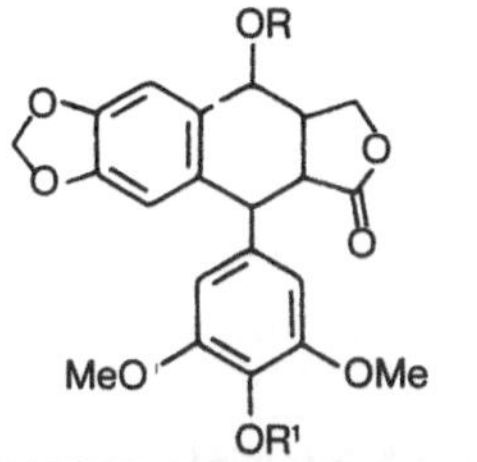

LXXVIII R=H, R¹=Me
XXIX R=R¹=H
XXX R=Glu, R¹=Me

testicular cancer and small cell lung cancer and is now commercially produced from **LXXVIII** [301, 302]

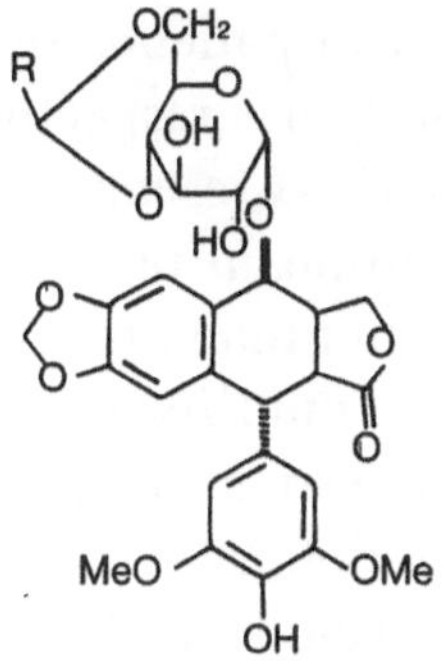

LXXXI R=Me

LXXXII R=

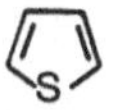

LXXXI and **LXXXII** possessed antitumor activity against several experimental animal tumors including Sarcoma-180, Ehrlich ascites carcinoma and Walker 256 carcinoma. They also showed activity against L-5178 Y and L-1210 murine leukemias [303–306]. Both compounds showed greatest activity when given in two or three doses/week or every 3 hrs on days 1,5 and 9 after tumor inoculation [304].

The toxicity in mice and rats given a single injection of **LXXXII** was approximately 50 mg/kg but is reduced to about 5 mg/kg when the drug is given daily for 6–12 days.

Avery *et al.* [306] reported the finding of severe form of delayed toxicity for **LXXXII** in mice carrying the L-5178 Y and L-1210 tumors. There was some evidence that it was dependent on the i. p. route of drug administration. Deaths for late toxicity occurred 1–3 months after the end of drug administration in 90–100% of mice cured by treatment with the highest dose (16 mg/kg) of **LXXXII**. Larsen *et al.* [307] reported toxic effects in the rhesus monkeys treated 6 days/week for four weeks with various doses of **LXXXII**. The most serious toxic effects found were bone marrow suppression and colitis with diarrhea.

LXXXI was relatively less effective in these tumors. It showed activity against acute myelogenous leukemia [308]. LXXXII has also been reported to be effective in the treatment of intracranial malignancies [309].

The pharmacokinetics of LXXXII and LXXXI differ in various aspects. After administering the tritiated forms of these compounds to cancer patients. Allen *et al.* [310] found that LXXXI had a biphasic plasma disappearance curve, whereas plasma decay kinetics of LXXXII followed a triphasic exponential curve with a terminal phase half-life of 11–38 hrs. Approximately 45% of the administered radioactivity was recovered within 72 hrs in urine of patients treated with either LXXXII or LXXXI of which 78% and 66% respectively were identified as parent compound. Although LXXXI resembled LXXXII in the extent to which it was excreted in the urine, its rate of excretion and renal clearance was some three-fold greater than that of LXXXII. It was suggested that this difference may account for the three-fold higher equitoxic dose of LXXXI. Both showed a high affinity for plasma proteins. At typical plasma concentration, 94% of LXXXI was bound to serum albumin, for LXXXII this value was 99%. Neither compound penetrates the blood-brain barrier well since only low concentrations of drugs were found in the cerebrospinal fluid [311].

Studies carried out to delineate the mechanism of action of LXXXII and LXXXI indicate that these compounds have diverse actions at the biochemical level. In contrast to many other plant derived compounds with antitumor activity (podophyllotoxin itself), LXXXII and LXXXI do not arrest dividing cells in metaphase, but rather block cells in the premitotic stage of the cell cycle [303, 304]. LXXXI incubated with various human hematopoietic cell lines inhibited cell growth and induced chromosomal aberrations in the G2 and S phases of cell cycle. Other effects of these compounds are the inhibition of respiration by Ehrlich ascites tumor cells and electron transport at the NADH dehydrogenase level by mitochondria and submitochondrial particles from rat liver [312].

The primary mechanism of action of LXXXI and LXXXII is believed to be *via* their interaction with DNA [313]. Dose-dependent single- and double-stranded breaks in DNA caused by LXXXI and LXXXII have been widely reported [314–317]. Zhang *et al.* [318] synthesized a series of orthoquinone analogs of **LXVIII** possessing various C-4a-aniline moieties. Evaluated for their inhibitory activity against human DNA topoisomerase II, their activity was found to cause cellular protein-linked DNA breakage and their cytotoxicity against KB cells.

Thurston *et al.* also [319 a] reported the mechanism of action of **LXXXI** and **LXXXII** by inhibiting catalytic activity of type-II DNA topo-isomerase and concurrent enzyme-mediated production of lethal DNA strand breaks.

11   Sesbania

It is commonly known as coffee bean, rattle brush or rattle box. The activity of seed extract against P-388 leukemia in mice and KB cells in culture was reported by Powell *et al.* [319 b]. Sesbanine [**LXXXXIII**] was isolated and initially presumed to be the active component [320, 321]. Several syntheses of sesbanine were accomplished [322, 325], but racemic **LXXXXIII** provided to NCl by Kande and Demuth was found inactive in the P-388 leukemia *in vivo* [322, 271]. Reexamination of recrystallized natural [**LXXXXIII**] showed that it was not the cytotoxic principle and the activity remained in the mother liquor. Concerted efforts to separate the active fractions finally resulted in the isolation of sesbanimide [**LXXXXIV**] (5 x 10-5% yield). It has now been established as major cytotoxic and antileukemic principle [326]. **LXXXXIV** was active against L-1210 leukemia at a dose of 128 μg/kg and highly active against M-5076 sarcoma and P-388 leukemia at a dose of 256 and 120 μg/kg respectively. **LXXXXIV** was inactive against B16 melanoma and MX-1 mammary xenograft. The activity shown against P-388 leukemia and M-5076 sarcoma system made the compound a potential candidate for advanced preclinical study. **LXXXXIV** has been renamed as sesbanimide A [327]. Synthesis of **LXXXXIV** was reviewed by Matsuda *et al.* [328].

LXXXIII

LXXXIV

12   Taxus

The toxicity of *Taxus baccata* L. (English Yew) (Taxaceae) has been known since antiquity. All parts of the tree are toxic except the red fleshy envelope of the fruit which is eaten by birds. Lucas [329] in 1856 for the first time isolated from the leaves a toxic alkaloid which was named taxine. The structure of taxine was not established at that time but degradation product of taxine was identified as S-3-dimethyl-amino-3-phenylpropionic acid [LXXXV] known as Winterstein's acid [330]. Later on taxine was shown to be a mixture of 3 alkaloids with an unusual diterpenoid skeleton-taxane [331] but the structure of only one major alkaloid was established as taxine-1. The structure of some other taxane compounds isolated from *T. baccata* and the Japanese yew *T. cuspidata* were established e. g.: taxinine [LXXXVI]-a decomposition product of taxine [332] and many others [333].

	R¹	R²	R³	R⁴
LXXXVI	O	H	COCH=CHPh	OAc
XCVI	OAc	OAc	H	OAc
CXII	OAc	H	Ac	H
CXIII	H	H	H	OAc

In the course of screening natural products for anticancer activity the novel diterpenoid-taxol [LXXXVII] isolated form the stem bark of *T. brevifolia* [334] showed remarkable activity against various leuke-mias, sarcoma 180, the Walker 256 carcinosarcoma, and the Lew's lung tumor [334]. With this major breakthrough in the natural prod-ucts chemistry almost all the available *Taxus* species were studied; *T. baccata* (Europe), *T. brevifolia* (North America), *T. cuspidata, T. wallchiana* and *T. mairei* (Asia) and *Austrotaxus spiccata* Compton (New Caledonia).

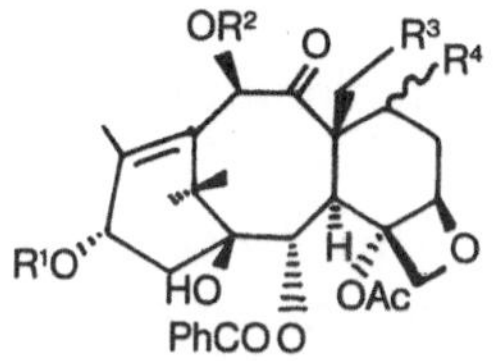

A = PhOCNH, O (structure)

B = (structure with CNH, O)

C = PhOCNH, O (structure)

D = nC5H11OCNH, O (structure)

E = BuᵗOOCNH, O (structure)

	R¹	R²	R³	R⁴
LXXXVII		Ac	H	β-OH
LXXXIX	H	Ac	H	H
XC	H	H	H	β-OH
XCI	H	Ac	OH	β-OH
XCII	B	H	H	β-OH
XCIII	A	H	H	β-OH
XCIV	A	H	H	α-OH
XCV	B	H	H	α-OH
CI	C	Ac	H	β-OAc
CII	C	H	H	β-OAc
CIII	A	H	H	β-Xylose
CIV	B	H	H	β-Xylose
CV	D	H	H	β-Xylose
CVI	A	Ac	H	β-Xylose
CVII	B	Ac	H	β-Xylose
CVIII	D	Ac	H	β-Xylose
CIX	A	MeCH (OH) CH₂CO	H	H
CX	B	MeCH (OH) CH₂CO	H	H
CXV	E	H	H	β-OH

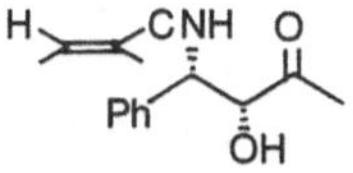

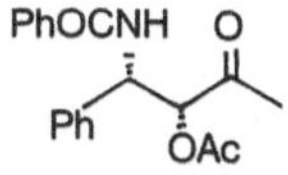

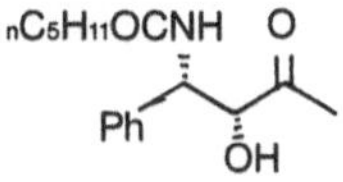

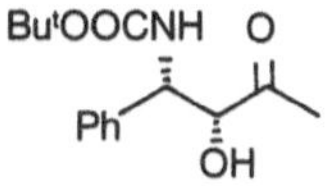

As described earlier **LXXXVII** has an unusual skeleton-taxane type which is composed of three [9.3.1.0 ^{3,8}] pentadecene rings [**LXXXVIII**]. The proposed nomenclature for this compound has been modified as shown in [**LXXXVIII**]. With the advent of nuclear magnetic resonance spectroscopy and X-ray crystallography at least 19 taxane derivatives were isolated including baccatin III [**LXXXIX**] (revised structure) [335].

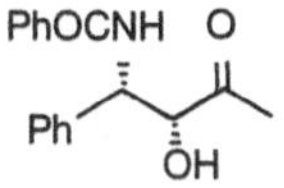

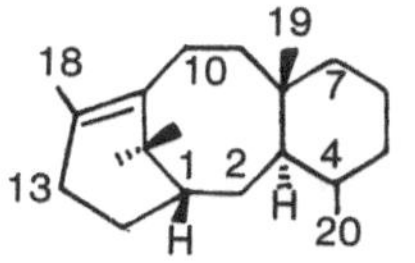

LXXXVIII

Excellent reviews dealing with the work on taxol have appeared [336–340, 76]. The highly cytotoxic and antileukemic compound taxol was isolated by bioassay-directed fractionation from the bark of *T. brevifolia* Nutt. [334] in 0.02% yield. The structure of taxol as [**LXXXVII**] is evidenced from 1H-NMR and X-ray crystallographic techniques of taxol and its degradation products.

Taxol can be differentiated structurally from other taxane diterpenoids by its ester side chain at C-13 and by its oxetane ring D and can be assumed to be the N-benzoyl-β-phenylisoserine ester of baccatin III. Taxol is represented by the chem-3D Plus program illustrating its 3D-shape [**LXXXVIIa**]. Taxol has also been isolated from *T. wallichiana* and *T. cuspidata* [341].

LXXXVIIa

More than one hundred compounds possessing taxane skeleton have been isolated from various Taxus species. The diterpenoid cephalomannine [**LIII**] isolated from *T. wallichiana* (syn. *Cephalotaxus manii)* [341, 342] and the structure [**LIII**] for cephalomannine was established by mild methanolysis to five compounds, **LXXXIX,** methylester, 10-deacetylbaccatin III [**XC**], 10-deacetylepibaccatin III and 7-epibaccatin III [342]. Compound **LIII** was also isolated from *T. baccata* [343]. The compounds isolated from *T. baccata* differing from taxol only in the nature of the N-acyl group were named as taxols B, C, D and so on. Taxol A was similar to taxol and taxol B to cephalomannine [343].

LIII is different from **LXXXVII** only in the location of amide group in the distal portion of C-13 ester unit. Other new active compounds isolated from this plant are 19-hydroxybaccatin III [**XCI**], 10-deacetylcephalomannine [**XCII**] and 10-deacetyl taxol [**XCIII**] [344]. A rapid epimerization in **XCII** and **XCIII** occurred to give the corresponding C-7 epimers, 7-epi-l0-deacetyltaxol [**XCIV**] and 7-epi-l0-deacetylce-phalomannine [**XCV**] [345]. Weekly cytotoxic in KB cell line – 1-beta-hydroxybaccatin I was also isolated from *T. wallichiana* Zucc [341]. The post-taxol fraction afforded new cytotoxic taxanes from *T. brevi-folia* and *T. baccata* [346–348]. The compounds isolated are decina-moyltaxine J [**XCVI**], 7-epi-taxol [**XCVII**], keto-taxol derivative [**XCVIII**], taxine A [**XCIX**] and taxagifine [**C**]. Compounds **XC** and **XCVI** showed ED50 28 and 1.0 μg/ml respectively against KB cells. The cytotoxicity of **C** was comparable to **LXXXVII** but **C** possesses two structural features that create quite substantial conformational changes in the molecule – (i) the lack of an oxetane-type bridge between C-5 and C-20 and (ii) the presence of a new ether bridge between C-12 and C-16 [348].

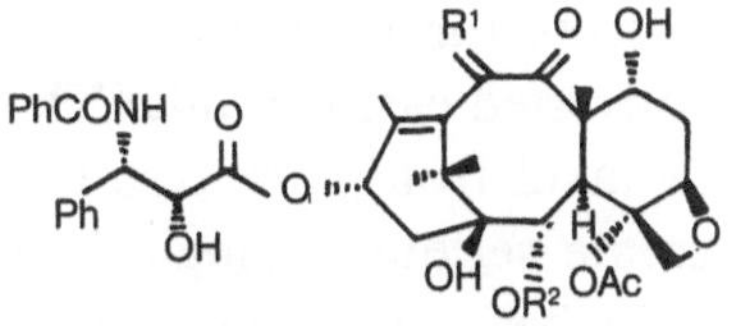

XCVII $R^1 = \beta$-OAc, $R^2 = $ Ac
XCVIII $R^1 = $ O, $R^2 = $ Bz
CXI $R^1 = $ O, $R^2 = $ Ac

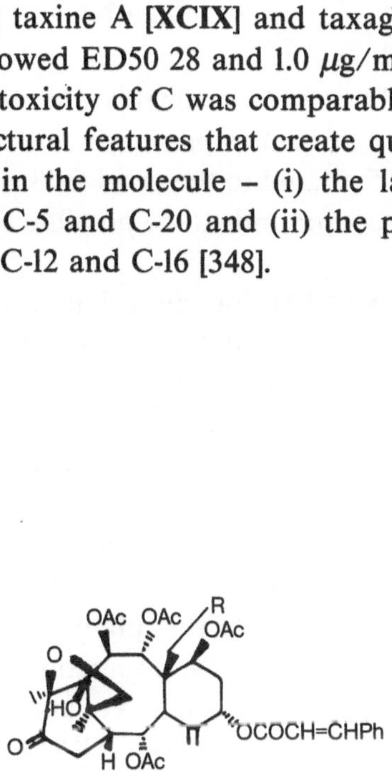

C   R = H
CXIV R = OCOPh

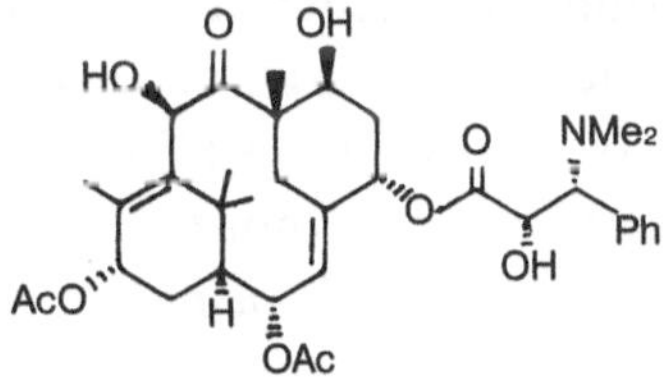

XCIX

Acetylation of crude post-taxol fraction yielded 2', 7-diacetyltaxol [**CI**] and 2', 7-diacetyl-l0-deacetyltaxol [**CII**] [347].
Bioactivity-directed fractionation of the trunk bark of *T. baccata* using a microtubule inhibition assay resulted in the isolation of six taxol derivatives [**CIII-CVIII**] with a xylose unit at C-7, two of which had an N-hexanoyl group in place of N-benzoyl group and were named as derivatives of taxol C. In two other derivatives, β-hydroxybutyryl groups replaced the 10-acetyl groups of taxol and cephalomannine.

Compounds **LXXXVII** and baccatin VI were also isolated from
T. baccata [343].

10-Deacetyl-10-oxo-7-epi-taxol [**CXI**] and **XCVII** were isolaed from
pre-taxol fraction of *T. brevifolia* bark [349]. Various hydroxylated or
acetylated derivatives of taxusin [**CXII**] have been isolated from
leaves, bark or wood of *T. baccata* [350–352]. X-Ray crystallography
confirmed the structure of taiwanxan [**CXIII**], isolated from *T. mairei*
[353]. Compounds **C** and **CXIV** were also isolated from *T. cuspidata*
[354].

More than thirty new taxanes have been isolated from *Austrotaxus*
spicata [355] without a side chain at C-13 as present in **LXXXVII,** but
many of them are acylated at C-5 related to the taxol C-13 side chain.
Potier [356] has suggested these compounds to be possible biogenetic
intermediates of taxol.

To fulfil the requirement of **LXXXVII** for clinical use, some new
sources, for its isolation or for **LXXXIX** and **XC,** both of which can be
converted easily into **LXXXVII,** were investigated. Since the isolation
of taxol from bark resulted in the death of the plant which would
create serious ecological problems. It is said that "if taxol proves
effective ... the yew population could be so severely depleted that
there would not be enough trees left to make treatment successful".
No successful total synthesis of taxol has yet been achieved. Compound **XC** was isolated from the leaves of this plant which can be
quickly regenerated without affecting the yew population. The presence of **LXXXIX** and **XC** has been reported in leaves and needles of
six *Taxus* species [357] and the highest amount of **LXXXIX** by weight
(0.01%) was found in *T. media* cv. *thicksii* needles with comparable
amounts in *T. cuspidata* cv. *capitata, T. canadiensis* and *T. brevifolia*
needles. But in stem, **LXXXIX** was found only one half of the
substance in the needles. The highest yield (0.02%) of **XC** was in
T. baccata cv. repandin needles.

Semiquantitative determination of taxol-like materials by ELISA
technique gave 0.05% (leaves) and 0.08% (stem bark) yield [358].
Further, from these studies it was suggested that **XC** may be slightly
more available than **LXXXVII** and also the yield of key intermediate
LXXXIX might be increased by chemical manipulations designed to
transform **LXXXVII** and **XC** into **LXXXIX** to make isolation easy
from the plant. Interestingly, while carrying out the transformation of
XC into **LXXXVII** [334] one of the derivatives obtained, named

taxotere [CXV], was found to have interesting pharmacological properties [359, 360]. Compound **CXV** had thus better bioavailability and also better pharmacological activities than **LXXXVII** itself and has a bright future to be developed as a new anticancer agent.

Pharmacological activity:

Taxol has a broad spectrum of antitumor activity in humans, particularly in drug-refractory ovarian [361] and breast [362] carcinomas and malignant melanoma [363]. Various reports are available in the literature describing the mechanism of action of **LXXXVII** [364–366]. Preferential binding of **LXXXVII** has been demonstrated to be microtubules rather than a tubulin dimer. This binding results in the formation of discrete bundles of stable microtubules, because of the reorganization of the microtubule cytoskeleton [367]. **LXXXVII** has different binding sites from those for exchangeable GTP, colchicine, vinblastine and podophyllotoxin [368]. Both the microtubule bundles and esters were present in human leukemic cell lines treated with **LXXXVII**. It has been shown in phase I clinical trials in leukemia that the response to **LXXXVII** was directly related to the ability of leukemic blasts to form microtubule bundles. Compound **LXXXVII** alters the normal equilibrium that exists between microtubules and the tubulin dimers thus resulting in the lowering of critical concentration of tubulin required to form microtubules [364] and ultimately disrupting the cell division and normal cellular activities in which microtubules are involved. Taxol-treated microtubules are stable to cold and $CaCl_2$ which normally disrupt the polymer. **LXXXVII** binds the cells in a specific and saturable manner with a single set of high-affinity binding sites [369].

Compound **LXXXVII** blocks cell cycle traverse in mitosis as demonstrated by studies with HeLa cells, BALB/c fibroblasts and with murine P-388 leukemia. By decreasing the intra cellular transport of cholesterol side-chain cleavage enzymes, **LXXXVII** inhibits steroidogenesis in human Y-1 adrenocortical and MLTC-1 Leydig tumors [370]. Some specific functions have also been inhibited by **LXXXVII** in various non-malignant cells such as chemotaxis, migration, cell spreading, polarizations, generation of hydrogen peroxide and killing of phagocytized microorganisms in human polymorphonuclear leukocytes [371]. Ding *et al.* [372] showed that compound **LXXXVII** mimics the effects of endotoxic bacterial lipopolysaccharide on macrophages resulting in a rapid decrement of tumor necrosis factor – alpha (TNF-alpha) receptors and TNF-alpha release. The inhibition of secretory functions of specialized cells e.g. insulin secretion in isolated rat islets of Langerhans and protein secretion in rat hepatocytes by **LXXXVII** has been reported [373, 374].

In preclinical antineoplastic activity, **LXXXVII** has been reported to be moderately active against murine L-1210, P-388 and P-1534 leukemias and Walker 256 carcinosarcoma, Sarcoma 180 and Lewis lung tumor [334], and good antitumor activity against several human tumor xenografts was also demonstrated.

Two distinct forms of resistance of **LXXXVII** have been characterized. First, a series of mutant Chinese hamster ovary cells with acquired **LXXXVII** resistance have altered α- and/or β-tubulin subunits and require **LXXXVII** for cell replication [375]. The second mechanism involves the multidrug resistant phenotype [376, 377]. Resistance to **LXXXVII** in human leukemia cell lines has been correlated with the development of polypoid cells, but very little information is available on the types of resistance that may develop in human tumors [378].

During the clinical pharmacology, taxol's insolubility in aqueous medium poses a problem with intravenous administration. Nowadays, it is dissolved in ethanol, and Cremophor (polyoxyethylated castor oil) is added which is toxic and can provoke allergy [379]. A triacetin-based emulsion has also been used for this purpose [380].

To carry out the detailed pharmacokinetic studies, various analytical assay methods have been developed and the most sensitive and specific was the reverse phase HPLC which can measure taxol concentration as low as 50 n mol/l [381–383]. After 24 hrs only 5% of **LXXXVII** was recovered in urine indicating that renal clearance is contributing minimally to systemic clearance [384]. No metabolite of **LXXXVII** in human blood and urine has been identified; however, the minor conversion of **LXXXVII** into 7-epi-taxol [XCVII] in normal saline solution and in tissue culture medium was observed [385, 383]. Monsarrat *et al.* [386] have demonstrated the recovery of 11.5% and 29% of injected taxol in rat bile as **LXXXVII** and metabolites respectively. The two hydroxylated metabolites were found to possess comparable activity to that of **LXXXVII** in preventing microtubule disassembly.

In one patient, **LXXXVII** has been measured in the ascites, 7 hrs post-infusion and maintained for at least 12 hrs at a concentration which was 40% of concurrent plasma levels, but there was no **LXXXVII** detected post-infusion in the cerebrospinal fluid of leukemia patients [384].

Phase I clinical trials have recommended to utilize a 24-hr continuous infusion schedule with a prophylactic antiallergic premedication regimen for all phase II taxol trials. A vast number of reports are available describing phase I clinical trials of **LXXXVII** [387–389]. The major dose limiting toxicity in all phase I solid tumor trials was the neutropenia [390, 383] and abdominal pain [391].

In early phase I trials antineoplastic activity has been observed in melanoma, adenocarcinoma of unknown origin, advanced and cisplatin-refractory ovarian, non-small cell lung, gastric, colon, head and neck carcinomas [382, 390, 388], with advanced non-small cell lung, breast, head and neck, colon, pancreatic and advanced ovarian carcinomas, and melanoma [392]. Adverse systemic effects including alopecia and sporadic neutropenia were also observed with a low concentration of **LXXXVII** in blood [391].

The phase II evaluation started with the side effects of **LXXXVII** in phase I trial. The study on a renal cell and advanced ovarian carcinoma showed a low level of activity of **LXXXVII,** and disparate responses of 6% and 18% have been noted in 2 phase II trials completed [393, 363]. Taxol has promising activity in advanced and refractory ovarian cancer [394]. Now, the phase II trials in breast, non-small cell and small cell lung, colon, prostate, cervical and head and neck carcinomas are avaiting the adequate supply of **LXXXVII**. Very exciting preliminary results have been obtained in breast carcinoma [395].

To overcome the problem **LXXXVII** supply as described earlier, a large number of analogs have been extracted or synthesized and in most of the cases, the primary baccatin III [**LXXXVIX**] framework is present. Three major classes of assay have been used – microtubule assembly assays, mammalian cell culture toxicity and assays in the mouse. The microtubule assembly promotion is carried out either by measuring the initial rate of microtubule assembly [396] or by measuring the initial rate of microtubule disassembly [397]. The cytotoxicity tests are carried out generally in three cell lines KB cells, J 774-2 cells (a mouse macrophase-like cell line) or P-388 cells. Assays in mouse have been carried out in P-388 leukemia, B16 melanoma and human tumors were used as xenografts in athymic mice.

The results of various studies can be summarized as follows:
The absolute requirement for the full activity is the C-13 ester side chain of **LXXXVII** as **LXXXVII** and **LIII** are both active while compounds lacking the side chain e.g. **LXXXVIX, XC** and **XCVI** are essentially inactive. Also the baccatin III [**LXXXVIX**] derivatives are all much less effective than **LXXXVII**. A taxol-type side chain, however, had activity. The N-acyl substituent on the C-13, side chain is not very important. For maximum biological activity the C-2'-hydroxyl group is very important. Compound **LXXXVII** has three hydroxyl groups at positions 1, 7 and 2'. The C-1 hydroxyl is tertiary and can not be readily acylated under mild condition, however, acetylation of **LXXXVII** afforded 2'-acetyltaxol, whereas vigorous conditions gave 2', 7-diacetyltaxol similar to **CI** isolated from *T. brevifolia*. Mild hydrolysis of **CI** yielded 7-acetyltaxol. 2'-acetyltaxol is almost 30-fold less active than **LXXXVII** and 2'-desoxy derivatives are 2-4-fold less active in the tubulin assembly assay and 12-fold less active in cytotoxic assay. Also the 2'-(t-butyldimethylsilyl) taxol derivative was less cytotoxic than **LXXXVII**. The 3'-phenyl group contributes overall activity of **LXXXVII** and the replacement of 3'-N-benzoyl group with other N-acyl groups leads to little loss of activity or an increase in activity. However, activity was lost on removal of the 3'-N-benzoyl group. The variations at C-2' and C-3' can be carried out without major loss of activity. If an amide function is present at C-3', the stereochemistry at C-2' results in a pronounced contribution to activity.

Thus in the 10-deacetyl series inversion at C-2' is ineffective to tubulin disassembly activity if there is an N-benzoyl group present, but the activity was reduced when there is an N-t-BOC group present. If 2'- and 3'-groups are interchanged stereochemically, the compound with the natural configuration is more active in the tubulin disassembly assay than the one with the unnatural configuration.

It has been concluded by a comparison of cytotoxicity data with tubulin assembly ar disassembly activity that the activities of most of the analogs broadly parallel their tubulin assembly or disassembly activities. 2'-acetyltaxol has similar cytotoxicity as **LXXXVII**: in contrast to the fact that the former was not able to promote microtubule assembly. These 2'-acyl derivatives are hydrolyzed *in vivo* to the corresponding 2'-hydroxy compounds and the cytotoxicity is reduced if 2'-hydroxy group is converted to some hydrolytically stable group e.g. t-butyl-dimethyl silyl ether.

Swindell *et al.* [396] concluded by molecular modelling that the conformation of the side chain is not strongly influenced by the taxane skeleton, and proposed that the taxol recognition site on microtubules possesses a hydrophobic cleft designed to accept a side chain with its functionality preorganized by stereochemistry and hydrogen bonding to resemble that of taxotere.

If the taxane ring is modified by acylation at C-7, or a polar sugar residue is attached at C-7, it is observed that the former does not reduce the tubulin disassembly inhibition whereas the latter slightly increases it. Also, the removal of C-10 acetyl group slightly reduces this activity and cytotoxicity. Attachment of polar groups at both C-7 and C-10, epimerization at C-7 slightly reduces the activity. The activity was reduced significantly by oxidation at C-7, although it is also possible that 7-oxotaxol under cell culture conditions underwent oxetane ring-opening [398]. A drastic reduction in cytotoxicity and tubulin disassembly inhibition activity was observed if the oxetane ring is opened; it was suggested that during this opening some conformational changes occur [399].

In a nutshell, we can say that changes in the taxane skeleton appear to reduce the activity of taxol. The activity of taxotere [CXV] is comparable to taxol but the former is more important because its precursor has been isolated from *T. baccata* leaves (a part which can be regenerated without harming the tree) and also CXV is approximately 25% more water soluble than LXXXVII. CXV is more potent than LXXXVII in polymerizing tubulin in the absence of GTP [400, 401]. Compound CXV also showed activity in many murine tumor models [402]. The pharmacokinetic data demonstrated the biphasic disposition of the drug. Recently Extra *et al.* [403] started phase I evaluation of CXV formulated in ethanol and polysorbate 80. Concluding to this it is observed that the investigations carried out so far in human tumors with LXXXVII indicate that LXXXVII has the potential to become an important new drug for the treatment of malignancies. Taxol can be used in combination with other drugs and/or radiation; in addition to this it also provides a tool for studying the microtubule assembly-disassembly regulation and the cellular functions of microtubules. Defining the role of LXXXVII in first and second line treatment for untreated as well as refractory and recurrent disease patients with ovarian cancer has become a goal in the development of this agent, and a phase III study of taxol and cisplatin versus cisplatin and cyclophosphoramide has started [404].

But to keep up the goal, an adequate supply of **LXXXVII** or identifying suitable analogs for wide-spread clinical use are required [405]. One may look for the hemisynthesis of **LXXXVII** or the active analogs from more abundant natural products e.g. **LXXXVIX,** which is derived from needles of *T. baccata*. Both **LXXXVII** and **CXV** have been successfully synthesized from **LXXXVIX** so it opens another area for exploration.

13   Thalictrum

Thalicarpine [**CXVI**] (thaliblastine) isolated from roots of *T. dasycarpum* [406] showed hypotensive effects in laboratory animals. In later studies it was seen that **CXVI** had antitumor activity against the rat Walker 256 carcinosarcoma over a wide dosage range [407]. Its several closely related compounds have also shown cytotoxic activity against human KB cells maintained in monolayer culture [408].

CXVI is a dimeric alkaloid and possesses a high level of biological activity in diverse systems, but the mechanism by which it produces these effects is not clear. Allen and Creaven [409] have shown that **CXVI** has profound effects on macromolecular biosynthesis in cultured mouse L-1210 cells inhibiting DNA, RNA and protein synthesis, although DNA synthesis was affected more rapidly than either RNA or protein synthesis.

They also found that tritiated **CXVI** binds to DNA and that this binding is completely reversible and **CXVI** did not bind to human serum albumin *in vitro* and it did bind to some unidentified human serum component *in vivo* [410]. Liao *et al.* [411] reported that **CXVI** and tetrandrine inhibited thymidine and uridine uptake in HeLa cells and the concentration of drug required for 50% inhibition is 5 μM for **CXVI.** Compound **CXVI** at single (270 and 380 mg/kg) or repeated (85 and 170 mg/kg) i.p. doses to normal rats or as a 90-day treatment (1.25–5 mg/kg) of pregnant animals had almost no toxic effects as revealed by body and organ weight [412]. Mircheva *et al.* [413] showed that the immunosuppressive effect of **CXVI** (250 mg/kg) on humoral and cellular immunity was smaller than that of vinblastine (4 mg/kg).

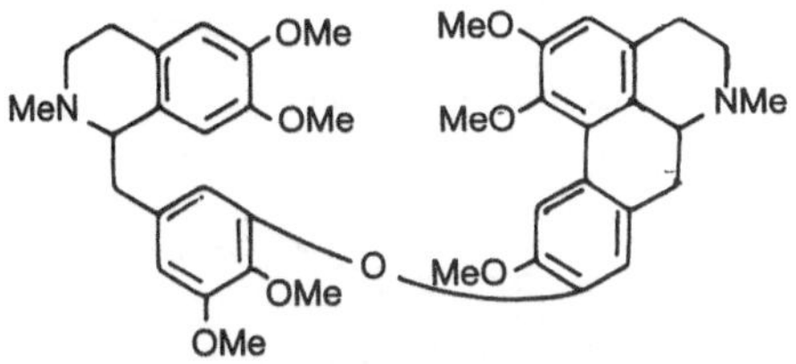

CXVI

On the basis of its activity against the Walker 256 carcinosarcoma, **CXVI** entered into initial trials but soon was found to possess serious toxicity at doses below those required for antitumor activity.

Thalmine [**CXVII**] isolated from *T. minus* at 250 mg/kg showed significant activity in mice and rats against ascites lymphoma NK/LY. **CXVII** (60–150 mg/kg) and thalmidine [**CXVIII**] (30–100 mg/kg) showed only weak inhibitory effects on the growth of lymphoma NK/LY, alveolar hepatoma PC-1 and Pliss lymphosarcoma [414].

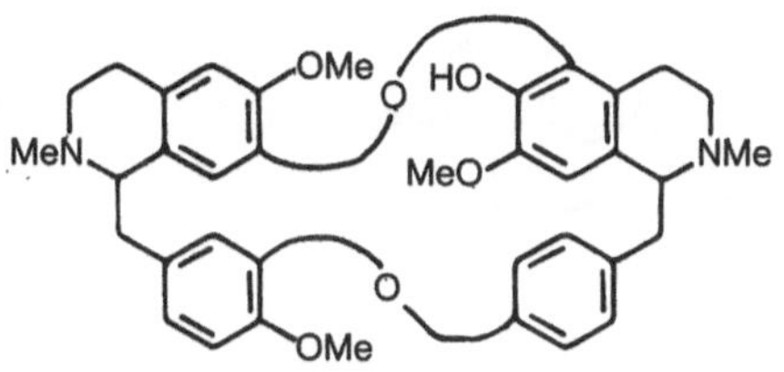

CXVII

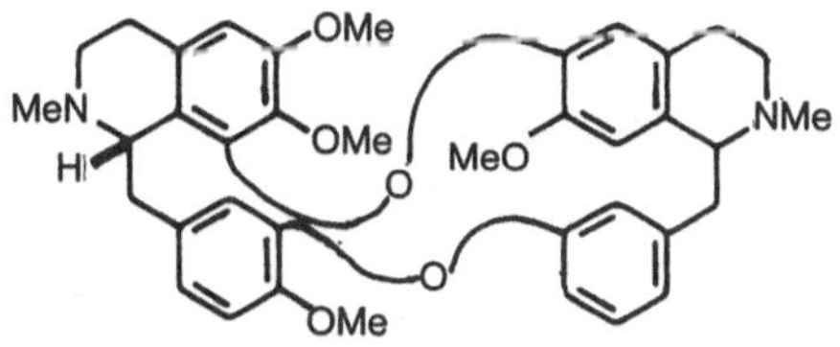

CXVIII

Thalictrine [**CXIX**] isolated from *T. foliolosum* DC. at a 30–150 mg/kg dose showed weak inhibitory effects in lymphoma NK/LY alveolar hepatoma, PC-1 and Pliss lymphosarcoma test system in mice or rat [414]. Zhou *et al.* [415] reported the isolation and antitumor activity of thalidasine [**CXX**] and thalifoetidin [**CXXI**] from the roots of *T. fargesii.*

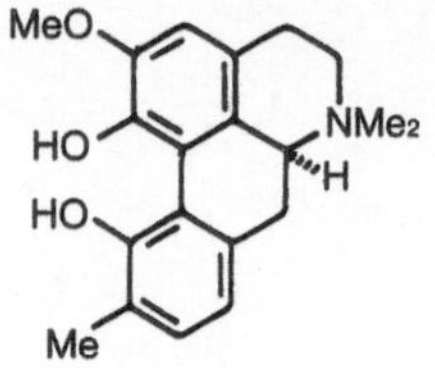

MeO
HO
HO
Me
NMe₂
H

CXIX

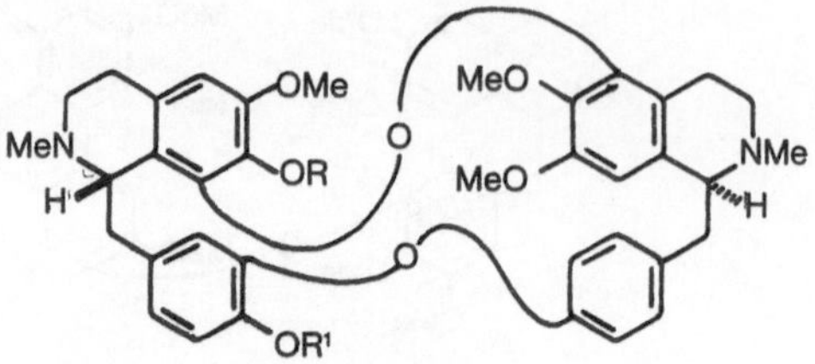

MeN
H
OMe
OR
O
MeO
MeO
NMe
H
O
OR¹

CXX   R = R¹ = Me
CXXI   R = Me, R¹ = H

Hernandezine [CXXII] isolated from *T. glandulosissium* was effective for treatment of mice bearing P-388 leukemia, S-180 ascites and C-26 colon cancer. Though CXXII inhibited the growth of mouse L-1210 cells and human oral cancer KB cells. Preliminary results showed that CXXII blocked cell cycle transfer from G1 to S phase and its cytocidal action might be cell cycle-specific. Thalidezine [CXXIII] and isothalidezine exerted a similar inhibitory effect on L-1210 cells [416].

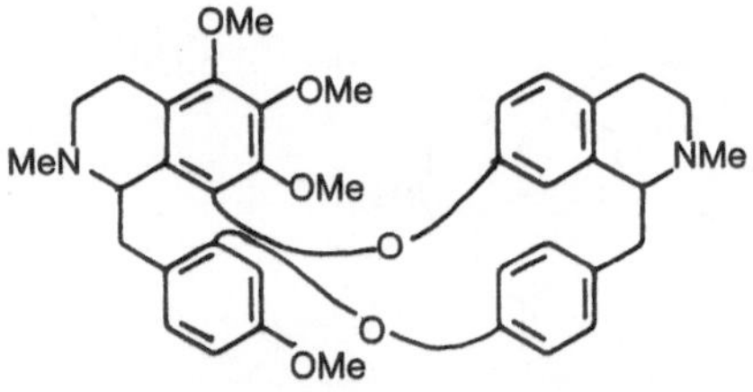

OMe
OMe
MeN
OMe
OMe
NMe
O
O
OMe

CXXII·

OH
OMe   MeO
⁺Me₂N
OMe
NMe
H
O
O
OMe

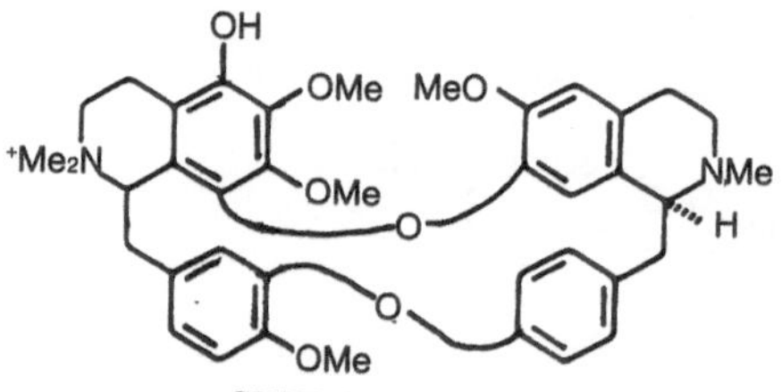

CXXIII

Miscellaneous Plants

Besides the above-described plants various other plant extracts and/or compounds were found to possess marked antitumor activity. The Table describes the important plants with active compounds reported along with the specific activity.

Plant name	Compounds*	Dose	Activity	Ref.
Abrus precatorius	Abrin A Abrin B	5 µg/ml (Ed50 10 µg/kg) 150 µg/kg (Ed50 25 µg/kg)	Sarcoma 180 and Ehrlich ascites tumor cells	417
Andenostemma larenia	Ent-11-hydroxy-15-oxo-kaur-16-en-19-oic acid [CXXIV] and adenostemmoic acid B [CXXV]	—	L-5178 Y cultured cell with prolonged survival of mice	418
Aglaia odorata	Odorinol [CXXVI] (leaves)	50 mg/kg/day, i.p.	*In vivo* P-388 lymphocytic leukemia in male T/C=136%	419
Ailanthus excelsa	Ailanthone [CXXVII] and glaucarubinone [CXXVIII]	0.12-400 mg/kg 0.12-0.5 mg/kg	P-388 lymphocytic leukemia and KB test in mice system.	420
Alpinia galanga	Galanol A [CXXIX] Galanol B [CXXX]	—	Cytotoxic	421
Angelica acutiloba	Polysaccharide (roots)	—	Sarcoma-180, IMC carcinoma solid form of MM-46 tumor	422
Annona bullata	Bullatacin [CXXXI] and bullatacinone [CXXXII] (bark), 16-hydroxy-(–)-kauranoic acid	ED50 10 µg/ml and 10 µg/ml ED50 8.25 × 10 µg/ml	Human tumor cell lines A-549 lung cell in human cells	423 424
Annona montana	Annomonicin [CXXXIII] and montanacin [CXXXIV]	—	L-1210, P-388 and MDA — MB 231 cell lines	425
Anthemis nobilis	Sesquiterpene lactone [CXXXV]	ED50 1.5 × 10 M ED50 3.5 × 10 M	HeLa cells KB cells	426
	Nobilin [CXXXVI] hydroxy nobilin, 10-epoxy, nobilin and 3-dehydronobilin [CXXXVII]	—	*In vitro* HeLa and nasopharynx carcinoma human tumor cells	427
Aristolochia indica	Aristolochic acid [CXXXVIII]	LD50 14.32 mg/kg i.p. in mice	P-388 lymphocytic leukemia and bronchial epider moid carcinoma	428
A. lonca	aritolactam	—	moid carcinoma	429

Plant name	Compounds*	Dose	Activity	Ref.
Artemisia absinthemum, A. sieversiana	Artemisetin and chrysoplenetin		Melanoma B16 and Pliss lymphorsarcoma	430
A. capillaris	Cappilarisin	—	*In vitro* L-929 and KB cells	431
Asclepias albicans	Uzarigenin 3-β-glucopyranosyl-(1–4)-β–D-glucoside [CXXXIX]	15-60 mg/kg	P-388 lymphocytic leukemia	432
Blumea balsamifera	Blumealactones A [CXL], B [XCLI] and C [CXLII] (Leaves)	50 μg/ml	Yoshida sarcoma cells in tissue culture	433
Bryophyllum pinnatum	Bryophyllin A [CXLIII],	ED50 14 ng/ml, 10 ng/ml, 30 ng/ml	KB cells, A549 and HCT-8 tumor cells.	435
	Bryophyllin B [CXLIV]	ED50<80 ng/ml	*In vitro* KB tissue culture cell	436
Caesalpinia pulcherrima	2,6-Dimethoxybenzoquinone and 4'-methylisoliquiritigenin	ED50 2.8 and 3.2 μg/ml	*In vitro* KB test system	437
**Camptotheca acuminata*	Camptothecin [CXLIVa] Camptothecin sodium [CXLIVb] 10-hydroxycamptothecin [CXLIVc]	0.79 mg/kg/injection with highest doses of 40 mg/kg/injection for camptothecin	All are active against variety of tumors including murine tumors, camptothecin very effective in bladder tumors.	437a
Carica papaya	Carpain [CXLV]	—	*In vitro* against mouse lymphoid leukemia L1210, lymphocytic leukemia, P-388 and ascites tumor cells	438
Cassia tora	Torosaol I [CXLVI] and torosaol II [CXLVII] (Roots)	—	KB cells	439
Castillea linariaefolia	Acetoside [CXLVIII] Isoacetoside [CXLIX]	ED50 2.6 μg/ml ED50 10 μg/ml	*In vivo* against murine P-388 lymphocytic leukemia	440
Centaurea alexandrina	Arctiin [CL] (Aerial parts)	ED50 2.6 μg/ml	KB cells	441

Plant name	Compounds*	Dose	Activity	Ref.
Cetraia laeirvigata	Polysaccharides	200 mg/kg, i. p.	Mouse sarcoma 180, Ehrlich ascites tumor and cervical cancer	442
		50 and 100 mg/kg	Increased phago-cytosis function of reticuloendothelial system	
Chrysoplenium grayanum	Chrysosplenol F and chrysos-plenol G	—	Marginal cytotoxic against KB cells *in vitro*	443
Cnidoscolus phyllacanthus	Faveline methyl ether [CLI], fave-line [CLII] and deoxofaveline [CLIII] (bark)	—	P-388 murine leukamia cells	444
Coleus forkohlii	Barbatusin [CLIV]	200 and 400 mg/kg	Lewis lung carci-noma and lympho-cytic leukemia P-388 in mice	445
Combretum caffrum	Combretastatin A-4 [CLV] (stemwood)	IC50 2-3 μM/ ED50<0.003 μg/ml ED50<0.01 μg/ml	Inhibition of tubu-lin polymerization L-1210 and P-388	446
Crossopterix febrifuga	Betulic acid (stem-bark)	LD50 0.375 μg/ml	Human colon carcinoma cell lines CO-115	447
Crotalaria assamica	Monocrotaline [CLVI]	LD50 700 mg/kg	Inhibited growth of transplanted tumor in white mice, affected protein synthesis and metabolism within cell	448
Cynanchum komarovii	7-Demethoxyxy-lophorine and desoxytylophorinin N-oxide [CLVII]	—	*In vitro* P-388 Leukemia cell	449
Dolabella auricularia	Dolastin B	ED50 13×10 μg/ml	Lymphocytic leu-kemia P-388 *in vitro*	450
Dolichos trilobus	Saponins (Roots)	i. p.	Sarcoma 37 *in vitro* in mice	451
Doronicum austriacum	Total extract	—	Inhibited prolifer-ation of mouse fibroblasts cell cultures	452

Plant name	Compounds*	Dose	Activity	Ref.
Dregea volubilis	Dregeoside Ap and dregeoside Ao	—	Ehrlich carcinoma *Melanoma B-16*	453
Elaeodendron buchananii	Root bark extract.	ED50 100 µg/ml	L-1210 leukemic cells	454
	Elabunin [CLVIII]	ED50 1 µg/ml	L-1210 leukemic cells	
Epilobium angusitifolium	Phytohemaggluti-nin	—	Antitumor	455
Eriodictyon californicum	Cirsimartin [CLIX] & chrysoeriol [CLX]	10 µg/ml	Inhibitors B(a)P metabolism 71 and 32%	456
Ervatamia heyneana	Leaves extract	—	B-16 melanoma in mice	457
Eupatorium breirpes	Brevipenin [CLXI]	—	Antitumor	458
Euphorbia kansui	Root extract	—	P-388 lymphocytic leuke in mice	459
	Kansuiphorin A [CLXII] and kansuiphorin B [CLXIII]	0.1 mg/kg 0.5 mg/kg	177%, P-388 lym-phocytic leukemia Human cancer melanoma renal cancer cells	
Euphorbia lagascae	Piceatannol [CLXIV]	ED50<0.01 µg/ml	*In vitro* 9 KB and 9 PS	460
Flammulina velutipes	Polysaccharide (fruits)	—	Sarcoma 180 solid	461
Foeniculum vulgare	Flavonoid (fruits)	—	Antitumor	462
Fomes japonicus	Polysaccharides	10 µg/ml 1 mg/kg/day	P3HR-I, MK-2 and HEP-2 Sarcoma 180 ascites tumor cells in mice	463
Genista	Genistein [CLXV]	IC50 6.5-12.0 µg/ml	MDA-468, MCF-7 and MCF-7-D-40	464
Gloriosa superba	Colchicine [CLXVI]	1-10 µg/ml	Malignant human gliomas	465
Gossypium barbadense	Gossypolone	20-31 µg/ml	50% inhibition of thymidine incorpo-ration and 50% decrease in nucleic acid content	466
			SW-13 tumor bear-ing nude mice	468
			Antitumor and anti-mitochondrial	468

Plant name	Compounds*	Dose	Activity	Ref.
Heliotropium indicum	Leaves extract	200 mg/kg	Schwartz leukemia	469
H. subulatum	Total extract	—	Nasopharynx in tissue culture and P-388 lymphocytic leukemia in mice	470
Hippophae salicifolia	Aqueous and alcoholic extract of bark	—	Inhibition against mouse fibrosarcoma and Yoshida sarcoma	471
Hydrangea dulcisfolium	Flavonoids	—	Inhibition against UV induced DNA mutation *in vitro* tests	472
Hypericum revolutum	Root bark extract	—	CD-115 human colon carcinoma cell line	473
Indigofera mysorensis	Aerial part extract	—	P-388 lymphocytic leukemia in mice and human epidermoid carcinoma of nasopharynx in tissue culture	474
Inula cuspidata	Total extract	—	Human epidermoid carcinoma of nasopharynx in tissue culture and P-388 lymphocytic leukemia in mice	475
Ipomoea indica	Ipolearoside [CLXVII]	—	WM system	476
Jatropha glandulifera	Total extract	—	Human epidermoid carcinoma of nasopharynx in tissue culture and P-388 lymphocytic leukemia in mice	477
Liriodendron tulipifera	Lipiferolide [CLXVIII] and epitulipinolide [CLXIX]	—	KB system	478
Luffa cylindrica	Seeds extract	4 and 8 mg/kg, i.p.	Ascitic form of Schwartz leukemia in transplanted tumor	479
L. acutangula	Seeds extract	4 and 8 mg/kg, i.p.	Prolong the life span of test animal by 16.6%	

Plant name	Compounds*	Dose	Activity	Ref.
L. graveolens	Fruits extract	—	Human epidermoid carcinoma of naso-pharynx tissue culture	480
Lychnophora antillana	Lychnostatin 1 [CLXX] and lych-nostatin [CLXXI]	ED50 2.0 and 0.19 μg/ml	P-388 lymphocytic leukemia cell line	481
Magnolia grandiflora	Peroxycostunolide [CLXXII] and peroxyparthenolide [CLXXIII]	2.7 and 2.8 μg/ml	Eagle's KB cells	482
M. officinalis	Magnolol [CLXXIV] (bark)	—	Mouse skin tumor promotion *in vivo*	483
Mallotus japonicus	Phloroglucinol derivatives	—	Cytotoxic in HeLa cells	484
Mammea americana	Mammein [CLXXV] and coumarins	—	Sarcoma 180 grown in stationary cell culture	485
Melodorum fruticosum	Melodorinol [CLXXVI], homo-melodienone [CLXXVII], 7-hydroxy-6-hydro-melodienone [CLXXVIII] and homoisomelidie-none [CLXXIX]	—	Cytotoxic to human tumor cell lines	486
Momordica charantia	Momorcharaside A [CLXXX] (seeds)	—	Inhibition of DNA and RNA syn-theses in S-180 tumor cells	487
Myrsine africana	Emodin and 2-hydroxy chry-sophanol (roots)	—	Cytotoxic	488
Narcissus tazetta	Pseudolycorine [CLXXXI]	i. p. LD50 110 mg/kg	Inhibited the growth of 256 carcinosarcoma	489
Nectandra rigida	Dehydrodiisoluge-nol [CLXXXII]	—	Cytotoxic	490
Nelumbo nucifera	Oxoushisunine [CLXXXIII]	—	Nasopharynx carcinoma	491
Nercicium erinaceum	Isoindolinone derivative [CLXXXIV] (seeds)	6.3 μg/ml	Cervix cancer cells *in vitro*	492

Plant name	Compounds*	Dose	Activity	Ref.
Nerium indicum	Non-volatile residue of leaves	30 mg/ml	Ehrlich ascites carcinoma	493
Nothopodytes nimmoniana	Total extract	—	Antitumor	494
Oldenlandia diffusa	Oldenlandosides I and II [CLXXXV, CLXXXVI]	—	Antitumor	495
Papaver somniferum	Papaverine	—	enhanced the cytotoxicity of nitrogen mustard in cell culture of C-1300 round cell neuroblastoma	496
Passiflora tetrandra	4-Hydroxy-2-cyclopenetone	IC50<1 μg/ml	P-388 murine leukemia cells	497
Plumbago zeylanica	Plumbagin [CLXXXVII]	2 mg/kg intratumorally and orally ED50 0.75 mg/kg, 4mg/kg	Decreased tumor growth 70 and 60% in rats P-388 lymphocytic leukemia	498
Plumeria rubra	Fulvoplumerin [CLXXXVIII], allamcin [CLXXXIX], allamancin [XCC], 2,5-dimethoxy-p-benzoquinone, plumericin [XCCI] and liriodendrin [XCCII]	—	P-388 murine leukemia cells	499
Podanthus mitigue	Ovatifolin [XCCIII] (stem and leaves)	—	KB cells	500
Polanisia dodecandra	Polacandrin [XCCIV]	ED50 0.60 μg/ml ED50 0.62 μg/ml ED50 6.06 μg/ml	P-388 cells RPMI-7951 cells HCT-8 colon	501
Polyalthia longifolia	Polyalthialdoic acid [XCCV] and Kolavenic acid [XCCVI]	ED50 6 × 10 μg/ml	Carcinoma human tumor cell culture and Crown gall tumors on potato disks	502
Polysticius vessicolor	Polysaccharides	—	Inhibited growth and pulmonary metastasis of melanoma B-16 on mice	503
Psoralea corylifolia	Bakuchiol [XCCVII]	—	Cytotoxic	504

Plant name	Compounds*	Dose	Activity	Ref.
Polygonum hydropiper	Burganal and polygodial	—	DMBA induced pappillomas in mice	505
Pogonopus speciosus	Tubulosine [XCCVIII]	—	Antitumor	506
Podocarpus gracilor	Podolide [XCCIX]	—	Tumor inhibiting activity	507
Pseudolarix kaempferi	Pseudolaric acid A and pseudolaric acid B	—	Inhibited growth of diesease-oriented human cancer cell lines	508
Psychotria rubra	Psychorubrin [CC]	ED50 30 µg/ml	KB cell system	509
Pterocarpus dalbergioides	Leaves extract	70 mg/kg/day, i.p. LD50 122 mg/kg, i.p.	Ehrlich ascites carcinoma in mice	510
Pulicaria crispa	2α-Hydroxyalantolactone 2α-hydroxy-5α, 6α-epoxyalantolactone [CCI] µg/ml and axillarin [CCII]	ED50 0.33 µg/ml ED50 0.4 µg/ml 25 µg/ml	KB cell in culture Decreased the metabolism of benzo(a)pyrone by 61.3% over DMSO controls	511
Rabdosia longituba	Longikaurin A [CCIIa] and longi-kaurin B [CCIIb]	—	Cytotoxicity *in vitro* against cultured rat mammary cancer	512
Rauwolfia serpentina	Serpentine [XXXIV] and alstonine [CCIII]	400 µg/day for 15 days	Mammary cancer MS 301	513
Rhazya stricta	Vallesiachotamine [CCIV], sewarine [CCV] and tetra-hydrosecamine [CCVI]	—	KB carcinoma of nasopharynx test system *in vitro*	514
Rhodococcus lentifragmentus	Arabinogalactam -peptidoglucan (AP) complex	—	Syngeneicfibrosarcoma Meth A cells in mice	515
Rodialoa henyi	Heterodendrin and 1,2,3,4,6-penta-O-galloyl-B-D-glucoside	0.2% 0.2%, i.p.	Suppressed growth of sarcoma cells by 25%	516
Rollinia sylvatica	Sylvaticin [CCVIIa]	—	Human tumor cells	517
Rubia cordifolia	Total extract Rubescensin A and rubescensin B [CCVIIb]	TCD50 µg/ml	P-388 lymphocytic leukemia Hepatosoma BFL-7402 cell in culture	519

Plant name	Compounds*	Dose	Activity	Ref.
Ruta graveolens	Rutacridone epoxide [CCVIII] (roots)	—	Antitumor	520
Sandoricum koetjake	3-oxo-olean-12-en-29-oic acid [CCIX] and katonic acid [CCX] (stem)	ED50 0.61 and 0.11 μg/ml	P-388 cultured cell	521
Saponaria officinalis	Protein SL (seeds)	1×10^{-12} Mol/l	50% Inhibition of protein synthesis	522
Securinega virosa	Virosecurinine [CCXI] and viroallosecurinine [CCXII] (leaves)	—	Cytotoxic	523
Semecarpus anacardium	Nuts extract	—	Increase life span of leukemias L-1210, P-388	524
Seseli mairei	Seselidiol [CCXIII] (roots)	—	*In vitro* KB, P-388, L-1210 and HCT-8 system	525
Strychnos potatorum	Quercetin	—	Inhibit growth of COLO320 DM cells of human colon	526
Styrax officinalis	Total extract	—	*In vivo* antitumor	527
Tagetes minuta	Flower extract	—	Lewis lung carcinoma *in vivo*	528
Tetragonia tetragonioides	β-Carotene	—	Inhibitor of skin carcinogenesis in mice	529
			Decrease adenylate cyclase activity in melanoma cells in culture	530
Trioanthes cucumeroides	Glycoproteins (Tubers)	—	Lung cancer cells	531
Volvariella volvacea	Polysaccharide	—	Sarcoma-180 in mice	532
Wedelia asperrima	Wedeloside [CCXIV]	LD100 1 mg/kg	Inhibited formation of aflatoxin B1-induced tumors in rats	533
Wistaria brachybotrys	Knots extract	—	Gastric cancer	534

Plant name	Compounds*	Dose	Activity	Ref.
	Afromosin [CCXV] and soyasaponin [CCXVI]	—	Mouse skin tumor and pulmonary tumor	535
Zephyranthes candida	Trans-Dihydronar-cidasine [CCXVII]	ED50 $3.2 \times 10 \, \mu g/ml$	P-388 lymphocytic	536

* Part of the plant/extract is given if reported.
** The other sources are *Nothapodytes foetida* Wight Sleum, *Merrilliodendron megacarpum* (Helmsl.) Sleum, *Ophiorrhiza mungos* L. and *Ervatamia heyneana* (Wall) T. Cooke.

CXXIV

CCXVII

References

1 G. K. Hughes, F. N. Lahey, J. R. Price and L. J. Webb: *Nature, 162,* 223 (1948).
2 F. N. Lahey and W. C. Thomas: *Aust. J. Sci. Res. 2*A, 423 (1949).
3 R. D. Brown, L. J. Drummond, F. N. Lahey and W. C. Thomas: *Aust. J. Sci. Res. 2*A, 662 (1949).
4 L. J. Drummond and F. N. Lahey: *Aust. J. Sci. Res. 2*A, 630 (1949).
5 R. D. Brown and F. N. Lahey: *Aust. J. Sci. Res. 3,* 593 (1950).
6 T. R. Govindachari, B. R. Pai and P. S. Subramanian: *Tetrahedron 22,* 3245 (1966).
7 J. G. Gougoutas and G. A. Kaski: *Acta Crystallogr. 26*B, 853 (1970).
8 G. H. Svoboda: *Lloydia 29* 206 (1966).
9 H. R. Sullivan, R. E. Billings, J. L. Occolowitz, H. E. Boaz, F. J. Marshell and R. F. McMohan: *J. Med. Chem. 13,* 904 (1970).
10 R. E. Belts, D. E. Walters and J. P. Rosazza: *J. Med. Chem. 17,* 599 (1974).
11 D. R. Brannon, D. R. Horton and G. H. Svoboda: *J. Med. Chem. 17,* 653 (1974).
12 J. Schneider, E. L. Evans, E. Grunberg and R. I. Fryer: *J. Med. Chem. 15,* 266 (1978).
13 S. M. Kupchan, R. W. Britton and M. F. Ziegler: *J. Org. Chem. 38,* 178 (1973).
14 S. M. Kupchan, R. W. Britton and J. A. Lacadie: *J. Org. Chem. 40,* 648 (1975).
15 M. Li, H. Liu, Y. Cong, H. Yu, X. Su, Q. Yu and H. Zhao: *Zhongcaoyao 14,* 361 (1983).

16 J. Zhang, R. Xu, Y. Li and Z. Chen: *Huaxue Xuebao 42*, 684 (1984).
17 X. Li and S. Tso: *Chung T'sao Yao 11*, 530 (1980).
18 I. H. Hall, K. H. Lee and S. A. Eigebaly et al.: *J. Pharm. Sci. 68*, 883 (1979).
19 J. D. Phillipson and F. A. Darwish: *Planta Med. 35*, 308 (1979).
20 K. H. Lee, Y. Imakura, Y. Sumida and R. Y. Wu et al.: *J. Org. Chem. 44*, 2180 (1979).
21 J. D. Phillipson and F. A. Darwis: *Planta Med. 41*, 209 (1981).
22 I. H. Hall, K. H. Lee, M. Okano, D. Sims and I. Ibuka et al.: J. Pharm. Sci. *70*, 1147 (1981).
23 K. H. Lee, M. Okano, I. H. Hall, D. A. Brent and B. Soltman: *J. Pharm. Sci. 71*, 338 (1982).
24 K. H. Lee, N. Hayashi, O. Masayoshi, H. Nozaki and M. Ju-ICHI: *J. Nat. Prod. 47*, 550 (1984).
25 R. Yu, S. Wang and X. Zhou et al.: *Zhoncaoyao 19*, 294 (1988).
26 L. Lin, J. Zhang, Z. Chen and R. Xu: *Huaxue Xuebao 40*, 73 (1982).
27 S. S. Handa, A. D. Kinghorn, G. A. Cordell and N. R. Farnsworth: *J. Nat. Prod. 46*, 359 (1983).
28 T. Takahashi and T. Tsuyuki: Jpn. Patent 187, 411 (1984): [*C. A. 106*, 47354 r (1987)].
29 T. Takahashi, T. Tsuyuki: Jpn. Patent 39, 404 (1985): [*C. A. 106*, 90159 t (1987).]
30 T. Takahashi, T. Tsuyuki: Jpn. Patent 62, 87, 591 (1987): [*C. A. 107*, 223369 v (1987)].
31 S. Toshiro, Y. Shin, T. Takahiko, T. Takeyoshi, H. Tadashi, and N. Toshihiro: *Tetrahedron Lett. 27*, 593 (1986).
32 T. Sakaki, S. Yoshimura and T. Tsuyuki et al.: *Chem. Pharm. Bull. 34*, 4447 (1986).
33 N. Fukamiya, M. Okano, M. Miyamote, K. Tagahara and K. H. Lee: *J. Nat. Prod. 55*, 468 (1992).
34 "The Alkaloids" (A. Brossi and M. Suffness Eds) Vol. 37, p., Academic Press, New York, 1990.
35 R. L. Noble, C. T. Beer and J. H. Cutts: *Ann. N. Y. Acad. Sci. 76* 882 (1956).
36 G. H. Svoboda, N. Neurs and M. Gorman: *J. Am. Pharm. Assoc. Sci. Ed. 48*, 659 (1959).
37 G. H. Svoboda: *Lloydia 24* 173 (1961).
38 N. Langlois and P. Potier: *Phytochemistry 11* 2617 (1972).
39 P. Rosoanaivo, N. Langlois and P. Potier: *Phytochemistry 11*, 2616 (1972).
40 Atta-ur-Rahman, M. Bashir, M. Hafeez, N. Perveen, J. Fatima and A. N. Mistry: *Planta Med. 47* 246 (1983).
41 S. Mukhopadhyay and G. A. Cordell: *J. Nat. Prod. 44*, 335 (1981).
42 N. Langlois, R. Z. Andriamialisoa and N. Neuss: *Helv. Chim. Acta 63*, 793 (1980).
43 R. Z. Andriamiailisoa, N. Langlois and P. Potier: *Tetrahedron Lett.* 2849 (1976).
44 G. H. Svoboda, M. Gorman, A. J. Barnes and A. T. Oliver: *J. Pharm. Sci. 51*, 518 (1962).
45 G. H. Svoboda, A. T. Oliver and D. R. Bedwell: *Lloydia 26* 141 (1963).
46 G. H. Svoboda: *J. Pharm. Sci. 52*, 407 (1963).
47 M. Gorman, G. H. Svoboda and N. Neuss: *Lloydia 28*, 269 (1965).
48 W. I. Taylor and N. R. Farnsworth eds, *"Catharanthus Alkaloids Botany, Chemistry Pharmacology and Clinical Uses"* Dekker, New York, 1975.
49 A. De Bruyn, L. De Taeye and M. J. O. Anteunis: *Bull Soc. Chim. Belg. 89*, 629 (1980).
50 E. Wenkert, E. W. Hagaman, B. Lal and G. E. Gutowski et al.: *Helv. Chim. Acta 58*, 1560 (1975).
51 D. E. Dorman and J. W. Paschal: *Org. Magn. Res. 8*, 413 (1986).

52   M. S. Morales-Rios, J. Espineira and P. J. Nathan: *Magn. Res. Chem. 25*, 376 (1987).
53   J. W. Moncrief and W. N. Lipscomb: *J. Am. Chem. Soc. 87*, 4963 (1965).
54   J. P. Kutney, D. E. Gregonis, R. Imhof and I. Itoh et al.: *J. Am. Chem. Soc. 97*, 5013 (1975).
55   N. Langlois, F. Gueritte, Y. Langlois and P. Potier: *J. Am. Chem. Soc. 98*, 7017 (1976).
56   J. P. Kutney, J. Cook, K. Juji and A. M. Treasurywala et al.: *Heterocycles 3*, 205 (1975).
57   N. Neuss, I. S. Johnson, J. G. Armstrong and C. J. Jansen Jr: "Advances in Chemotherapy" (A. Goldin, F. Hawking and R. Schnitzer eds.), Vol. 1, Academic Press, New York, 1964).
58   G. H. Svoboda and A. J. Barnes: *J. Pharm. Sci. 53*, 1227 (1964).
59   K. Mislow and J. Siegel: *J. Am. Chem. Soc. 106*, 3319 (1984).
60   G. Richter CO: Ger. Patent 2,259,388 (1974): [*C. A. 81*, 82369 m (1974)].
61   G. Richter CO: Neth. Patent Appl. 17,069 (1972): [*C. A. 83* 84848 (1975)].
62   A. El-Sayed and G. A. Cordell: *J. Nat. Prod. 44*, 289 (1981).
63   G. H. Svoboda, I. S. Johnson, M. Gorman and N. Neuss: *J. Pharm. Sci. 51*, 707 (1962).
64   A. El.-Sayed, G. A. Handy and G. A. Cordell: *J. Nat. Prod. 46*, 517 (1983).
65   A. El-Sayed, G. A. Handy and G. A. Cordell: *J. Nat. prod. 43*, 157 (1980).
66   S. Mukhopadhyay and G. A. Cordell: *J. Nat. Prod. 44*, 611 (1981).
67   S. S. Tafur, W. E. Jones, D. E. Dorman, E. E. Logsdon and G. H. Svoboda: *J. Pharm. Sci. 64*, 1953 (1975).
68   M. Beljanski, J. Bugiel: Fr. Demande 2,419,725 (1975): [*C. A. 92*, 140721 k (1980)].
69   P. J. Kruegger, D. P. Carew, J. H. C. Lui and E. J. Staba: *Planta Med. 45*, 56 (1982).
70   I. S. Wright, G. H. Svoboda and J. Vlantis: *Cancer Res. 20*, 1016 (1960).
71   W. A. Creasey, A. C. Sartorelli and D. G. Johns: Antineoplastic and Immunosuppressive Agents II *38*, 232 (1975).
72   C. W. Taylor, S. E. Salmon, W. G. Satterle and A. B. Robertson et al.: *Inv. New Drugs 8*, 51 (1990).
73   D. R. Budman, W. Kreis, J. Behr and P. Schulman et al.: *Invest. New Drugs 8*, 268 (1991).
74   E. A. Rowinsky and R. C. Donehower: *Pharmacol. Ther. 52* 35 (1991).
75   I. S. Johnson, J. G. Armstrong, M. Gorman and J. P. Burnett: *Cancer Res. 23*, 1390 (1963).
76   P. Potier: *Chemical Society Reviews 44*, 113 (1992).
77   W. T. Beck: "Alkaloids In Antitumor Drug Resistance, 1984, B. W. Fox and M. Fox eds.) p. 589, Springer Verlag, Berlin.
78   R. J. Owellen and C. A. Hartke: *J. Med. Chem. 15*, 894 (1972).
79   A. B. Huang, C. M. Lin and E. Hamel: *Biophys. Res. Commun. 128*, 1239 (1985).
80   J. J. Manfredi and S. B. Horwitz: *Exp. Cell. Res. 150*, 205 (1984).
81   K. G. Bensch and S. E. Malawista: *J. Cell Biol. 40*, 95 (1969).
82   F. Rosner, Y. Hirshaut, H. W. Grundwald and M. Dietrich: *Cancer Res. 35*, 700 (1975).
83   M. A. Johnson, H. F. Wright and G. H. Svoboda: *J. Lab. Clin. Med. 54*, 830 (1959).
84   H. Madoc-Jones and F. Mauro: *J. Cell. Physiol. 72*, 185 (1968).
85   A. R. Safa, C. J. Glover and R. L. Felsted: *Cancer Res. 47*, 5149 (1987).
86   W. T. Beck: *Adv. Enz. Regul. 22*, 207 (1984).
87   F. Brewer and J. R. Warr: *Cancer Treat Rep. 71*, 353 (1987).
88   T. Truruo: *Cancer Treat. Rep. 67*, 889 (1983).
89   S. I. Akiyama, N. Shiratshi and Y. Kuratomi et al.: *J. Natn. Cancer Inst. 76*, 834 (1986).

90   M. Inaba and E. Earuyama: *Cancer Res. 48,* 2064 (1988).
91   M. P. Gosland, B. L. Lum and B. I. Sikic: *Cancer Res. 49,* 6901 (1989).
92   A. Gruber, C. Peterson and P. Reizenstein: *Int. J. Cancer 41,* 224 (1988).
93   P. R. Twentyman: *Brit. J. Cancer 57,* 254 (1988).
94   K. Veda, C. Cardarelli, M. M. Gottesman and I. Pastan: *Proc. Natl. Acad. Sci. U.S.A. 84,* 3004 (1987).
95   J. H. Horton, P. J. Houghton and J. A. Houghton: *Cancer Res. 44,* 582 (1984).
96   G. B. Henderson and J. M. Tsuji: *Cancer Res. 48,* 5995 (1988).
97   R. A. Bender and B. A. Chabner in "Pharmacological Prinziples of Cancer Treatment" (B. A. Chabner ed.). p. 256, Saunders, Philadephia, Pennsylvania, 1982.
98   R. A. Bender, M. C. Castle, D. A. Margileth and V. T. Oliverio: *Clin. Pharmac. Ther. 22,* 430 (1977).
99   S. M. Et. Dareer, V. M. White, F. P. Chen. L. B. Mellett and D. L. Hill: *Cancer Treat. Rep. 61,* 1269 (1977).
100 M. C. Castle: "The Vinca alkaloids" (P. V. Wooley eds.) p. 147, Klvwer Academic Publishers Dordrecht, 1984.
101 R. L. Nelson, R. W. Dyke and M. A. Root: *Cancer Chem. Pharmacol 2,* 243 (1979).
102 R. Rahmani, J. P. Kleisbauer, J. P. Cano, M. Martin and J. Barbet: *Cancer Treat. Rep. 69,* 839 (1985).
103 S. P. Labinjoki, H. M. Verajan Korva and A. E. Huthikangas et al.: *J. Immunoassay 7,* 113 (1986).
104 M. J. Ratain and N. J. Vogelzang: *Cancer Res. 46,* 4827 (1986).
105 W. A. Creasey, A. I. Scott and C. C. Wei et al.: *Cancer Res. 35,* 1116 (1975).
106 C. J. Barnett, G. J. Cullinan and K. Gerzon et al.: *J. Med. Chem. 21,* 88 (1978).
107 M. J. Sweeney, G. B. Boder, G. J. Cullinan and H. W. Culp et al.: *Cancer Res. 38,* 2886 (1978).
108 J. A. Houghton, L. G. Williams and P. J. Hougthon: *Cancer Res. 45,* 3761 (1985).
109 R. A. Conrad, G. J. Cullinan, K. Gerzon and G. A. Poore: *J. Med. Chem. 22,* 391 (1979).
110 K. S. P. B. Rao, M. P. M. Collard and J. P. C. Dejonghe et al.: *J. Med. Chem. 28,* 1079 (1985).
111 M. Inaba and E. Maruyama: *Cancer Res. 48,* 2066 (1988).
112 R. A. Bender, M. C. Castle, D. A. Margileth and V. T. Oliverio: *Clin. Pharmacol. Ther. 22,* 430 (1977).
113 V. D. Jackson, M. C. Castle and R. A. Bender: *Cancer Res. 39,* 4346 (1978).
114 K. N. Thimmaiah and V. S. Sethi: *Microchemical J. 41,* 320 (1990).
115 V. S. Sethi, M. C. Castle, P. Surratti, D. V. Jackson and C. L. S. Purr: *Proc. Am. Ass. Cancer Res. 22,* 173 (1981).
116 J. A. Houghton, L. G. Williams, P. M. Torrance and P. J. Houghton: *Cancer Res. 44,* 582 (1984).
117 V. S. Sethi, V. D. Jackson, D. R. White, Z. F. Richards et al.: *Cancer Res. 41,* 3551 (1981).
118 J. A. Houghton, L. G. Williams, P. M. Torrance and P. J. Houghton: *Cancer Res. 44,* 582 (1984).
119 G. C. Todd, W. R. Gibson and D. M. Morton: *J. Toxicol. Environ. Health 1,* 843 (1976).
120 F. Norido, M. Finesso and C. Fiorito et al.: *Toxicol. Appl. Pharmacol. 93,* 433 (1988).
121 L. J. Muller, C. M. Moorer-Van Delft and E. W. Roubos: *Cancer Res. 48,* 7184 (1988).
122 W. J. Thomas, M. T. Bailony and A. T. Lightsey et al.: *Am. J. Ped. Hematol Oncol. 8,* 266 (1986).

123   A. J. Gottlieb, V. Weinberg, R. R. Ellison and E. S. Henderson et al.: *Blood 64*, 267 (1984).

124   S. Rosenthal, G. P. Canellos, J. Whang-Peng and H. R. Gralnick: *Am. J. Med. 63*, 542 (1977).

125   W. Crist, A. Carroll and J. Shuster et al.: *Blood. 76*, 489 (1990).

126   H. Glucksberg, M. A. Cheever and V. T. Farewell et al.: *Cancer 48*, 1073 (1981).

127   H. Priesler, R. B. Davis and J. Krishner et al.: *Blood 68*, 1441 (1987).

128   C. H. Diggs, P. H. Wiernik, J. A. Levi and L. K. Kvols: *Cancer 39*, 1949 (1977).

129   J. Wagstaff, W. Steward and M. Jones et al.: *Hematol Oncol. 4*, 135 (1986).

120   P. Selby, P. Patel and S. Milan et al.: *Brit. J. Cancer 62*, 279 (1990).

131   B. W. Dana, S. Dahlberg and T. P. Miller et al.: *J. Clin Oncol. 8*,. 1155 (1990).

132   D. B. Boyd, M. Coleman and S. Papish et al.: *J. Clin Oncol. 6*, 425 (1988).

133   D. L. Longo, V. T. Devita and P. L. Duffey et al.: *J. Clin. Oncol. 9*, 25 (1991).

134   P. S. Schein, B. A. Chabner and G. P. Canellos et al.: Cancer 35, 354 (1975).

135   D. C. Case: *Oncology 41*, 159 (1984).

136   R. C. Young, D. L. Longo and E. Glatstein et al.: *Proc. Am. Soc. Clin. Oncol. 6*, 790 (1987).

137   M. Lipeman and M. L. Votaw: *Cancer 41*, 1664 (1978).

138   G. Palmieri, R. Laurie and F. Caponigro et al.: *Hematol Oncol. 8*, 179 (1990).

139   E. Rapp, J. L. Pater and A. Willian et al.: *J. Clin Oncol. 6*, 633 (1988).

140   B. J. Takasugi, A. E. Robertson and S. E. Salmon et al.: *Invest. New Drugs 2*, 387 (1984).

141   R. G. Aitchison, I. A. Reilly, A. G. Morgan and N. H. Russell: *Brit. J. Cancer 61*, 765 (1990).

142   M. L. Samuels, D. E. Johnson and P. Y. Holoye: *Cancer Chemother. Rep. 59*, 563 (1975).

143   P. J. Loehrer, S. D. Williams and L. H. Einhorn: *J. Nat. Cancer Inst. 80*, 1373 (1988).

144   J. A. Neidhart, S. A. Anderson and J. E. Harris et al.: *J. Clin. Oncol. 9*, 832 (1991).

145   N. Murray, D. Osoba and A. Shah et al.: *J. Nat. Cancer Inst. 83*, 190 (1991).

146   I. C. Henderson: in "Chemotherapy for advanced disease in Breast Diseases" (J. R. Harris, S. Hellman, I. C. Henderson and D. W. Kinne Lippincott, eds.) Vol. *42*B, Philadelphia (1987).

147   R. Hart, M. Perloff and J. Holland: *Cancer 48*, 1522 (1981).

148   V. A. Levin, G. E. Sheline and P. H. Gutin: "Canner Principles and practice of oncology" 1557 editted by V. T. Devita, S. Hellman and S. A. Rosenberg New York.

149   P. Fenaux, I. Quinguandon and M. T. Caulier et al.: *BLUT 60*, 238 (1990).

150   J. L. Welborn, P. Emrick and M. Acevedo: *Am. J. Hematol. 35*, 18 (1990).

151   T. R. Jenkins and A. J. Zaloznik: *Cancer 64*, 1362 (1989).

152   P. S. Gill, B. Akil and P. Colletti et al.: *Am. J. Med. 87*, 57 (1989).

153   M. Azab, J. P. Droz, C. Theodore, J. P. Wolff and J. L. Amiel: *Cancer 64*, 1829 (1989).

154   R. C. Spain: *Sem. Oncol. 15*, 6 (1988).

155   R. D. Dillman, S. L. Seagren and K. J. Propert et al.: *New Engl. J. Med. 323*, 940 (1990).

156   D. D. Von-Hoff, P. J. Goodman and C. A. Preasont et al.: *Eur. J. Cancer 26*, 405 (1990).

157   D. S. Kim, H. Moon, Y. Y. Swang and M. I. Park: *Gynecol. Oncol. 38*, 144 (1990).

158 G. A. Gomez and J. E. Sokal: *Cancer Treat. Rep. 63*, 1385 (1979).
159 K. A. Starling, M. H. Donaldson and M. E. Haggard et al.: *Am J. Dis. Child. 123*, 105 (1972).
160 C. Erlichman, G. Bjurnason, P. Bunting et al.: *Proc. Am. Soc. Clin. Oncol. 10*, 314 (1991).
161 B. L. Lum. S. Kaubish and M. P. Gosland et al.: *Proc. Am. Soc. Clin. Oncol. 10*, 277 (1991).
162 H. J. Durivage, A. C. Buzzaid and M. B. Todd et al.: *Proc. Am. Soc. Clin. Oncol. 10*, 335 (1991).
163 R. L. Nelson, R. W. Dyke and M. A. Root: *Cancer Treatment Rev. 7*, 17 (1980).
164 M. J. Ratain, N. J. Vogelsang and J. A. Sinkule: *Clin. Pharmacol. Therap. 41*, 61 (1987).
165 H. D. Weiss, M. D. Walker and P. H. Wiernik: *N. Eng. J. Med. 291*, 127 (1974).
166 P. Potier: *Sem. Oncol. 16*, 2 (1989).
167 S. Binet, A. Fellous and H. Lataste et al.: *Sem. Oncol. 16*, 5 (1989).
168 A. Fellous, R. Ohayon and T. Vacassin et al.: *Sem. Oncol. 16*, 9 (1989).
169 S. Binet, E. Chaineau and A. Fellous et al.: *Int. J. Cancer 46*, 262 (1990).
170 S. Cros, M. Wright and M. Morimota et al.: *Sem. Oncol. 16*, 15 (1989).
171 M. Spielman, M. Jouve and F. Turpin et al.: *Breast Can. Res. Treat. 16*, 17 (1990).
172 A. Dieras, J. M. Morvan and E. Bellissant et al.: *Breast Cancer Res. Treat 16*, 161 (1990).
173 R. Rahmani, M. Martin, J. Barbet and J. P. Cano: *Cancer Res. 44*, 5609 (1984).
174 F. Jehl, E. Quoix, H. Montell, G. Pauli and A. Krikorian: *Proc. Am. Soc. Clin. Oncol. 9* 252 (1990).
175 F. Jehl, E. Quoix and D. Leveque et al.: *Cancer Res. 51*, 2073 (1991).
176 A. Kirkorian, R. Rahmani, M. Bromet, P. Bore and J. P. Cano: *Sem. Oncol. 16*, 21 (1989).
177 P. Bore, R. Rahmani, J. Van Cantfort, C. Focan and J. P. Cano: *Cancer Chemother. Pharmocol. 23*, 247 (1987).
178 M. Besenval, M. Delgado, J. P. Demarez and A. Krikorian: *Sem. Oncol. 16*, 37 (1989).
179 A. Depierre, E. Lemarie and G. Dabouis et al.: *Am. J. Clin. Oncol. 14*, 115 (1991).
180 R. G. Powell, D. Weisleder, C. R. Smith and I. A. Wolff: *Tetrahedron Lett.* 1081 (1969).
181 R. G. Powell, D. Weisleder, C. R. Smith and W. K. Rohwedder: *Tetrahedron Lett.* 815 (1970).
182 Cephalotoxus Research Coordinating Group: *Chinese Med. J. 2*, 263 (1976).
183 W. W. Pandler and J. McKay: *J. Org. Chem. 38*, 2110 (1973).
184 K. L. Mikolajezak, R. G. Powell and C. R. Smith: *J. Pharm. Sci. 63*, 1280 (1974).
185 K. L. Mikolajezak, R. G. Powell and C. R. Smith: *Tetrahedron* 1995 (1972).
186 R. G. Powell, D. Weisleder and C. R. Smith: *J. Pharm. Sci. 61*, 1227 (1972).
187 K. L. Mikolajezak, R. G. Powell and C. R. Smith: *J. Med. Chem. 18*, 63 (1975).
188 S. Takeda, N. Yajima, K. Kitasato and N. Unemi: *J. Pharmacobio. Dyn. 5*, 841 (1982).
189 K. Lin, W. M. Chao, R. Han and Z. K. Pan: *Zhonghua Yixue Zazhi 63*, 29 (1983).
190 T. L. Jiang, R. H. Liu and S. E. Salmon: *Invest. New Drugs 1*, 21 (1983).
191 W. R. Cobb, A. E. Bogden, S. D. Reich, T. W. Griffin, D. E. Kelton and D. J. Lepage: *Cancer Treat Rep. 67*, 173 (1983).

192 K. L. N. Savaraj, L. G. Feun, G. Zhanggang and T. L. Loo: *Proc. Am. Assoc. Cancer Res. 24,* 289 (1983).

193 T. Okano, T. Ohnuma, J. F. Holland, H. P. Koeffler and H. Jui: *Invest. New. Drugs 1,* 145 (1983).

194 M. P. Hacker, J. A. Stewart, R. A. Newman and I. H. Krakoff: *Proc. Am. Soc. Cancer Res. 24,* 325 (1983).

195 Y. Yan, X. Ding, S. Lu and W. Liu et al.: *Zhonghua Xueyexue Zazhi 11,* 69 (1990).

196 Y. Liu: Eur. Patent 203,386 (1986): [*C. A. 106,* 90,209 j (1987)].

197 Y. Liu: Can. Patent 1,267,845 (1990): [*C. A. 113,* 197998 m (1990)].

198 L. Ren and Z. Xue: *Zhongcaoyao 12,* 1 (1981).

199 R. G. Powell, R. W. Miller and C. R. Smith: *Chem. Commun.* 102 (1979).

200 R. W. Miller, R. G. Powell and C. R. Smith: U.S. Patent 0739 (1979): [*C. A. 92,* 28557 k (1980)].

201 R. W. Miller, R. G. Powell and C. R. Smith: U.S. Patent 4,206,221 (1980): [*C. A. 93,* 168465 z (1980)].

202 M. Hayat, G. Mathe, M. M. Janot, P. Potier, N. Dat-Xuong, A. Cave, T. Sevenet, C. Kan-Fan, J. Poisson, J. Miet, J. Le Men, F. Le Goffic, A. Gouyette, A. Ahond, L. K. Dalton and T. A. Connors: *Biomedicine 21,* 101 (1974).

203 D. Pelaprat, R. Oberlin, B.-P. Roques and J.-B. Le Pecq.: C. R. Hebd. Seances Acad. Sci., Ser D *283,* 1109 (1976).

204 G. H. Svoboda, G. A. Poore and M. L. Montfort: *J. Pharm. Sci. 57,* 1720 (1968).

205 S. Goodwin, A. F. Smith and E. C. Horning: *J. Am. Chem. Soc. 81,* 1903 (1959).

206 J. Bruneton and A. Cave: *Ann. Pharm. Fr. 30,* 629 (1972).

207 K. N. Kilminster, M. Sainsburg and B. Webb: *Phytochemistry 11,* 389 (1972).

208 S. Michel, F. Tillequin and M. Koch: *Tetrahedron Lett. 21,* 4027 (1980).

209 S. Michel, F. Tillequin, M. Koch and L. Ake Assi: *J. Nat. Prod. 46,* 489 (1983).

210 V. K. Kansal and P. Potier: *Tetrahedron 42,* 2389 (1986).

211 L. K. Dalton, S. Demerac, B. C. Elmes, J. W. Loder, J. M. Swan and T. Teitei: *Aust. J. Chem. 20,* 2715 (1967).

212 J.-B. Le Pecq, C. Gosse, N. Dat-Xuong and C. Paoletti: *C. R. Hebd. Seances Acad. Sci.,* Ser. D, *277,* 2289 (1973).

213 A. Gouyette, R. Reynaud, J. Sadet, M. Baillarge, C. Ganssu, S. Cros, F. Le Goffic, J.-B. Le Pecq, C. Paoletti and C. Viel: *Eur. J. Med. Chem. 15,* 503 (1980).

214 J.-B. Le Pecq, C. Gosse, N. Dat-Xuong and C. Paoletti: *C. R. Hebd. Seances Acad. Sci.,* Ser. D., *281,* 1365 (1975).

215 M. Suffness and G. A. Cordell: in "The Alkaloids" (A. Brossi, ed.) Vol. XXV, P. 89 Academic Press, New York, 1985.

216 M. Suffness and J. Douros: in "Anticancer Agents Based on Natural Product Models" (J. M. Cassady and J. D. Douros, eds.) p. 465, Academic Press, New York, 1980.

217 C. Paoletti. J.-B. Le Lecq, N. Dat-Xuong, P. Juret, H. Garnier, J.-L. Amiel and J. Rouesse: *Recent Res. Cancer Res. 74,* 107 (1980).

218 G. H. Svoboda and R. W. Kattau: *Lloydia 30,* 364 (1967).

219 C. Kan-Fan, B. C. Das, P. Potier and M. Schmid: *Phytochemstry 9,* 1351 (1970).

220 A. Goldin, A. A. Sperpick and N. Mentel: *Cancer Chem. Rep. 50,* 173 (1966).

221 G. W. Gribble: in "The Alkaloids" (A. Brossi and M. Suffness, eds.) Vol. 37, p. 239, 1990.

222   P. Rigaudy, J.-Y. Charcosset, C. Garbay-Jaurequiberry, A. Jacquemin-Sablon and B. P. Roques: *Cancer Res. 49*, 1836 (1989).
223   M. Samadi-Baboli, G. Favre, E. Blancy and G. Soula: *Eur. J. Cancer Clin. Oncol. 25*, 233 (1989).
224   G. F. Alberici, M. Pallardy, L. Manil, J.-J. Dessaux, J. Fournier, J.-M. Mondesir, C. Bohuon and P. Gros: *Int. J. Cancer 41*, 309 (1988).
225   A. M. Sautereaul, S. Cros and J. F. Tocanne: *Biopharm. Drug Dispos. 7*, 357 (1986).
226   F. Ali-Osman, M. L. Rosenblum, D. D. Giannini and V. A. Levin: *Cancer Res. 45*, 2988 (1985).
227   W. L. Alworth and T. J. Staga: *Carcinogenesis 6*, 487 (1985).
228   J. Benard, L. Bettan-Renaud, A. Gavoille, J.- L. Pico, F. Beaujean, M. Lpez and G. Riou: *Eur. J. Cancer Clin. Oncol. 24*, 1561 (1988).
229   T. Honda, M. Kato, M. Inoue, T. Shimamoto, K. Shima, T. Nakanishi, T. Yoshida and T. Noguchi: *J. Med. Chem. 31*, 1295 (1988).
230   T. Honda, T. Shimamoto and S. Kato: Japan Patent 63,215,690; *Chem. Abstr. 111*, 7660 j (1988); T. Honda, S. Kato and T. Shimamoto: Japan Patent 63,215,691; *Chem. Abstr. 111*, 7661 k (1988).
231   J. C. Ruckdeschel and S. Archer: *Proc. Meet. Am. Assoc. Cancer Res. 30*, A2420 (1989).
232   C. Auclair, A. Pierre, E. Voisin, O. Pepin, S. Cros, C. Colas, J.-M. Saucier, B. Verschuere, P. Gros and C. Paoletti: *Cancer Res. 47*, 6254 (1987).
233   V. Pierson, A. Pierre, Y. Pommier and P. Gros: *Cancer Res. 48*, 1404 (1988).
234   G. Atassi, P. Dumont, O. Pepin, O. Gros and P. Gros: *Proc. Annu. Meet. Am. Assoc. Cancer Res. 30*, A2458 (1989).
235   W. E. Ross: *Biochem. Pharmacol. 34*, 4191 (1985).
236   S. Douc-Rasy, J. F. Riou, J. C. Ahomadegbe and G. Riou: *Biol. Cell 64*, 145 (1988).
237   Y. Pommier, R. E. Schwartz, L. A. Zwelling and K. W. Kohn: *Biochemistry 24*, 6406 (1985); Y. Pommier, J. K. Minford, R. E. Schwartz, L. A. Zwelling and K. W. Kohn: *Biochemistry 24*, 6410 (1985).
238   L. H. Li and C. H. Cowie: *Biochem. Biophys. Acta 353*, 375 (1974).
239   V. S. Sethi: *Biochem. Pharmacol. 30*, 2026 (1981).
240   W. E. Ross, D. L. Glaubiger and K. W. Kohn: *Biochem. Biophys. Acta 519*, 23 (1978).
241   W. E. Ross and M. O. Bradley: *Biochem. Biophys. Acta 654*, 129 (1981).
242   L. A. Zwelling, S. Michaels, D. Kerrigan, Y. Pomier and K. W. Kohn: *Biochem. Pharmacol. 31*, 3261 (1882).
243   E.-S. M. El Mashak and J. F. Tocanne: *Eur. J. Biochem. 105*, 573 (1980).
244   F. Terce, J.-F. Tocanne and G. Laneelle: *Biochem. Pharmacol. 32*, 2189 (1983).
245   F. Terce, J.-F. Tocanne and G. Laneelle: *Eur. J. Biochem. 133*, 349 (1983).
246   P. Lesca, P. Lecointe, D. Pelaprat, C. Paoletti and D. Mansuy: *Biochem. Pharmacol. 29*, 3231 (1980).
247   P. Lesca, E. Rafidinarivo, P. Lecointe and D. Mansuy: *Chem. Biol. Interact. 24*, 189 (1979).
248   P. Lesca, P. Beaune and B. Monsarrat: *Chem. Biol. Interact. 26*, 299 (1981).
249   Y. Pommier, R. E. Schwartz, L. A. Zwelling, D. Kerrigan, M. R. Mattern, J. Y. Charcosset, A. Jacquemin-Sablon and K. W. Kohn: *Cancer Res. 46*, 611 (1986).
250   J.-Y. Charcosset, J.-M. Saucier and A. Jacquemin-Sablon: *Biochem. Pharmacol. 37*, 2145 (1988).
251   G. Renuault, C. Malvy, W. Venegas and A. K. Larsen: *Toxicol. Appl. Pharmacol. 89*, 281 (1987).
252   B. Dugue, C. Auclair and B. Meunier: *Cancer Res. 46*, 3828 (1986).
253   M. M. Moore, K. H. Brock, C. L. Doerr and D. M. DeMarini: *Environ. Mutagen. 9*, 161 (1987).

254 E. T. Sakamoto-Hojo, C. S. Takahashi, I. Ferrari and M. Motidome: *Mutat. Res. 199*, 11 (1988).

255 D. M. DeMarini and B. K. Lawrence: *Teratog. Carcinog. Mutagen 8*, 293 (1988).

256 P. Lecointe, P. Lesca, S. Cros and C. Paoletti: *Chem. Biol. Interact. 20*, 113 (1978).

257 M. Pinto, M. Guerineau and C. Paoletti: *Biochem. Pharmacol. 31*, 2161 (1982).

258 C. Paoletti, P. Lecointe, P. Lesca, S. Cros, D. Mansuy and N. Dat-Xuong: *Biochimie 60*, 1003 (1978).

259 B. Meunier, C. Auclair, J. Bernadou, G. Meunier, M. Maftouh, S. Cros, B. Monsarrat and C. Paoletti: *Dev. Pharmacol. 3*, 149 (1983).

260 G. Mathe, M. Hayat, F. De Vassal, L. Schwarzenberge, M. Schneider, J. Schulmberger, C. Jasmin and C. Rosenfeld: *Rev. Eur. Etud. Clin. Biol. 15*, 541 (1970).

261 P. Juret, Y. Le Talaer, J. E. Couette and T. Delozier: in "Breast Cancer, Experimental and Clinical Aspects" (H. T. Mourid and T. Palschof, eds.) p. 277, Pergamon Oxford, 1980.

262 P. Juret, A. Tanguy, A. Girard, J. Y. Le Talaer, J. S. Abbatucci, N. Dat-Xuong, J.-B. Le Pecq and C. Paoletti: *Eur. J. Cancer 14*, 205 (1987).

263 P. Juret, J. F. Heron, J. E. Couette, J. Delozier and J. Y. Le Talaer: Cancer Treat Rep. *66*, 1909 (1982).

264 J. R. Beck, R. N. Booher, A. C. Brown, R. Kwock and A. Pohland: *J. Am. Chem. Soc. 89*, 3934 (1967).

265 J. R. Beck. R. Kwok, R. N. Booher, A. C. Brown, L. E. Patterson, P. Pranc, B. Rockey and A. Pohland: *J. Am. Chem. Soc. 90*, 4706 (1968).

266 W. M. Bandaranayake, L. Crombie and D. A. Whiting: *J. Chem. Commun.* 970 (1969).

267 C. S. Oh and C. V. Greco: *J. Heterocycl. Chem. 7*, 261 (1970).

268 J. W. Loder and R. H. Nearn: *Aust. J. Chem. 28*, 651 (1975).

269 J. W. Loder and R. H. Nearn: *Tetrahedron Lett.* 2497 (1975).

270 J. W. Loder, C. C. J. Culvenor, R. H. Nearn, G. B. Russell and D. W. Stanton: *Aust. J. Chem. 27*, 179 (1974).

271 Screening Data Files, National Cancer Institute 1983.

272 S. M. Y. Kupchan, Y. Komoda, W. A. Court, G. J. Thomas, R. M. Smith, A. Karim and C. J. Gilmore; *J Am. Chem. Soc. 94*, 1354 (1972).

273 S. M. Kupchan, Y. Komoda, G. J. Thomas and H. P. J. Hintz: *Chem. Commun.* 1065 (1972).

274 M. C. Wani, H. L. Taylor and M. E. Wall: *Chem. Commun.* 390 (1973).

275 S. M. Kupchan, Y. Komoda, G. J. Thomas and W. A. Court: U.S. Patent 3,896,111 (1975): [*C. A. 83*, 209396 s (1975)].

276 Y. Komoda: *Kagaku No Ryoiki, 28* 887 (1974).

277 L. J. Hanka and M. S. Barnett: *Antimicrob. AG Chemother. 6*, 651 (1974).

278 S. M. Kupchan, A. R. Branfman, A. T. Sneden, A. K. Verma, R. G. Dailey, Y. Komoda and Y. Nagao: *J. Am. Chem. Soc. 97* 5294 (1975).

279 S. L. Remillard, I. Rebun, G. A. Howe and S. M. Kupchan: *Science 189* 1002 (1975).

280 M. K. Wolpert-Defilippes, R. H. Adamson, R. L. Cysyk and D. G. Johns: *Biochem. Pharmacol. 24*, 751 (1975).

281 T. E. Connor, C. Aldrich, A. Haddi, N. Lomax, P. Okano, S. Sethi and H. B. Wood: Proceedings of 66th Annual Meeting of American Association of Cancer Researchers 29 (1975).

282 R. Chen. Z. Hua, Z. Lu, L. Wang and B. Xu: *Yaoxue Tangbao 17*, 303 (1982).

283 H. Nozaki, Y. Matsuura, S. Hirono, R. Kasai, J. J. Chang and K. H. Kuo: *J. Nat. Prod. 53*, 1039 (1990).

284 Y. H. Kuo, C. H. Chen, L. M. Kuo, M. L. King, T. S. Wu, S. T. Lu, I. S. Chen, D. R. McPhail, and K. H. Lee: *Heterocycles 29*, 1465 (1989).
285 Y. H. Kuo, C. H. Chen, L. M. Kuo, M. L. King, T. S. Wu, M. Harura and K. H. Lee: *J. Nat. Prod. 53*, 422 (1990).
286 S. Arichi: Fr. 2,430,234 (1980): [*C. A. 93*, 53959 w (1980)].
287 S. Arichi and T. Hayashi et al.: Ger. 2,828,851 (1980): [*C. A. 92*, 209179 j (1980)].
288 M. Maeda, K. Yuki, O. Takahide, M. Masayo: *Kanazawa Ika Digaku Zasshi 15*, 163 (1990).
289 L. Xu, B. Wang, J. Gao: *Huaxi Yike Daxue Xuebao 22*, 124 (1991).
290 K. D. Lee and R. P. Huemer: *Jap. J. Pharmacol. 21*, 299 (1971).
291 H. Kim. Y. H. Lee, S. Kim: *Hanguk Saenghwa Hakoechi 23*, 179 (1990).
292 H. Matsunga, M. Katano, H. Yamamoto, M. Mori and K. Takatu: *Chem. Pharm. Bull. 37*, 1279 (1989).
293 K. Mitsou, Y. Hiroshi, M. Hisashi, M. Masato, T. Katsumi and N. Mitsunasi: *Gan to Kagaku Ryoho 17*, 1045 (1990).
294 W. Kim and N. P. Jung: *Koryo Insam Hakhoechi 13*, 24 (1989).
295 J. L. Hartwell and M. J. Shear: *Cancer Res. 7*, 716 (1947).
296 I. W. Kaplan: *N. Orleans Med. Surg J. 94*, 388 (1942).
297 L. S. King and M. Sullivan: *Science 105*, 433 (1947).
298 R. A. Miller: *Int. J. Dermatol 24*, 491 (1985).
299 B. J. Sullivan and H. I. Wechsler: *Science 105*, 433 (1947).
300 A. G. Heyenga, J. A. Lucas and P. M. Dewich: *Plant Cell Rep. 9*, 382 (1990).
301 D. E. Jackson: *Phytochemistry 24*, 2407 (1985).
302 A. J. Broomhead and P. M. Dewick: *Phytochemistry 29*, 3831 (1990).
303 C. Keller-Juslen, M. Kuhn and A. Wartburg et al.: *J. Med. Chem. 14*, 936 (1971).
304 H. Stahelin: *Eur. J. Cancer 6*, 303 (1970).
305 H. Stahelin: *Eur. J. Cancer 9*, 215 (1973).
306 T. L. Avery, D. Roberts and D. A. Price: *Cancer Chemother. Rep. 57*, 165 (1973).
307 D. N. Dombernowsky, N. I. Nissen and V. Larsen: *Cancer Chemother. Rep. 56*, 769 (1972).
308 G. Mathe, L. Schwarzenberg and P. Pouillart et al.: *Cancer 34*, 460 (1974).
309 B. D. Sklansky, R. S. Mann-Kaplan and A. F. Reynolds et al.: *Cancer 33*, 460 (1974).
310 L. M. Allen and P. J. Creaven: *Eur. J. Cancer 11*, 697 (1975).
311 C. C. Huang, Y. Hou and J. J. Wang: *Cancer Res. 33*, 3123 (1973).
312 M. Gosalvez, J. Perez-Garcia and M. Lopez: *Eur. J. Cancer 94*, 471 (1972).
313 P. I. Clark and M. L. Slevin: *Clin. Pharmacokinet. 12*, 223 (1987).
314 D. J. Loike and S. B. Horwitz: *Biochemistry 24*, 321 (1976).
315 B. H. Long and A. Minocha: *Proc. Am. Assoc. Cancer Res. 24*, 321 (1983).
316 W. Ross, T. Rowe, B. Glisson, J. Yalowich and L. Liu: *Cancer Res. 44*, 5857 (1984).
317 A. J. Woznaik and W. E. Ross: *Cancer Res. 43*, 120 (1983).
318 Y. L. Zhang, Y. C. Shen, Z. Q. Wang, H. X. Chen, X. Guo, Y. C. Cheng and K. H. Leo: *J. Nat. Prod. 55*, 1100 (1992).
319a L. S. Thurston, Y. Imakura, M. Harura, D. H. Li, Z. C. Liu, S. Y. Liu, Y. C. Cheng and K. H. Lee: *J. Med. Chem. 32*, 6 (1989).
319b R. G. Powell, C. R. Smith and R. V. Madrigal: *Planta Med. 30*, 101 (1976).
320 R. G. Powell, C. R. Smith, D. Weisleder, D. A. Muthard and J. C. Clardy: *J. Am. Chem. Soc. 101*, 2784 (1979).
321 R. G. Powell and C. R. Smith: *J. Nat. Prod. 44*, 86 (1981).
322 A. S. Kende and T. P. Demuth: *Tetrahedron Lett. 21*, 715 (1980).
323 J. C. Bottaro and G. A. Berchtold: *J. Org. Chem. 45*, 1176 (1980).

324 M. J. Wanner, G. Koomer and U. K. Pandit: *Heterocycles 15*, 377 (1981).
325 K. Tomioka and K. Koga: *Tetrahedron Lett. 21*, 2321 (1980).
326 R. G. Powell, C. R. Smith, D. Weisleder, G. K. Matsumoto, J. Clardy and J. Kozlowski: *J. Am. Chem. Soc. 105*, 3739 (1983).
327 R. G. Powell, R. D. Plattner and M. Suffness: *Weed. Sci. 38*, 148 (1990).
328 F. Matsuda, S. Terashima: *Stud. Nat. Prod. Chem. 1*, 305 (1988).
329 H. Lucas: *Arch. Pharm. 95*, 145 (1956).
330 E. Winterstein and A. Guyer: *Z. Physiol. Chem.* 175 (1923).
331 E. Graf: *Angew. Chem. 68*, 249 (1956).
332 M. Kurono, Y. Nakadaira, S. Onuma, K. Sasaki and K. Nakanishi: *Tetrahedron Lett.* 2153 (1963).
333 B. Lythgoe: in "The Alkaloids" (R. H. F. Manske, ed.) Vol. X, p. 597, Academic Press, New York, 1968.
334 M. C. Wani, H. L. Taylor, M. E. Wall, P. Coggon and A. T. McPhail: *J. Am. Chem. Soc. 93*, 2325 (1971).
335 D. P. Della Casa De Marcano and T. G. Halsall: *Chem. Commun.* 365 (1975).
336 R. W. Miller: *J. Nat. Prod. 43*, 425 (1980).
337 M. Suffnes and G. A. Cordell: in "The Alkaloids" (A. Brossi, ed.) Vol. XXV p. 3, Academic Press, New York, 1985.
338 S. Blechert and D. Guenard: in "The Alkaloids" (A. Brossi, ed.) Vol. 39, p. 195, Academic Press, San Diego, 1990.
339 D. G. I. Kingston: *Pharmacol. and Ther. 52*, 1 (1991).
340 S. B. Horwitz: TIPS *13*, 134 (1992).
341 R. W. Miller, R. G. Powell, C. R. Smith, R. Arnold, Jr and J. Clardy: *J. Org. Chem. 46*, 1469 (1981).
342 R. G. Powell, R. W. Miller and C. S. Smith Jr: *Chem. Commun.* 102 (1979).
343 V. Senilh, S. Blechert, M. Colin, D. Guenard, F. Picot, P. Potier and P. Varenne: *J. Nat. Prod. 47*, 131 (1984).
344 K. M. Witterup, S. A. Look, M. H. Stasko, T. J. Ghiorzi, G. M. Mieschik and G. M. Cragg: *J. Nat. Prod. 53*, 1249 (1990).
345 J. L. McLaughlin, R. W. Miller, R. G. Powell and C. R. Smith Jr.: *J. Nat. Prod. 44*, 312 (1981).
346 M. Shiro and H. Koyama: *J. Chem. Soc.* B 1342 (1971).
347 D. I. Kingston, G. Samaranayake and C. A. Ivey: *J. Nat. Prod. 53*, 1 (1990).
348 G. Chauviere, D. Guenard, C. Pascard, F. Picot, P. Potier and T. Prange: *Chem. Commun.* 495 (1982).
349 C. H. O. Huang, D. G. I. Kingston, N. F. Magri, G. Samaranayake and F. E. Boettner: *J. Nat. Prod. 49*, 665 (1986).
350 D. P. Della Casa de Marcano and T. G. Halsall: *Chem. Commun.* 1282 (1969).
351 IUPAC, Commission on Nomenclature of Organic Chemistry *86*, 1 (1978).
352 T. I. Ho, Y. C. Lin, G. H. Lee, S. M. Peng, M. K. Yeh and F. C. Chen: *Acta Crystallogr.*, Sect. C: *Cryst. Struct. Commun. 43*, 1378 (1987).
353 T. I. Ho, Y. C. Lin, G. H. Lee, S. M. Peng, M. K. Yeh and F. C. Chen: *Acta, Crystallogr,.* Sect. C: *Cryst. Struct. Commun. 43*, 1380 (1987).
354 F. Yoshi Zaki, M. Fukuda, S. Hisamichi, T. Ishida and I. Yasuko: *Chem. Pharm. Bull. 36*, 2098 (1988).
355 L. Ettouati, A. Ahond, O. Convert, D. Laurent, C. Poupat and P. Potier: *Bull. Soc. Chim. Fr.* 749 (1988); L. Ettouati, A. Ahond, O. Convert, C. Poupat and P. Potier: *Bull. Soc. Chim. Fr. 5*, 687 (1989).
356 F. Gueritte-Voegelein, D. Guenard and P. Potier: *J. Nat. Prod. 50*, 9 (1987).
357 K. M. Witherup, S. A. Look, M. W. Stasko, T. J. Gheorzi and G. M. Muschik: *J. Nat. Prod. 53*, 1249 (1990).
358 M. Jaziri, B. M. Diallo, M. H. Vanhaelen, R. J. Vanhaelen-Fastre, A. Zhiri, A. G. Becu and J. Homes: *J. Pharm. Belg. 46*, 93 (1991).

359 M. Colin, D. Guenard, I. Gueritte-Voegelein and P. Potier: *Eur. Pat. Appl.* EP253738 (Cl: CO7D305/14), 20th June 1988; Fr. Appl. 86.

360 M. Colin, D. Guenard, F. Gueritte-Voegelein and P. Potier: *Eur. Pat. Appl.* EP253739 (Cl: CO7D305/140, 20th Jan. 1988; Fr. Appl. 86/10401, 17th Jul. 1986; *Chem. Abstr. 109,* 22763 x (1988).

361 W. P. McGuire, E. K. Rowinsky, N. B. Rosenshein, F. C. Grumbine, D. S. Ettinger, D. K. Armstrong and R. C. Donehower: *Ann. Intera. Med. 111,* 273 (1989).

362 F. A. Holmes, R. S. Walters, R. L. Therault, A. D. Forman, L. K. Newton, M. N. Raber, A. U. Buzdar, D. K. Frye and G. N. Hortobagyi: *J. Natl. Cancer Inst. 83,* 1797 (1991).

363 A. I. Einzig, H. Hochster, P. H. Wiernik, D. L. Trump, J. P. Dutcher, E. Garowski, J. Sasloff and T. J. Smith: *Invest New Drugs 9,* 59 (1991).

364 P. B. Schiff, J. Fant and S. B. Horwitz: *Nature 277,* 665 (1979).

365 J. Parness, C. F. Asnes and S. B. Horwitz: *Cell. Motil. 3,* 123 (1983).

366 J. J. Manfride and S. B. Horwitz: *Pharmac. Ther. 25,* 83 (1984).

367 P. B. Schiff and S. B. Horwitz: *Proc. Natl. Acad. Sci.* USA *77,* 1561 (1980).

368 P. B. Schiff and S. B. Horwitz: *Biochemistry 20,* 3247 (1981).

369 J. Parness and S. B. Horwitz: *J. Cell Biol. 91,* 479 (1981).

370 W. E. Rainey, R. E. Kramer, J. I. Mason and J. W. Shay: *J. Cell Physiol. 123,* 17 (1985).

371 A. I. Annone, G. Wolberg, R. Reynolds-Vaughn and T. P. Zimmermon: *Agents and Actions 21,* 278 (1987).

372 A. H. Ding, F. Porteu, E. Sanchez and C. F. Nathan: *Science 248,* 370 (1990).

373 S. L. Howell, C. S. Hii, S. Shaikh and M. Trhurst: *Bioscience Rep. 2,* 795 (1982).

374 S. S. Kaufman, D. J. Tiema and J. A. Vanderhoof: *Toxicol. Appl. Pharmac. 82,* 233 (1986).

375 M. J. Schibler and F. Cabral: *J. Chell Biol. 102,* 1522 (1986).

376 R. Gupta: *J. Cell Physiol. 114,* 137 (1983); R. S. Gupta: *Cancer Treat. Rep. 69,* 515 (1985).

377 J. A. Moscow and K. H. Cowan: *J. Natn. Cancer Inst. 80,* 14 (1988).

378 J. R. Roberts, D. C. Allison, R. C. Donehower and E. K. Rowinsky: *Cancer Res. 50,* 710 (1990).

379 M. Lassus, D. Scott and B. Leyland-Jones: *Proc. Asco 4,* 268 (1985).

380 B. D. Darr, T. G. Sambandan and S. H. Yalkowsky: *Pharm. Res. 4,* 162 (1987).

381 S. M. Longnecker, R. C. Donehower, A. E. Cates, T. Chen., R. B. Brundrett, L. B. Grochow, D. S. Ettinger and M. Colven: *Cancer Treat. Rep. 71,* 53 (1986).

382 E. K. Rowinsky, P. J. Burke, J. E. Karg, R. W. Tucker, D. S. Ettinger and R. C. Donehower: *Cancer Res. 49,* 4640 (1989).

383 T. Brown, K. Havlin, G. Weiss, J. Cagnola, J. Koeller, J. Kuhn, J. Rizzo, J. Craig, J. Philipps and D. Von Hoff: *J. Clin. Oncol. 9,* 1261 (1991).

384 P. H. Wiernik, E. L. Schwartz, J. J. Straumann, J. P. Dutcher, R. B. Lipton and E. Paietta: *Cancer Res. 47,* 2486 (1987).

385 I. Ringel and S. B. Horwitz: *J. Pharmac. Exptl. Ther. 242,* 692 (1987).

386 B. Monsarrat, E. Mariel, S. Coris, M. Gares, D. Guenard, F. Gueritte-Voegelein and M. Wright: *Drug Met. Disp. 18,* 895 (1990).

387 M. S. Kris, J. P. O'Connell, R. J. Gralla, M. S. Wertheim, R. M. Parente, P. B. Schiff and C. W. Young: *Cancer Treat. Rep. 70,* 605 (1986).

388 P. H. Wiernik, E. L. Schwartz, A. Enzig, J. J. Straumann, R. B. Lipton and J. P. Dutcher: *J. Clin, Oncol. 5,* 1232 (1987).

389 J. L. Grem, K. D. Tusch and K. J. Simon: *Cancer Treat Rep. 71,* 1179 (1987).

390 T. Ohnuma, A. S. Zimet, V. A. Coffey, J. F. Holland and E. M. Greenspan: *Proc. Am. Assoc. Cancer Res. 26,* 662 (1985).

391 M. Markman, E. Rowinsky, T. Hakes, B. Reichman, W. Jones, S. Rubin, J. L. Lewis, M. Phillips Jr., L. Almadrones and W. Hoskins: *Proc. Am. Soc. Clin. Oncol. 10*, 601 (1991).

392 E. K. Rowinsky, M. Gilbert, W. P. McGuire, D. A. Noe, L. B. Grochow, A. Forastiere, D. S. Ettinger, B. G. Lubejko, B. Clark, S. E. Sartorius, D. R. Cornblath, C. B. Hendricks and R. C. Donehower: *J. Clin. Oncol. 9*, 1692 (1991).

393 S. S. Legha, S. Ring, N. Papadopoulos, M. Raber and R. Benjamin: *Cancer 65*, 2478 (1990).

394 T. Thigpen, J. Blessing, H. Ball, S. Hummel and R. Barret: *Proc. Am. Soc. Clin. Oncol. 9*, 604 (1990).

395 F. A. Holmes, D. Frye, R. L. Ther Rault, R. S. Walters, A. D. Forman, L. K. Newton, A. U. Buzdar and G. N. Hortobagyi: *Proc. Am. Soc. Clin. Oncol. 10*, 113 (1991).

396 C. S. Swindell, N. E. Krauss, S. B. Horwitz and I. Ringel: *J. Med. Chem. 34*, 1176 (1991).

397 H. Lataste, V. Senilh, M. Wright, D. Guenard and P. Potier: *Proc. Natn. Acad. Sci.* USA *81*, 4090 (1984).

398 N. F. Magri and D. G. I. Kingston: *J. Org. Chem. 51*, 797 (1986).

399 G. Samaranayake, N. F. Magri, C. Jitragsri and D. G. I. Kingston: *J. Org. Chem. 56*, 5114 (1991).

400 I. Barasosain, C. de Ines, F. Diaz, J. M. Andreu, V. CSC Madrid Peyrot, D. Leynadier, P. Garcia and C. Briond: *Proc. Am. Assoc. Cancer Res. 32*, 1952 (1991).

401 I. Ringel and S. B. Horwitz: *J. Nata Cancer Inst. 83*, 288 (1991).

402 M. C. Bissery, D. Guenard, F. Gueritte-Voegelein and F. Lavell: *Cancer Res. 51*, 4845 (1991).

403 J. M. Extra, F. Rousseau, J. Bourhis, V. Dieras and M. Marty: *Proc. Am. Assoc. Cancer Res. 32*, 1225 (1991).

404 E. Wilthshaw, S. Subramarian, C. Alexopoulos and G. H. Barker: *Cancer Treat. Rep. 63*, 1545 (1979); E. Wilthshaw, B. Evans, G. Rustin, E. Gilbey, J. Baker and G. Barker: *J. Clin. Oncol. 4*, 4093 (1988).

405 S. Boreman: *Chem. Engng. New 69*, 11 (1991).

406 S. M. Kupchan, R. Chakravarti and N. Yokoyama: *J. Pharm. Sci. 52*, 985 (1963).

407 S. M. Kupchan: *Trans NY Acad. Sci. 32*, 85 (1970).

408 N. M. Mollov, H. B. Dutschewska and K. Siljanovska: *Dokl. Bolg. Akad. Nauk 21*, 605 (1968).

409 L. M. Allen and P. J. Creaven: *Cancer-Res. 33*, 3112 (1973).

410 L. M. Allen and P. J. Creaven: *J. Pharm. Sci. 63*, 474 (1974).

411 L. H. Liao: *Proc. Natl. Sci. Counc. repub. China 4*, 245 (1980); [*C. A. 93*, 197567 u, (1980)].

412 D. Todorou, Kh. Getov and M. Ilarionova: *Dokl. Bolg. Akad. 34*, 445 (1981): [*C.A. 95*, 73635, (1981)].

413 I. Stoichkkov and I. Mircheva: *Probl. Onkol. 7*, 60 (1979): [*C. A. 93*, 142973 p (1980)].

414 S. Sh. Shakhabutdinov and S. F. Fakhrutdinov: *Farmakol. Alkaloidov Ikh Proizvod* 171, 1972: [*C. A. 80*, 103857 r, (1974)].

415 Y. Zhou, Y. Guo and X. Men: *Shenyang Yaoxueyan Xuebao 7*, 45, 1990: [*C. A. 113*, 158513 f (1990)].

416 C. X. Xu, L. Liu, R. H. Sun, X. Liu and R. Han: *Yaoxue Xeubao 25*, 330 (1990).

417 J. W. Lin, T. C. Lee and T. C. Tung: *Indian J. Pap. Protein Res. 2*, 311 (1978).

418 S. Schimizu, T. Miayse, K. Umehara and A. Veno: *Chem. Pharm. Bull. 38*, 1308 (1990).

419 N. Hayashi, K. H. Lee, I. H. Hall, A. T. McPhail and H. C. Huang: *Phytochemistry 21*, 2371 (1982).
420 M. Ogura, G. A. Cordell, A. Douglas and N. R. Farnsworth: *Lloydia 40*, 579 (1977).
421 M. Hiroshi and H. Hidechi: *Planta Med. 54*, 117 (1988).
422 Y. Haruki, K. Kanki, K. Hiroaki, C. Jongchol, H. Yumiko and O. Yasuo: *Planta Med. 56*, 182 (1990).
423 Y. H. Hui, J. K. Rupprecht, J. E. Anderson, D. L. Smith, C. J. Chang and J. L. McLaughlin: *J. Nat. Prod. 52*, 463 (1989).
424 Y. H. Hui, C. J. Chang, D. L. Smith, J. C. McLaughlin: *Pharm. Res. 7*, 376 (1990).
425 A. Jossan, A. Cave, B. M. Helene and B. Helene: *Tetrahedron Lett. 31*, 1861 (1990).
426 H. Grabarcyzk, B. Drozdz, H. Boguslaw and W. Jaina: *Pol. J. Pharmacol. 29*, 419 (1977).
427 M. Holub and Z. Samek: *Collect. Czech. Chem. Commun. 42*, 1053 (1977).
428 B. Xing, L. Zhao, B. Luo and L. Jin: *Guangxi Yixue 2*, (1982).
429 J. Hinou, C. Demetzos, C. Harvala and C. Roussakis: *Inter. J. Crude Drug. Res. 28*, 149 (1990).
430 I. I. Cemosova, L. M. Belenovskaya and A. N. Stukov: *Rastit. Resur 23*, 100 (1987).
431 Q. Xu, H. Mori, O. Sakamoto, A. Koda and H. Nishioka: *Wakan Igaku Gakkaishi 6*, 1 (1989).
432 K. Koike, C. Bevelle, S. K. Talapatra, G. A. Cordell and N. R. Farnsworth: *Chem. Pharm. Bull. 28*, 401 (1980).
433 Y. Fujimoto, S. Angusteine and S. Made: Jpn. Patent 6,287,589 (1987): [*C. A. 107*, 233371 q (1987)].
434 Y. Fujimoto, S. Angusteine and S. Made: *Phytochemistry 27*, 1109 (1988).
435 Y. Takashi, Y. Xiuzhen and K. Hsiung: *Chem. Pharm. Bull. 36*, 1615 (1988).
436 Y. Takashi, H. Mitsumasha, Y. Xiuzhen, C. J. Jang and L. K. Hsiung: *J. Nat. Prod. 52*, 1071 (1989).
437 H. Siegfried and W. Steglich: *Phytochemistry 22*, 2835 (1983).
437a M. Suffness in "The Alkaloids" (A. Brossi, ed.) Vol. XXV, p. 73, Academic Press, New York, 1985; T. Hsieh, C. C. Yang, H. Y. Chang and K. M. Ling: *Chin. Med. J. (Peking, Engl. Ed.) 92*, 57 (1979).
438 O. B. Luz, M. Victoria, C. Victoria, L. Lilia, D. V. Fe, D. C. Fliseo and V. Ed'na: *Asian J. Pharm. 80*, (1974).
439 S. Kitanaka and M. Takida: *Chem. Pharm. Bull. 38*, 1291 (1990).
440 G. R. Pettit, A. Numata, T. Takemura, R. H. Odo, J. M. Schmidt, M. G. Cragg and C. P. Pase: *J. Nat. Prod. 54*, 456 (1990).
441 F. M. Harraz and M. E. Amer: *Alexandria J. Pharm. Sci. 2*, 168 (1988).
442 G. Wang, Y. Z. Li, B. Wang, J. Gao, Z. Yan and X. Li; *Zhenggyo Zazhi 16*, 242 (1991).
443 A. Munehisa, H. Tashimitsu, S. Mineo, M. Naokata, B. Hua, K. Shougo and I. Yusuke: *J. Nat. Prod. 54*, 898 (1991).
444 E. Yuichi, O. Tomihisa and N. Shigeo: *Tetrahedron Lett. 32*, 3083 (1991).
445 Z. Raymond, L. David, C. L. Elile and A. H. J. Wang: *Tetrahedron 33*, 1457 (1977).
446 P. R. George and S. B. Sing: U.S. Patent 4,996,237 (1991): [*C. A. 115*, 189740 (1991)].
447 B. Thomas, A. Francisco and K. Hosteltmann: *Planta Med. 54* (1988).
448 Tumor Research Group: *Chung-Hua I Hsueh Tsa Chih* 472 (1973).
449 S. Fang, R. Zhang, Y. Chen, C. Xu and S. Lu: *Zhiwu Xuebao 31*, 934 (1989).
450 G. R. Pettit, Y. Kamano: Eur. Patent 399,668 (1990) [*C. A. 115*, 782 z (1991)].
451 H. Huang and C. Cheng: *Zhongguo Yaoli Xuebao 3*, 286 (1982).
452 J. Petricic, M. Osmak, M. Hadzija, Z. Kalodera and M. Slijepceirc: *Acta Pharm. Jugosl. 41*, 169 (1991).

453 S. Yoshimura, H. Narita, K. Hayashi and H. Mitsuhashi: *Chem. Pharm. Bull. 31*, 3971 (1983).
454 I. Kubo and K. Fukuhara: *J. Nat. Prod. 53*, 968 (1990).
455 E. Ch. Pukhal 'skaya, M. F. Petrova, P. N. Denisova and S. I. Denisova et al.: USSR Patent 396,040 (1974) [*C. A. 81*, 140866 j (1974)].
456 Y. L. Liu, D. K. Ho and J. M. Cassady: *J. Nat. Prod. 55*, 357 (1992).
457 M. P. Chitnis, K. G. Bhatia and M. K. Pathak: *Indian J. Exp. Biol. 17*, 212 (1979).
458 C. Guerrero, G. Campos and J. Taboada: *Rev. Latinoam. Quim. 19*, 147 (1988).
459 W. Tiang Shung, L. Yun-Meei, H. Mitsumasa and S. Tetsuro: *J. Nat. Prod. 54*, 823 (1991).
460 M. T. Gill, R. Baja, C. J. Chang, D. E. Nichols and J. L. McLaughlin: *J. Nat. Prod. 50*, 36 (1987).
461 P. Cao, Z. Wu and R. Wang: *Shenzwu Huaxue Zazhi 6*, 176 (1990).
462 N. Kawai, Y. Nishibe, Y. Ando and Y. Ando: Jpn. Patent 03,215,434 (1991): [*C. A. 115*, 263454 t (1991)].
463 Y. F. Liou and K. H, Lin: *T'ai-wan T Hsueh Hui Tsa Chih 18*, 549 (1979).
464 G. Peterson and S. Barnes: *Biochem. Biophys. Res. Commun. 179*, 661 (1991).
465 L. W. Haynes and R. O. Weller: *Acta Neuropathol. 44*, 21 (1978).
466 N. N. Kuznetsova and S. S. Nuridzhanyants et al.: *Deposited Doc.* 409 (1979): [*C. A. 92*, 140463 c (1980)].
467 M. R. Flack, R. Knazek and M. Reidenberg: U.S. Patent 551,353 (1991) [*C. A. 115*, 85409 f (1991)].
468 C. C. Benz, M. A. Kenisy and J. M. Ford et al.: *Mol. Pharmacol. 37*, 840 (1990): [*C. A. 113*, 90941 m (1990)].
469 S. Pal, S. K. Banerjee and B. Mukherji: *Indian J. Med. Res. 56*, 445 (1968).
470 B. S. Aswal, D. S. Bhakuni, A. K. Goel, K. Kar, B. N. Mehrotra and K. C. Mukherjee: *Indian J. Exp. Biol. 22*, 312 (1984).
471 R. Y. Ambaye, V. R. Khanolkar and T. B. Panse: *Proc. Indian Acad. Sci. 56B*, 123 (1962).
472 N. Kawai, Y. Nishibe, Y. Ando and Y. Ando: Jpn. Patent 03,215,433 (1991) [*C. A. 115*, 263453 a (1991)].
473 L. A. Decosterd, E. H. Stoeckli, J. C. Chapuis, J. D. Msonthi, B. Sordat and K. Hostettman: *Helv. Chim Acta 72*, 464 (1989).
473 B. N. Dhawan, G. K. Patnaik, R. P. Rastogi, K. K. Singh and J. S. Tandon: *Indian J. Exp. Biol. 15*, 208 (1977).
475 B. S. Aswal, D. S. Bhakuni, A. K. Goel, K. Kar, B. N. Mehrotra and K. Mukherjee: *Indian J. Exp. Biol. 22*, 312 (1984).
476 J. P. S. Sarin, H. S. Garg, N. M. Khanna and M. M. Dhar: *Phytochemistry 12*, 2461 (1973).
477 B. S. Aswal, D. S. Bhakuni, A. K. Goel, K. Kar, B. N. Mehrotra and K. C. Mukherjee: *Indian J. Exp. Biol. 22*, 312 (1984).
478 R. W. Doskotch, S. L. Keely, C. D. Hufford and F. S., El-Feraly: *Phytochemistry 14*, 769 (1975).
479 S. Pal, S. K. Chakraborty, A. Banerjee and B. Mukerjii: *Indian J. Med. Res. 56*, 445 (1968).
480 D. S. Bhakuni, M. L. Dhar, M. M. Dhar, B. N. Dhawan, B. Gupta and R. C. Srimal: *Indian J. Exp. Biol. 9*, 91 (1971).
481 G. R. Pettit, D. L. Herald, M. G. Cragg, J. A. Rideont and P. Brown: *J. Nat. Prod. 53*, 382 (1990).
482 F. S. El-Feraly and Y. M. Chan: *Tetrahedron Lett.* 1973 (1977).
483 T. Konoshima, M. Kozuka and H. Tokuda, et al.: *J. Nat. Prod. 54*, 816 (1991).
484 M. Arisawa, A. Fujita, T. Hayashi, K. Hayashi, H. Ochiai and N. Morita: *Chem. Pharm. Bull. 38*, 1624 (1990).

485   R. A. Finnegan, K. E. Merkel and N. Back: *J. Pharm. Sci. 61,* 1599 (1972).
486   J. H. Jung, C. J. Chang, D. L. Smith, J. L. McLaughlin, S. Pummangusa, C. Chaichantipyuth and C. Patarapanich: *J. Nat. Prod. 54,* 500 (1991).
487   Z. J. L. Zhu, Z. C. Zhong, Z. Y. Luo and Z. Y. Xiao: *Yaoxue Xuebao 25,* 898 (1990).
488   X. H. Li and J. L. McLaughlin: *J. Nat. Prod. 52,* 660 (1989).
489   Q. C. Pan and C. C. Pan et al.: *Hsueh Hsueh Pao 14,* 705 (1979).
490   P. W. LeQuesne and J. E. Larrahondo et al.: *J. Nat. Prod. 43,* 353 (1980).
491   T. H. Yang, C. M. Chen., C. S. Lu and C. L. Liao: *J. Chinese Chem. Soc. 19,* 143 (1972).
492   T. Mizuno, H. Kawagishi, T. Sveda, T. Yoshia and C. Suzuki: Jpn. Patent 03,157,367 (1991) [*C. A. 115,* 239699 q (1991)].
493   S. Pal, S. K. Chakraborti, A. Banerjee and B. Mukerji: *Indian J. Med. Res. 56,* 445 (1968).
494   J. S. Agarwal and R. P. Rastogi: *Indian J. Chem. 13,* 758 (1975).
495   J. T. Huang: *Arch. Pharm. 314,* 831 (1981).
496   K. W. West and J. M. Careskey et al.: *Surg. Forum. 32,* 444 (1981).
497   N. B. Perry, G. D. Albertson, J. W. Blunt, A. L. J. Cole, M. H. G. Munro and J. R. L. Walker: *Planta Med. 57,* 129 (1991).
498   M. Krishnaswamy and K. K. Purushotthaman: *Indian J. Exp. Biol. 18,* 876 (1980).
499   K. B. Kardono, S. Tsauri, K. Padmawinata, J. M. Pazzuto and A. D. Kinghorn: *J. Nat. Prod. 53,* 1447 (1990).
500   M. Hoeneisen, M. Silva and W. H. Watson: *Rev. Lationoam Quim 11,* 63 (1980).
501   K. C. Qianshi, F. Toshihiro and K. Yoshiki: *J. Nat. Prod. 55,* 1488 (1992).
502   J. J. H. Geng Xiang, D. L. Smith, K. V. Wood and J. L. McLaughlin: *Planta Med. 57,* 880 (1991).
503   Q. Hu, H. Wang, W. Shen, R. Chen and M. Zou: *Zhongguo Kangshengsu Zazhi 13,* 425 (1988).
504   I. Junichi, D. Tamae, T. Hiroyuki, O. Tsutomu and K. Michinori: *Yakugaku Zasshi 109,* 962 (1989).
505   T. Matsumoto and H. Tokuda: *Basic Life Sci.* 423 (1990).
506   W. W. Ma, J. E. Anderson, A. T. McKenzie, S. R. McLaughlin and M. S. Hudson: *J. Nat. Prod. 53,* 1009 (1990).
507   S. M. Kupchan, R. L. Baxter, M. F. Ziegler, P. M. Smith and R. F. Bryan: *Experientia 31,* 137 (1975).
508   D. J. Pan, Z. L. Li, C. G. Hu, K. Chen, J. J. Chang and K. H. Lee: *Planta Med. 56,* 363 (1990).
509   T. Hayashi, F. T. Smith and K. H. Lee: *J. med. Chem. 30,* 2005 (1987).
510   M. Endo and Y. Miyazaki: *Eisei Shikensho Hokuku* 69 (1972).
511   M. A. Al-Yahya, A. M. El-Sayed and J. S. Mossa et al.: *J. Nat. Prod. 51,* 621 (1988).
512   T. Fujita and Y. Takeda et al.: *Chem. Commun.* 205 (1980).
513   M. Beljanski and J. Bugiel: Fr. Patent 2,419,725 (1979): [*C. A. 92,* 140721 k (1980)].
514   G. A. Handy, S. Funayama and G. A. Coradell: *J. Nat. Prod. 44,* 696 (1981).
515   O. Hirai, T. Fujitsu, J. Mori and K. Kikuchi et al.: *J. Gen. Microbiol. 133,* 369 (1987).
516   H. Lou and C. Zuo: *Zhongcaoyao 21,* 194 (1990).
517   K. J. M. Mikolajczak, R. V. Madrigal, J. K. Rupprecht, Y. H. Hui and Y. M. Lin et al.: *Experientia 46,* 324 (1990).
518   M. K. Adwankar, M. P. Chitnis, D. D. Khandalekar and C. G. Bhadsavale: *Indian J. Exp. Biol. 18,* 102 (1980).
519   G. Ming, Y. E. Ma and Z. Zhang et al.: *Yao Hsueh T'ung Pao 16,* 6 (1981).
520   A. Nahrstedt, U. Eilert, B. Wolters and V. Wray: *Z. Naturforsch. 37C,* 200 (1981).

521   N. Kaneda, J. M. Pezzuto, A. D. Kinghorn and N. R. Farnsworth: *J. Nat. Prod. 55*, 654 (1992).
522   B. Shen and Y. Bai: *Shengwu Huaxue Zazhi 6*, 301 (1990).
523   H. Tatematsu, M. Mori, T. H. Yang, J. J. Chang, T. T. Lee and K. H. Lee: *J. Pharm. Sci. 80*, 325 (1991).
524   M. P. Chitnis, K. G. Bhatia, M. K. Pathak and K. V. Kesava Rao: *Indian J. Exp. Biol. 18*, 6 (1980).
525   C. Q. Hu, J. J. Chang and K. H. Lee: *J. Nat. Prod. 53*, 932 (1990).
526   N. Hosokawa, Y. Hosokawa, T. Sakai, M. Yoshida, N. Marui, H. Nishino, K. Kawai and A. Aoike: *Int. J. Cancer 45*, 1119 (1990).
527   A. Vlubelen and N. Goeren: *Planta Med. 24*, 290 (1973).
528   G. R. Iches, H. H.S. Fong, P. L. Schiff, R. E. Perdue and N. R. Farnsworth: *J. Pharm. Sci. 62*, 1009 (1973).
529   H. H. Steinel and R. S. V. Baker: *Cancer Lett. 51*, 163 (1990).
530   M. B. Hazuka, P. J. Edwards, F. Newman, J. J. Kinzie and K. N. Prasad: *J. Am. Coll. Nuts 9*, 143 (1990).
531   B. Wu, X. Wang, W. Yang, R. Huan, Y. Luo and J. Liu: *Jinan Daxue Xuebao 11*, 79 (1990).
532   E. Kishida, Y. Sone, S. Shibata and A. Misaki: *Agric. Biol. Chem. 53*, 1849 (1989).
533   P. B. Oelrichs and P. J. Vallely et al.: *J. Nat. Prod. 43*, 414 (1990).
534   T. S. Kyokai: "Shin Joyo Wakanyaku" Nauko-do Publication, Tokyo, 120 (1973).
535   K. Takao, K. Midori, K. Mutsuo, T. Harukuni, N. Hoyoku and I. Akio: *J. Nat. Prod. 55*, 1776 (1992).
536   G. R. Petit, G. M. Cragg, S. B. Singh, J. A. Duke and D. L. Doubek: *J. Nat. Prod. 53*, 176 (1990).

Progress in Drug Research, Vol. 42
Edited by Ernst Jucker
© 1994 Birkhäuser Verlag Basel (Switzerland)

Carcinogenicity, mutagenicity and cancer preventing activities of flavonoids: A structure-system-activity relationship (SSAR) analysis

By A. Das[1], J. H. Wang[2] and E. J. Lien[1,3]

[1] Department of Pharmaceutical Sciences, School of Pharmacy, University of Southern California, 1985 Zonal Avenue, Los Angeles, CA-90033, USA, and [2] Visiting Research Scholar from School of Pharmacy, Beijing Medical University, China; [3] To whom correspondence should be addressed.

1   Introduction

Flavonoids and related phenolic compounds are widely distributed among vascular plants and are found in numerous fruits, grains vegetables and other parts of higher plants [1–3]. Isolation and structural determination of flavonoids have been employed in plant taxonomy [1, 2]. Because of the wide range of chemical structures of flavonoids, coupled with a variety of test systems and different dose levels used, sometimes conflicting reports have been published in the literature regarding their numerous pharmacological and toxicological activities. This prompted us to conduct a literature survey and a structure-system-activity-relationship (SSAR) analysis of existing data, with particular emphasis on the carcinogenicity/mutagenicity and cancer preventive aspects of the flavonoids.

Since the past decade, researchers have shown considerable interest in flavonoids as human dietary components and as pharmacological agents with significant activity exhibited in a variety of animal cell systems. About three thousand flavonoids have already been reported and new compounds are being reported at an ever-increasing rate [4].

2   Structures of flavonoids

Flavonoids are conjugated aromatic systems originating from their precursors, chalcones and can be categorized into different classes according to their structures (Figure 1).

The most widely occurring flavonoids are flavones and flavonols which are generally present in plants with O-glycosidic linkage at the A and/or C ring hydroxyl groups [1, 2, 4]. As components of fruits and vegetables, flavonoids serve as part of the human diet, with daily intake amounting to almost 1 gram. A large variety of pharmacological activities have been attributed to them such as:

(i) Inhibition of lipid peroxidation in rats and antioxidant activity [4–7].

(ii) Cytotoxic and/or antimutagenic and anticarcinogenic activity by inhibition of liver enzymes and/or receptor-mediated estrogenic activity [8, 12].

(iii) Antiallergic and antiinflammatory activity by inhibition of immunoglobulin-mediated histamine and allergic mediator release from mast cells [9].

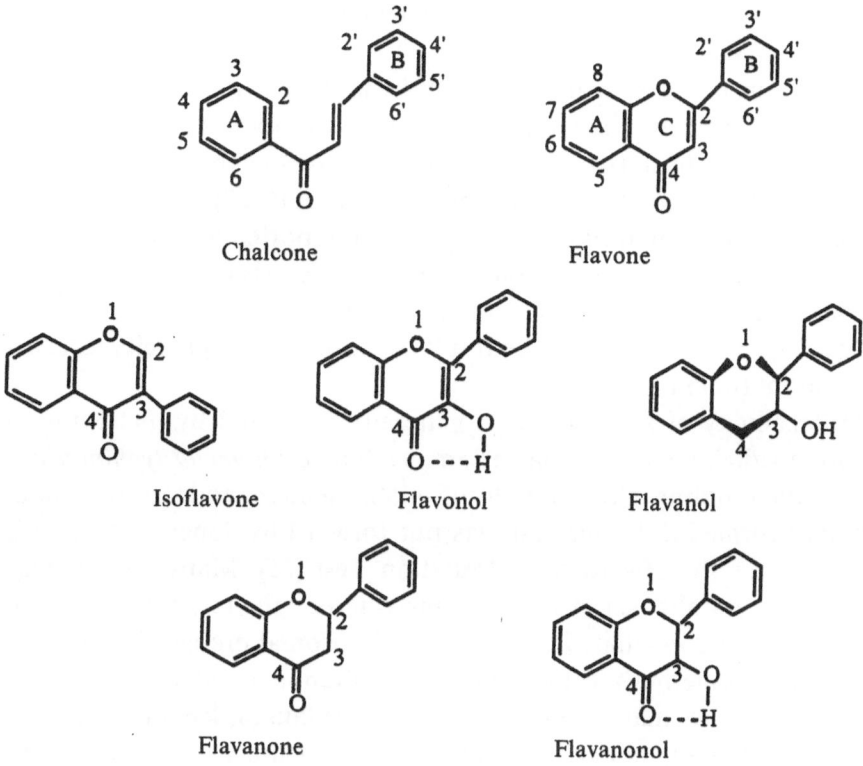

Fig. 1
Flavonoids and related compounds

(iv) Mutagenicity, carcinogenicity and genotoxic effects of flavonoids [10, 11].

(v) Inhibition of aldose reductase in the rat lens, and potential agent for attenuating diabetic complications [4, 13].

(vi) Antiviral activity against certain serotypes of rhinovirus and inhibition of reverse transcriptase of avain myeloblastosis, Rous-associated virus-2' and Maloney murine leukemia virus [14, 15].

(vii) Antibacterial and fungitoxic effects of isoflavonoid phytoalexins and related chalcones like phlorizin [4].

This survey will focus mainly on the structure-system-activity relationship (SSAR) analysis of mutagenic and carcinogenic flavonoids and also discuss the various mechanisms involved in the antitumor activity of flavonoids and related compounds tested in various biological systems.

3   Mutagenicity studies of flavonoids

Numerous researchers have studied the mutagenicity of synthetic and naturally occurring flavonoids and related compounds using various strains of the bacteria *Salmonella typhimurium* as the test system for screening mutagens and carcinogens [10, 11, 16–22]. Quercetin and some closely related flavonoids have been reported to induce specific locus mutations, chromosomal aberrations, sister chromatid exchanges (SCE's), DNA strand breaks and weak cellular transformations [4, 23, 24]. Details of the results of various mutagenicity tests are listed in Table I.

Mutagenicity of a substance is generally measured by incubating it with a suitable strain of bacterium, such as *Salmonella typhimurium*, and then noting the number of histidine-independent (revertant) clones formed [16]. This test was put forward by Ames et al. and is popular as the His Reverse Mutation Test [25]. Many studies also include a parallel set of experiments whereby the test substance and bacterium are incubated with a liver microsomal preparation, the S-9 fraction, sometimes called the mammalian microsomal activation system. In fact many flavonoids such as galangin, kaempferol, myricetin, wogonin, norwogonin and others do not exhibit any mutagenicity unless activated with the 'S-9 mix' [10, 18, 21, 22]. In many cases the mutagenicity values reported in Table I were the initial linear slopes of the dose-response curves, fitted by a least squares linear regression.

Jurado et al. had developed an alternative bacterial assay for determining mutagenicity of various substances, and called it the L-arabinose resistance test of *Salmonella typhimurium* (abbreviated as the Ara Test) [21]. In this test, the tester strain of bacteria is unable to use L-arabinose as the sole carbon source, and fails to grow in the presence of L-arabinose plus another carbon source such as glycerol. This forward mutation assay is based upon changes from L-arabinose sensitivity to L-arabinose resistance and is a sensitive assay for detection of weak mutagens.

4   Structural requirements necessary for the mutagenicity of flavonoids

(1) Molecular planarity is a requirement (as seen with flavones and flavonols) since non-planar flavonoids (such as flavanones hesperetin,

Table 1
Data on *in vitro* mutagenicity tests of flavonoids on bacteria *Salmonella Typhimurium*

Structure of compound	Test	Strain	Amount of compound in μg	Mutagenic activity	S–9 Mix[a]	Ref.[b]
I. Flavonols	Ames Test	TA 98	20	High 11.6 His+ revertants/nM	+	10
(i) Quercetin		TA 100		Moderately high	+	
		TA 1537, TA 1538		Low	+	
		TA 98	10	Comutagen with 2-AAF[c] (2-AAF, 7.9- fold synergism)	+	11
		TA 100		1.7 His+ revertants/nM	−	17, 18
				6.1 His+ revertants/nM	+	18
		TA 98		2.8 His+ revertants/nM	−	17, 18
				12.4 His+ revertants/nM	+	
		TA 1537		0.75 His+ revertants/nM	−	18
				1.0 His+ revertants/nM	+	
	Ara[d] Test	BA 13		Mutagenic Potency = 1/MMD[e] = 250	+	21
	Ames Test	TA 98		19.0 His+ revertants/nM	+	22
				3.1 His+ revertants/nM	−	
		TA 100		6.0 His+ revertants/nM	+	
				4.2 His+ revertants/nM	−	

Table I (continued)

Structure of compound	Test	Strain	Amount of compound in µg	Mutagenic activity	S-9 Mix[a]	Ref.[b]
(ii) Kaempferol	Ames Test	TA 100	25	Moderately High 7.3 His+ revertants/nM	++	10
		TA 98		Moderately High	++	
		TA 1537		Low	++	
		TA 98	10	Comutagen with 2-AAF[c] (2-AAF, 5.1- fold synergism)	++	11
	Ara[d] test	TA 100		7.7 His+ revertants/nM	++	18
		BA 13		Mutagenic Potency = 1 / MMD[e] = 66.67	++	21
	Ames Test	TA 98		9.7 His+ revertants/nM	++	22
		TA 100		5.9 His+ revertants/nM	++	
(iii) Morin	Ames Test	TA 98		Very Low	++	10
		TA 100		Very Low	++	
		TA 1537	280	Very Low 0.05 His+ revertants/nM	++	
		TA 98	10	Comutagen with 2-AAF[c] (2-AAF, 3.27- fold synergism)	+	11
	Ara[d] Test	BA 13		Mutagenic Potency = 1 / MMD[e] = 6.71	+	21
	Ames Test	TA 98		0.6 His+ revertants/nM	++	22
		TA 100		0.5 His+ revertants/nM	++	

Table I (continued)

Structure of compound	Test	Strain	Amount of compound in μg	Mutagenic activity	S-9 Mix[a]	Ref.[b]
(iv) Rhamnetin	Ames Test	TA 98, TA 100 TA 1537	100	Moderate Low 0.45 His+ revertants/nM	+ +	10
		TA 98		Moderately High 12.6 His+ revertants/nM 0.1 His+ revertants/nM	+ −	22
		TA 100		5.6 His+ revertants/nM 1.2 His+ revertants/nM	+ −	
		TA 97, TA 98, TA 100		Low	+	20
(v) Isorhamnetin	Ames Test	TA 98		1.8 His+ revertants/nM 0.6 His+ revertants/nM	+ −	22
		TA 100		2.2 His+ revertants/nM	+	
		TA 97, TA 98, TA 100, TA 102, TA 1535, TA 1538		None	+, −	20
(vi) Kaempferide	Ames Test	TA 1537	100	Low 0.24 His+ revertants/nM	+ +	10
		TA 98		Moderate 6.7 His+ revertants/nM	+ +	22
		TA 100		5.3 His+ revertants/nM	+ +	

Table I (continued)

Structure of compound	Test	Strain	Amount of compound in μg	Mutagenic activity	S-9 Mix[a]	Ref.[b]
(vii) Galangin	Ames Test	TA 98	20	Low 2.0 His+ revertants/nM	++	10
		TA 100, TA 1537		Low	++	11
		TA 98	10	Comutagen with 2-AAF[c] (2-AAF, 4.69-fold synergism)	++	11
	Ara[d] Test	BA 13		Mutagenic Potency = 1 / MMD[e] = 31.25	++	21
	Ames Test	TA 98		Moderate 4.3 His+ revertants/nM	++	22
		TA 100		4.4 His+ revertants/nM	++	
(viii) 8-Hydroxy Galangin	Ames Test	TA 98		Moderate 5.8 His+ revertants/nM	++	18
		TA 100		Low 0.67 His+ revertants/nM	++	
		TA 1537		0.97 His+ revertants/nM	++	
(ix) 2'-Hydroxy Galangin	Ames Test	TA 98	10	None Comutagen with 2-AAF[c] (2-AAF, 1.28-fold increase in activity)	+	11

Table I (continued)

Structure of compound	Test	Strain	Amount of compound in µg	Mutagenic activity	S-9 Mix[a]	Ref.[b]
(x) Myricetin	Ames Test	TA 100	250	Very Low 0.12 His+ revertants/nM	++	10
		TA 98	10	Almost None Comutagen with 2-AAF[c] (2-AAF, 10.16-fold synergism)	+	11
	Ara[d] Test	BA 13		Mutagenic Potency = 1 / MMD[e] = 4.22	+	21
	Ames Test	TA 98		0.14 His+ revertants/nM	++	22
		TA 100		0.4 His+ revertants/nM	++	22
(xi) Robinetin	Ames Test	TA 100	500	Very Low 0.06 His+ revertants/nM	++	10
		TA 98		None	+	22
		TA 100		0.3 His+ revertants/nM	-	22
(xii) Fisetin	Ames Test	TA 98	100	Very Low 0.14 His+ revertants/nM	+	10
		TA 100, TA 1537		Very Low	+	
		TA 98	10	Almost None Desmutagenic to 2-AAF[c] (2-AAF, 0.64-fold decrease in activity)	+	11
	Ara[d] Test	BA 13		Mutagenic Potency = 1 / MMD[e] = 7.58	-	21
	Ames Test	TA 98		0.1 His+ revertants/nM	+	22
		TA 100		0.28 His+ revertants/nM	+	22

Table I (continued)

Structure of compound	Test	Strain	Amount of compound in μg	Mutagenic activity	S-9 Mix[a]	Ref.[b]
(xiii) Flavonol	Ames Test	TA 98, TA 100, TA 1537, TA 1538	500	None <0.01 His+ revertants/nM	+, −	10
		TA 98	10	None Comutagen with 2AAF[c] (2AAF, 6.69-fold increase in activity)	+	11
		TA 98, TA 100		None	+, −	22
II. Flavones						
(xiv) Chrysin	Ames Test	TA 98, TA 100, TA 1537, TA 1538	500	None <0.01 His+ revertants/nM	+	10
		TA 98, TA 100, TA 1537		None	+, −	18, 22
(xv) Apigenin	Ames Test	TA 98, TA 100, TA 1537, TA 1538	500	None <0.01 His+ revertants/nM	+, −	10, 18 22
		TA 97, TA 98		Almost None	+, −	20

Table I (continued)

Structure of compound	Test	Strain	Amount of compound in μg	Mutagenic activity	S-9 Mix [a]	Ref. [b]
(xvi) Wogonin	Ames Test	TA 98	10	None Desmutagenic to 2-AAF [c] (2-AAF, 0.54-fold decrease in activity)	+	11
		TA 98		Low 0.39 His$^+$ revertants/nM	+ +	18
		TA 100		Very High 13.8 His$^+$ revertants/nM	+ +	
		TA 1537		Low 1.6 His$^+$ revertants/nM	+ +	
		TA 98		Very High 9.8 His$^+$ revertants/nM	+ +	22
(xvii) Norwogonin	Ames Test	TA 98		Low 1.2 His$^+$ revertants/nM	+ +	18
		TA 100		Very High 17 His$^+$ revertants/nM	+ +	
		TA 1537		Low 1.7 His$^+$ revertants/nM	+ +	
(xviii) Isowogonin	Ames Test	TA 100		Moderate to Low 3.4 His$^+$ revertants/nM	+ +	18
		TA 1537		Low 1.1 His$^+$ revertants/nM	+ +	

Table I (continued)

Structure of compound	Test	Strain	Amount of compound in μg	Mutagenic activity	S-9 Mix[a]	Ref.[b]
(xix) Flavone	Ames Test	TA 98, TA 100, TA 1535, TA 1537, TA 1538	500	None <0.01 His+ revertants/nM	+, –	10
		TA 98	10	None Comutagen with 2-AAF[c] (2-AAF, 1.19-fold increase in activity)	+	11
	Ara[d] Test	BA 13		Mutagenic Potency = 1 / MMD[e] = 1.04	+	21
	Ames Test	TA 98, TA 100, TA 1537		None	+, –	18, 22
(xx) Luteolin	Ames Test	TA 98, TA 100, TA 1537		None	+, –	18, 22
		TA 98, TA 100, TA 1535, TA 1538		None	+, –	20
(xxi) Primetin	Ames Test	TA 98 TA 100		None Low 1.4 His+ revertants/nM	++ ++	18
		TA 1537		Low 0.35 His+ revertants/nM	++	

Table I (continued)

Structure of compound	Test	Strain	Amount of compound in μg	Mutagenic activity	S-9 Mix[a]	Ref.[b]
III. Flavanones (xxii) Hesperetin	Ames Test	TA 98, TA 100, TA 1537, TA 1538	500	None <0.01 His+ revertants/nM	+, -	10
	Ara[d] Test	BA 13		Mutagenic Potency = 1 / MMD[e] = 3.39	+ +	21
	Ames Test	TA 98, TA 100		None	+, -	22
(xxiii) Naringenin	Ames Test	TA 98, TA 100, TA 1537, TA 1538	500	None <0.01 His+ revertants/nM	+, -	10
	Ara[d] Test	BA 13		Mutagenic Potency = 1 / MMD[e] = 3.55	- -	21
	Ames Test	TA 98, TA 100		None	+, -	22
(xxiv) Eriodictyol	Ames Test	TA 98, TA 100, TA 1537, TA 1538	100	None <0.01 His+ revertants/nM	+, -	10
		TA 98, TA 100		None	+, -	22

Table I (continued)

Structure of compound	Test	Strain	Amount of compound in μg	Mutagenic activity	S–9 Mix[a]	Ref.[b]
(xxv) 7,4'-Dihydroxy Flavanone	Ames Test	TA 100		Low 0.3 His+ revertants/nM	+	22
IV. Flavanonols (xxvi) Taxifolin	Ames Test	TA 98, TA 1537	500	Yes Very Low 0.08 His+ revertants/nM	+ +	10
	Ara[d] Test	BA 13		Mutagenic Potency = $1 / MMD^e = 0.62$	–	21
	Ames Test	TA 100		Low 0.3 His+ revertants/nM	–	22
(xxvii) Hydrorobinetin	Ames Test	TA 100		Low 0.7 His+ revertants/nM	–	22

Table I (continued)

Structure of compound	Test	Strain	Amount of compound in µg	Mutagenic activity	S–9 Mix[a]	Ref.[b]
V. Flavonol Glycosides						
(xxviii) Quercitrin	Ames Test	TA 98	2000	Very Low <0.01 His+ revertants/nM	–	10
		TA 98	50	3.3 His+ revertants/nM	f	
		TA 100, TA 1537		Very Low	f	
(xxix) Rutin	Ames Test	TA 98	2000	Almost None <0.01 His+ revertants/nM	–	10
		TA 98	100	1.14 His+ revertants/nM	f	
		TA 98	20	None	+	11
				Desmutagenic to 2-AAF[c] (2-AAF, 0.95- fold decrease in activity)		
	Ara[d] Test	BA 13		Mutagenic Potency = 1 / MMD[e] = 3.10	±	21
	Ames Test	TA 98, TA 100		Very Low	g	22
(xxx) Isoquercitrin	Ames Test	TA 98, TA 100		Very Low	g	22

Table I (continued)

Structure of compound	Test	Strain	Amount of compound in μg	Mutagenic activity	S-9 Mix[a]	Ref.[b]
(xxxi) Kaempferitrin	Ames Test	TA 98, TA 100		Very Low	g	22
VI. Flavanols						
(xxxii) (+)-Catechin	Ames Test	TA 98, TA 100, TA 1535, TA 1538	500	None <0.01 His+ revertants/nM	+, −	10
	Ara[d] Test	BA 13		Mutagenic Potency = 1 / MMD[e] = 1.57	−	21

(a) Mammalian microsomal activation system (see text and references). Preparations (liver S9 fractions) were obtained from Aroclor 1254 induced rat livers in most cases. (+) indicates enhanced mutagenicity; (−) indicates no activation by S9 (ref. 5) or absence of S9 (ref. 17) or diminished mutagenicity in presence of S9 (ref. 16); (+ +) indicates metabolic activation was obligatory for mutagenicity; (− −) indicates absence of S9 was obligatory for mutagenicity; (±) indicates the need for metabolic activation depends on the mutagenesis protocol; (+, −) indicates both in the presence and in the absence of S9.
(b) References.
(c) 2-acetylaminofluorene, a well-known mutagen.
(d) L-arabinose resistance test of *Salmonella typhimurium* abbreviated as the Ara test.
(e) MMD = minimum mutagenic dose.
(f) indicates treatment with cecal cell free extract containing many glycosidase enzymes.
(g) indicates flavonol glycosides have no mutagenicity in the absence of "hesperidinase", a crude extract of *Aspergillus niger* containing various hydrolyzing glycosides. However, in presence of "hesperidinase", their mutagenicity is similar to those of their aglycones.

eriodictyol and 7,4-dihydroxy flavone; flavanol catechin, and flavano-
nols taxifolin and hydrorobinetin) exhibit very weak or no mutagenicity [16]. Thus the double bond at 2–3 position is required for
conjugation of the lone-pair electrons on the ring oxygen with the
carbonyl group $(C = O)$, and is important for mutagenicity as can be
seen from a comparison of quercetin with taxifolin [17, 21] (see Table I).

(2) Presence of free phenolic groups is also necessary since permethyl
quercetin has no mutagenicity whereas quercetin is a strong mutagen
[16]. However quercetin pentaacetate has equivalent mutagenicity to
quercetin in the presence of 'S-9 mix' probably because deacetylation
occurs as the first step in metabolic activation [16, 22].

(3) Flavonols with a free hydroxyl group at position 3 are the most
mutagenic among the flavonoid family (like quercetin, kaempferol,
galangin, rhamnetin, kaempferide) especially in *S. typhimurium* strain
98 [10, 21, 22]. Furthermore, flavonoids which are only A-ring hydroxylated and/or methoxylated, such as wogonin and norwogonin were
also highly mutagenic in the Salmonella strain TA 100 upon metabolic
activation [18]. Thus it appears that there are two groups of flavonoids
with different structural features determining their mutagenic activity
and strain sensitivity, that is, either a 3-hydroxyl group or an 8-
hydroxyl/methoxyl group is necessary for the mutagenic activity of
the flavonoids (compare quercetin/luteolin/norwogonin) [17, 18, 20].

(4) Among flavonols (that is 3-hydroxy flavones), the number and
position of the hydroxyl group(s) on the phenolic ring B appear
critical for mutagenicity: (a) the 2'-hydroxyl group appears to retard
the mutagenic potency as observed by comparing quercetin/morin
and galangin/2'-hydroxy galangin [11]. It is probable that the 2'-
hydroxyl group interacts with the C-ring (see Fig. 1) thereby distorting
the structural planarity of the flavonoids required for exhibiting
mutagenicity. (b) hydroxyl groups at 3' and 4' position are necessary
for exhibiting mutagenicity in the absence of 'S-9 mix' [17, 21, 22]. In
other words flavonols lacking the 3' and/or the 4'-hydroxyl groups
(such as galangin, kaempferol, morin, 8-hydroxy galangin, kaempferide) are non-mutagenic in the absence of the mammalian activation
system. As to the number of hydroxyl groups, it seems that too many
hydroxyl groups in the phenolic ring B, reduce the mutagenic activity
drastically (compare quercetin/myricetin), whether this is due to
altered redox potential, unfavorable lipophilicity and/or metal binding ability remains to be studied.

(5) Flavonols with a free hydroxyl group at position 5 exhibit marked mutagenic activity such as quercetin, kaempferol, galangin, rhamnetin and kaempferide, but mutagenic potency is very poor for fisetin and robinetin [17, 22]. Ogawa et al. had postulated that the 5-hydroxyl group is essential for enhancing the mutagenicity of 2AAF (2-acetyl-amino fluorine) [11].

(6) Flavonol glycosides such as rutin, isoquercitrin, kaempferitrin, quercitrin and others essentially require hydrolysis of the 3-O-sugar moieties by mixed glycosidases or 'hesperidinase' to become active mutagens [10, 22].

(7) The 7-hydroxyl group in flavonols is not essential for mutagenic activity [17] although comparison of the pairs kaempferol/kaemp-feride and quercetin/rhamnetin suggest that substitution with a meth-oxyl group reduces the mutagenic potency of the parent compounds [17, 22]. In fact McGregor and Jurd have suggested that the 7-position hydroxyl group may be responsible for metabolic activation of the compound while the 5-hydroxyl group is more important for muta-genicity [17].

Although structure-activity relationship (SAR) studies regarding mu-tagenicity of flavonoids on various strains of *Salmonella typhimurium* have been undertaken, analogous SAR studies have not been carried out in mammalian cells. Quercetin is the only compound studied in detail that exhibited weak mutagenicity in *Escherichia coli*, no muta-genicity in *Bacillus subtilis*, some mutagenic activity in *Drosophila melanogaster* and caused gene conversion in yeast [26–28]. Quercetin induced chromosomal anomalies in culture cells *in vitro* but conflict-ing results were obtained in the micronucleus test *in vivo* [23, 29, 30]. Recently Pennie and Campo reported the synergism of quercetin with bovine papillomavirus type 4 (BPV-4) in causing full oncogenic trans-formation of cells *in vitro* and suggested that quercetin may be a probable *in vivo* cocarcinogen with BPV-4 [31].

5   Carcinogenicity studies of flavonoids

The *in vivo* genotoxicity and carcinogenicity studies of flavonoids in mammals are predominantly negative. The first such study was by Ambrose et al. who reported a low toxicity of quercetin in rats and rabbits in short- and long-term studies with a diet containing 1% quercetin [32]. Subsequently a number of studies have been conducted to investigate the carcinogenic potential of flavonoids, especially quercetin. Data from different sources are presented in Table II.

While quercetin was reportedly non-carcinogenic in *in vivo* studies with ddY mice, strain A mice, ACI rats and golden hamsters following oral administration of 1 to 10% quercetin in diet for short and long durations of time, Pamucku et al. reported it to be a rat intestinal and bladder carcinogen at a level of 0.1% in diet [34]. Similarly Sahu et al. reported that quercetin, kaempferol and neohesperidin dihydrochalcone (NHDC) were clastogenic in Swiss male mice, while McGregor et al. failed to confirm these findings even after performing detailed experiments with these flavonoids [30, 29].

Quercetin, rhamnetin, NHDC and hesperetin dihydrochalcone did not increase the micronucleus frequency significantly under various exposures and sampling conditions within the dose range of 100 to 1000 mg/kg, either in the bone marrow or in the peripheral blood erythrocytes, in male or female Swiss Webster mice upon oral or intraperitoneal (i.p.) administration [29]. McGregor et al. did however report that galangin in highly toxic doses significantly increased the micronucleus frequency in the bone marrow and peripheral blood erythrocytes, although no other studies reporting the carcinogenicity of galangin are available to date [29].

In a two-stage carcinogenesis study *in vivo,* a 5% quercetin diet under various conditions did not exhibit any initiation (after 4 weeks) or promotion (after 25 weeks) of carcinogenesis in the urinary bladder of male F344 rats [38]. Recently Sakai et al. examined the effect quercetin (15–45µM) on the two-stage transformation of BALB/3T3 cells *in vitro* and reported that it acted as an initiator only when 0.49 µM of 12-O-tetradecanoyl-phorbol-13-acetate (TPA), a well-known tumor promoter, was used in a subsequent stage to induce complete transformation [39]. However, 15–30 µM of quercetin reportedly restrained the tumor promoting activity of TPA in the same study, when the same cells were initiated with the standard carcinogen, 3-methylcholanthrene.

Very recent studies consider quercetin to be a controversial carcinogen, especially among Japanese researchers who appear concerned at the technical report of the National Toxicology Program (NTP) which concluded that there was "some evidence of carcinogenic activity of quercetin in male F344/N rats" [40–42]. Researchers caution about the lack of substantial experimental evidence and also point out the

Table II
Data on *in vivo* carcinogenicity tests of flavonoids and related compounds

Compound	Test animal	Amount in diet	Tissue	Tumor development M	F	Carcinogenic?	Ref.
Quercetin	ddY mice	2% w/w in pellet diet, for 842 days	(a) Lung	21/37	18/33		
			(b) Liver	4/37	–		
			(c) Forestomach	–	1/33		
			(d) Salivary gland	–	2/33	NO	33
			(e) Uterus	–	3/33		
			(f) Ovary	–	1/33	(No statistical difference in tumor incidence between the treated and the control groups)	
			(g) Heart	1/37	–		
			(h) Leukemia	7/37	15/33		
			(i) Lymph node	1/37	–		
			(j) Soft tissues	1/37	1/33		
			(k) Adrenal gland	1/37	–		
			(l) Breast	–	1/33		
	strain A mice	5% in diet for 161 days	Lung	3/23	1/24	NO	35

Table II (continued)

Compound	Test animal	Amount in diet	Tissue	Tumor development M	Tumor development F	Carcinogenic?	Ref.
Quercetin (cont.)	Albino rats of local stock derived from Norwegian strain	0.1% in diet for 406 days	(a) Intestine	6/7	14/18	YES	34
			(b) Urinary bladder	2/7	3/18		
	Swiss male mice	200 mg/kg i.p.[a]	Bone marrow erythrocytes	P/N[b] ratio = 0.71		MAYBE	30
		400 mg/kg i.p.[a]		P/N[b] ratio = 0.51			
	ACI rats, inbred strain	1% in diet for 540 days	Testis	1/10	–		36
		5% in diet for 540 days	(a) Testis	3/8	–	NO	
			(b) Adrenal cortex	1/8	–		
			(c) Cecum	1/8	–		
			(d) Pancreas	1/8	–		
		10% in diet for 850 days	(a) Testis	6/19	–	(No statistical difference in tumor incidence between the treated and the control groups)	
			(b) Adrenal cortex	3/19	1/18		
			(c) Cecum	3/19	–		
			(d) Pituitary gland	–	2/18		
			(e) Uterus	–	1/18		
			(f) Pancreas	1/19	–		
			(g) Thigh	–	1/18		

Table II (continued)

Compound	Test animal	Amount in diet	Tissue	Tumor development M	F	Carcinogenic?	Ref.
Quercetin (cont.)	Non inbred golden hamsters	10% in diet for 735 days	(a) Forestomach	3/16	2/16		
			(b) Adrenal cortex	2/16	–		
			(c) Ileum	–	1/16		
		4% in diet for 709 days	(a) Forestomach	–	2/12		
			(b) Uterus	–	1/12	NO	37
		1% in diet for 351 days followed by basal diet for 350 days	Forestomach	2/7	–		
Kaempferol	Swiss male mice	200 mg/kg i.p.[a]	Bone marrow erythrocytes	P/N[b] ratio = 0.88			
		400 mg/kg i.p.[a]		P/N[b] ratio = 0.71		NO	30
Rutin	Swiss male mice	100 mg/kg i.p.[a]	Bone marrow erythrocytes	P/N[b] ratio = 0.98			
		200 mg/kg i.p.[a]		P/N[b] ratio = 0.92		NO	30
	ACI rats, inbred strain	5% in diet for 540 days	(a) Adrenal cortex	2/11	–		
			(b) Pituitary gland	–	1/9		
			(c) Urinary bladder	–	1/9	NO	36
			(d) Testis	3/11	–		

Table II (continued)

Compound	Test animal	Amount in diet	Tissue	Tumor development M	Tumor development F	Carcinogenic?	Ref.
Rutin (cont.)	ACI rats, (cont.)	10% in diet for 850 days	(a) Ileum	1/20	–		
			(b) Colon	1/20	–		
			(c) Adrenal cortex	1/20	–	NO	36
			(d) Pancreas	–	1/19		
			(e) Breast	–	1/19		
			(f) Testis	6/20	–		
			(g) Uterus	–	1/19		
			(h) Heart	–	1/19		
	Non inbred golden hamsters	10% in diet for 735 days	(a) Forestomach	1/17	–		
			(b) Adrenal cortex	2/17	2/14	NO	37
			(c) Uterus	–	1/14		
Neo-Hesperidin-Dihydro-Chalcone[c] (NHDC)	Swiss male mice	200 mg/kg i.p.[a]	Bone marrow erythrocytes	P/N[b] ratio = 1.11		NO	30
		400 mg/kg i.p.[a]		P/N[b] ratio = 0.84			

(a) i.p. indicates intraperitoneal injection.
(b) P/N ratio indicates the ratio of percentage of micronuclei in polychromatic cells to the percentage of micronuclei in normochromatic cells in the bone marrow.
(c) The structure of NHDC is very similar to that of flavonoids as shown:

possible involvement of α_{2u}-globulin in quercetin renal carcinogenicity observed only in male rats [41, 42]. From all the available data it seems reasonable to accept the authors' suggestion that "it is still too premature to label quercetin a carcinogen, and that its risk potential in man is at best negligible". It becomes all the more convincing, especially when we discuss (in the next section) the anti-tumorpromoting activity and the anticarcinogenic nature of a number of flavonoids.

6   Flavonoids as anti-tumorpromoting agents

Concurrent with the studies of mutagenicity and carcinogenicity of flavonoids were reports about their antitumor and anti-mutagenic activity. Numerous researchers have reported the inhibitory activity of some flavonoids on the mutagenicity and carcinogenicity of polycyclic aromatic hydrocarbons (PAH) such as Benzo[a]pyrene (B[a]P) and its 7,8-dihydrodiol [43–47] and other carcinogens such as aflatoxin [48], 2-aminoanthracene (2AA), [8], TPA [49], azoxymethanol [50], 4-(methylnitrosamino)-1-(3-pyridyl)-1-butanone (NNK) [51]. A survey of the antitumor activity of some flavonoids and related compounds is presented in Table III.

A number of flavonoids inhibit the metabolism of B[a]P to the ultimate carcinogen B[a]P 9, 10-diol epoxide. Huang et al. had suggested that the probable mechanisms of action were: (a) inhibition of the cytochrome P450 (cP450) monooxygenase system that metabolizes B[a]P, and (b) antagonistic interaction with the ultimate mutagenic metabolites, the diol epoxides [43]. Shah and Bhattacharya showed that many flavonoids inhibit the adduct formation of B[a]P and B[a]P diol epoxide with DNA *in vitro,* and it is this adduct of DNA which initiates carcinogenesis in case of a number of genotoxic chemicals [45]. A recent study agrees with Huang's suggested mechanisms of action and concludes that flavones are much more efficient inhibitors of cP450 than their corresponding isoflavone or flavanone analogs [47].

Deschner et al. found significant activity of quercetin and its glycoside rutin, in reducing azoxymethanol (AOM)-induced colonic neoplasia and AOM-induced focal areas of dysplasia in CFI mice fed with 2% quercetin or 4% rutin [50]. It was suggested that quercetin inhibits the tumor promotion stage rather than the initiation stage of carcinogenesis. Another structurally related polyphenol, (+)-catechin, a flavonol

Table III
Anti-carcinogenic and/or antimutagenic properties of some flavonoids

Compound	Test system	Concentration	Activity	Reference
(i) Quercetin	Bacteria S.typhimurium, TA 100 strain	ID_{50} = 5 nm	Inhibits mutagenicity of 0.05nm Benzo[a]pyrene 7,8 diol 9,10 epoxide.	43
	In-vitro binding of Benzo[a]pyrene to DNA[a]	ID_{50} = 17.5 nm	Inhibition of B[a]PDNA adduct formation.	45
(ii) Kaempferol	Bacteria S.typhimurium, TA 100 strain	ID_{50} = 10 nm	Inhibits mutagenicity of 0.05 nm Benzo[a]pyrene 7,8 diol 9,10 epoxide.	43
	In-vitro binding of Benzo[a]pyrene to DNA[a]	ID_{50} = 40 nm	Inhibition of B[a]PDNA adduct formation.	45
	In-vitro metabolism of 3.17 nm Benzo[a]pyrene by S-9 liver homogenate	IC_{50} = 4.7 μg/ml	Inhibits the oxidative metabolism of B[a]P to water soluble carcinogenic derivatives.	47
(iii) 5,7-Methoxy Quercetin	Bacteria S.typhimurium, TA 100 strain	ID_{50} = 5 nm	Inhibits mutagenicity of 0.05 nm Benzo[a]pyrene 7,8 diol 9,10 epoxide.	43
(iv) Quercitrin	Bacteria S.typhimurium, TA 100 strain	ID_{50} = 5 nm	Inhibits mutagenicity of 0.05 nm Benzo[a]pyrene 7,8 diol 9,10 epoxide.	43

Table III (continued)

Compound	Test system	Concentration	Activity	Reference
(v) Rutin	Bacteria S.typhimurium, TA 100 strain	ID_{50} = 5 nm	Inhibits mutagenicity of 0.05 nm Benzo[a]pyrene 7,8 diol 9,10 epoxide.	43
(vi) Galangin	In-vitro metabolism of 3.17 nm Benzo[a]pyrene by S-9 liver homogenate	IC_{50} = 3.6μg/ml	Inhibits the oxidative metabolism of B[a]P to water soluble carcinogenic derivatives.	47
(vii) Myricetin	Bacteria S.typhimurium, TA 100 strain	ID_{50} = 2 nm	Inhibits mutagenicity of 0.05 nm Benzo[a]pyrene 7,8 diol 9,10 epoxide.	43
(viii) Robinetin	Bacteria S.typhimurium, TA 100 strain	ID_{50} = 2.5 nm	Inhibits mutagenicity of 0.05 nm Benzo[a]pyrene 7,8 diol 9,10 epoxide.	43
	In-vitro binding of Benzo[a]pyrene to DNA[a]	ID_{50} = 3.75 nm	Inhibition of B[a]PDNA adduct formation.	45
(ix) Luteolin	Bacteria S.typhimurium, TA 100 strain	ID_{50} = 5 nm	Inhibits mutagenicity of 0.05 nm Benzo[a]pyrene 7,8 diol 9,10 epoxide.	43
(x) Morin	Bacteria S.typhimurium, TA 100 strain	ID_{50} = 10 nm	Inhibits mutagenicity of 0.05 nm Benzo[a]pyrene 7,8 diol 9,10 epoxide.	43
(xi) Myricitrin	Bacteria S.typhimurium, TA 100 strain	ID_{50} = 10 nm	Inhibits mutagenicity of 0.05 nm Benzo[a]pyrene 7,8 diol 9,10 epoxide.	43

Table III (continued)

Compound	Test system	Concentration	Activity	Reference
(xii) Apigenin	Bacteria S.typhimurium, TA 100 strain	ID_{50} = 10 nm	Inhibits mutagenicity of 0.05 nm Benzo[a]pyrene 7,8 diol 9,10 epoxide.	43
	In-vitro metabolism of 3.17 nm Benzo[a]pyrene by S-9 liver homogenate	IC_{50} = 3.6 μg/ml	Inhibits the oxidative metabolism of B[a]P to water soluble carcinogenic derivatives.	47
(xiii) Diosmetin	Bacteria S.typhimurium, TA 100 strain	ID_{50} = 10 nm	Inhibits mutagenicity of 0.05 nm Benzo[a]pyrene 7,8 diol 9,10 epoxide.	43
(xiv) Fisetin	Bacteria S.typhimurium, TA 100 strain	ID_{50} = 10 nm	Inhibits mutagenicity of 0.05 nm Benzo[a]pyrene 7,8 diol 9,10 epoxide.	43
(xv) Isorhamnetin	In-vitro binding of Benzo[a]pyrene to DNA[a]	ID_{50} = 57.5 nm	Inhibition of B[a]PDNA adduct formation.	45
(xvi) Acacetin	In-vitro metabolism of 3.17 nm Benzo[a]pyrene by S-9 liver homogenate	IC_{50} = 3.6 μg/ml	Inhibits the oxidative metabolism of B[a]P to water soluble carcinogenic derivatives.	47
(xvii) 4', 5-Dihydroxy Flavone	In-vitro metabolism of 3.17 nm Benzo[a]pyrene by S-9 liver homogenate	IC_{50} = 3.2 μg/ml	Inhibits the oxidative metabolism of B[a]P to water soluble carcinogenic derivatives.	47

Table III (continued)

Compound	Test system	Concentration	Activity	Reference
(xviii) 4', 5-Trimethoxy Flavone	In-vitro metabolism of 3.17 nm Benzo[a]pyrene by S-9 liver homogenate	$IC_{50} = 3.2 \mu g/ml$	Inhibits the oxidative metabolism of B[a]P to water soluble carcinogenic derivatives.	47
(xix) Chrysin	Bacteria S.typhimurium, TA 100 strain	$ID_{50} > 100$ nm	Inhibits mutagenicity of 0.05 nm Benzo[a]pyrene 7,8 diol 9,10 epoxide.	43
	In-vitro metabolism of 3.17 nm Benzo[a]pyrene by S-9 liver homogenate	$IC_{50} = 4.6 \mu g/ml$	Inhibits the oxidative metabolism of B[a]P to water soluble carcinogenic derivatives.	47
(xx) Chrysin 5,7 Dimethylether	In-vitro metabolism of 3.17 nm Benzo[a]pyrene by S-9 liver homogenate	$ID_{50} = 2.9 \mu g/ml$	Inhibits the oxidative metabolism of B[a]P to water soluble carcinogenic derivatives.	47
(xxi) Genistein	Bacteria S.typhimurium, TA 100 strain	$ID_{50} = 100$ nm	Inhibits mutagenicity of 0.05 nm Benzo[a]pyrene 7,8 diol 9,10 epoxide.	43
	In-vitro metabolism of 3.17 nm Benzo[a]pyrene by S-9 liver homogenate	$IC_{50} = 12 \mu g/ml$	Inhibits the oxidative metabolism of B[a]P to water soluble carcinogenic derivatives.	47

(a) Microsome mediated binding of 60 μM [³H]Benzo[a]pyrene to 0.5 mg DNA for 30 min.

compound with both catechol and resorcinol moieties, reportedly inhibits the formation of DNA damaging intermediates by selectively blocking the enzymatic activation of the tobacco-specific procarcinogen, NNK [51]. The probable mechanisms of chemoprevention by (+)-catechin and flavonoids include: (a) inhibition of the cP450 monooxygenase system that causes metabolic activation of a number of procarcinogens including NNK; (b) scavenging of reactive electrophilic species generated by procarcinogen activation and preventing its interaction with the DNA, and (c) inhibition of tumor promotion by modulating the tumor promoter receptor. One of these receptors is Protein Kinase C (PKC) which gets activated by tumor promoters, TPA and teleocidin.

A number of reports are available concerning the inhibitory effects of quercetin, fisetin, luteolin, kaempferol and morin on the *in vitro* and *in vivo* effects of TPA and teleocidin [49, 52, 53]. Experiments *in vitro* revealed that quercetin acted like a typical calmodulin antagonist, N-[6-aminohexyl]-5-chloro-1-naphthalene-sulfonamide (W-7), which inhibits TPA, teleocidin, PKC and modulates the phorbol ester receptors in the mouse skin [53]. In a two-stage carcinogenesis experiment of female ICR mice, initiation with 50 μg of 7,12-dimethylbenz[a]anthracene (DMBA) and promotion with 2.5 μg of TPA were antagonized by 5 μM of morin, kaempferol and flavonol glycosides rutin, myricitrin and mauritianin [49]. While flavanones like naringenin did not inhibit tumor promotion by TPA, only the flavonol glycosides antagonized the cell-mediated immunosuppression by tumor promoters. Thus apparently the flavonoid glycosides differ in their antitumor effect from those of the aglycones by inhibiting different pharmacological actions of TPA and teleocidin.

A literature search regarding receptor-mediated activity of flavonoids revealed the estrogenic nature of a number of isoflavonoids. One of the early reports is that of coumestrol and related compounds [54]. Although coumestrol is a coumarin-like compound isolated from clover, it exhibits striking structural similarity with the estrogenic isoflavone, genistein [54]. Fig. 2 shows the structural similarity of these estrogenic natural products, all of which contain a similar pharmacophore as found in estradiol and the synthetic diethylstilbestrol.

While coumestrol and the phytoestrogen-isoflavonoids genistein, daidzein and equol have been shown to interact with the mammalian estrogen receptor [ER], bioflavonoids such as quercetin and related

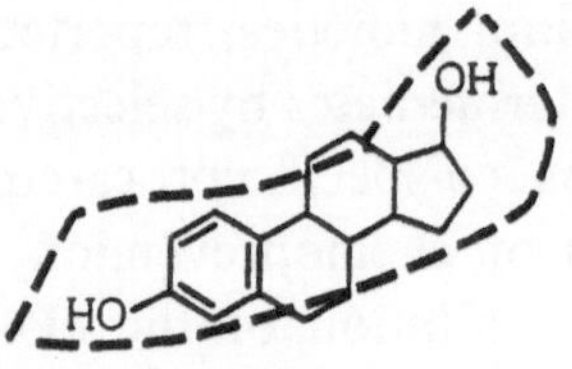

Estradiol (natural)

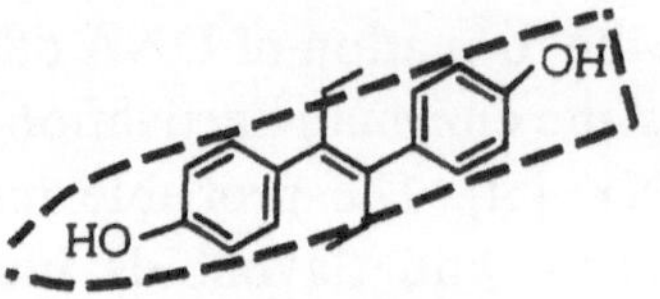

Diethylstilbestrol (synthetic)

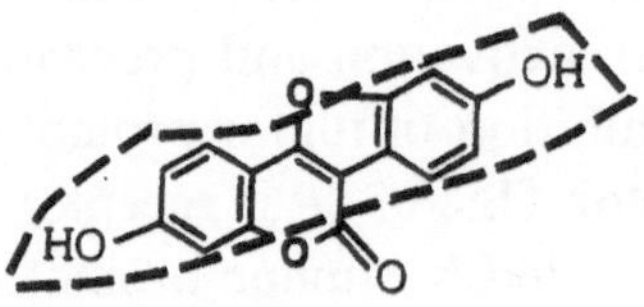

Coumestrol
(Found in: *Medicago sativa,
Taraxacum mongolicum* Ref. 62)

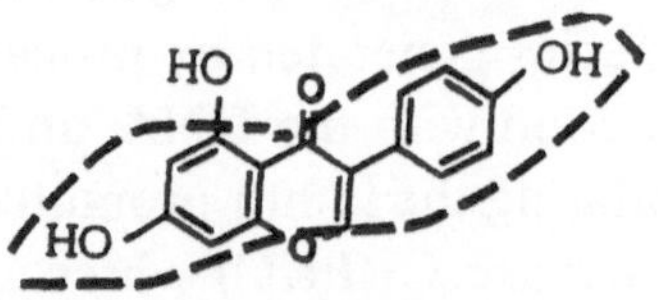

Genistein (Isoflavone)
(Found in: *Sophora japonica, S. subprostrata Pueraria thunbergiana, Glycine
max* Ref. 63)

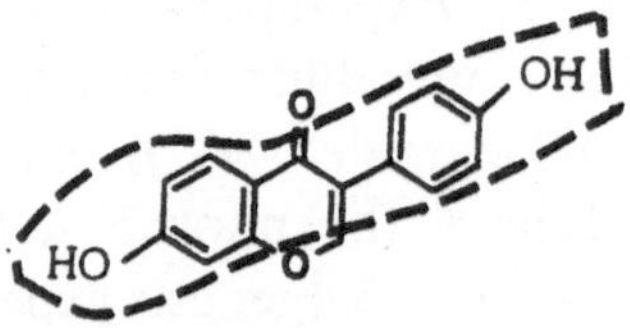

Daidzein (Isoflavone)
(Found in: *Sophora subprostrata,
Pueraria thunbergiana, P. pseudo-
hirsuta, P. thomsonii, Trifolium
pratense* Ref. 63)

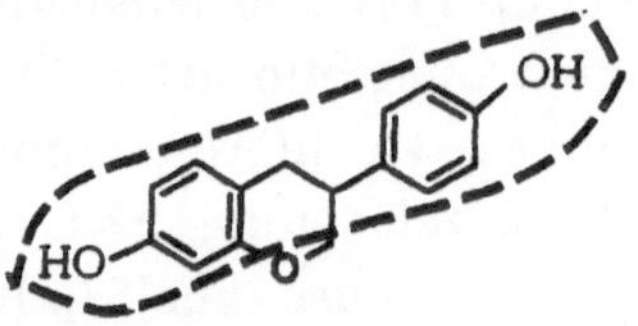

Equol (Isoflavandiol)
(Found in the urine of mares, humans and
goats)

Fig. 2
Structural similarity of estrogen and phytoestrogen-isoflavonoids

flavones do not interact with the ER [55–57]. However, flavonoids
such as quercetin, rutin and luteolin have been shown to compete with
[³H]estradiol in occupying type II estrogen binding sites (EBS) found
in the nucleus and cytosol of rat uterine preparations, in normal and
neoplastic hematopoietic cells, in acute lymphoid leukemia (ALL),
acute myeloid leukemia (AML) cells, and in human breast cancer cell
line MCF-7 [57–60]. In fact quercetin and luteolin were found to have
higher binding affinity than estradiol for the type II EBS and it has
been postulated that the physiological function of the type II sites
might not be to bind estrogen, but rather to bind to a type II ligand
which, some evidence suggests, maybe a plant flavonoid-like molecule
of dietary origin [57–60]. The type II EBS receptor appears to have
antagonistic activity on cell growth, acting as an anti-estrogen whose

levels are dramatically elevated in rapidly proliferating cell populations and which when occupied by bioflavonoids such as luteolin and quercetin bring about cell growth inhibition [57, 61]. A recent article points out an interesting theory that the binding of flavonoids to vertebrate proteins may represent an evolutionary linkage between the actions of steroids in mammals and communication between plants and the nitrogen-fixing bacteria, *rhizobia* [61].

7   Conclusion

While extensive research still continues in the area of isolation, structural elucidation and determination of physiological and pharmacological activity of new flavonoids in animal systems, a number of physiological functions have already been identified for flavonoids in the higher plants. Pollination by insects and birds is essential for plant reproduction, and flavonoids impart color and high visibility to attract bird and insect pollinators [2]. They may also play a role in plant growth and development by regulating respiration since many of them act as uncouplers and inhibitors of ATP formation. Their physiological activities are strongly affected by their glycosylation and hydroxylation pattern as well as the type of C2–C3 bond. Josette Tronchet (University of Besançon) says that 'The level of flavonoids accumulating in the epidermal cells in plants is controlled by light and they in turn provide a screen against the ultraviolet light' [2]. Indeed it is postulated that at higher altitudes or in the desert, flavonoids protect pines, cacti and other desert plants from ultraviolet light, thereby preventing mutations and other harmful effects of the radiant energy. Flavonoids may also be involved in imparting resistance in varietal plants against diseases such as fungal infection in Leguminosae, where isoflavonoids such as pisatin, phaseollin, medicarpin and others are implicated to act as antifungal agents [2].

The beneficial effects of flavonoids in the human diet has been a subject of bitter argument during the last two decades. As can be seen from the data presented earlier, the carcinogenic activity of quercetin is still a matter of controversy [34, 40–42]. But reports about the cancer preventive nature and the anti-estrogenic nature of flavonoids and isoflavonoids overwhelmingly point out that not only are the vast majority of flavonoids completely innocuous but that they may be beneficial in a variety of human disorders, and thus provide benefits in addition to fibers and vitamins which are found in fresh fruits and vegetables.

From a consideration of the chemical nature of flavonoids, one can see that the presence or absence of the C2–C3 double bond or a change in the number and pattern of hydroxylation, methylation and glycosylation will lead to variations in their solubility, absorptivity, resonance contributions, ionization constants, metal chelation and thereby biological activity. Thus a slight variation in their chemical structure may result in varying degrees of reactivity and/or failure to react or interfere with a biological receptor site such as a membrane, an enzyme or another low molecular weight component. In general flavonoids have a phenolic nature, sufficient water solubility, can interact with various specific receptor groups primarily by hydrogen bonding and dipolar/hydrophobic interactions, and can easily cross the biological membranes. Hence they may have relatively weak influences over a broad range of biological systems, and have overall proven to be beneficial to humans over a long period of time.

References

1   T. A. Geissman, Chemistry of the flavonoid compounds, Pergamon press, Oxford (1962).
2   J. B. Harborne, T. J. Mabry, and H. Mabry, The Flavonoids, Chapman and Hall, London (1975).
3   N. M. Ferguson and E. J. Lien, J. Nat. Prod., 45: 523–524 (1982).
4   V. Cody, E. Middleton, Jr. and J. B. Harborne, Plant Flavonoids in Biology and Medicine. Biochemical, Pharmacological and Structure-Activity Relationships, Alan R. Liss Inc., NY, (1986).
5   M. Amella, C. Bronner, F. Briancon, M. Haag, R. Anton and Y. Landry, Planta Medica, 52: 16–20 (1985).
6   H. Gao and E. J. Lien, Int. J. Oriental Med., 15: 70–76 (1990).
7   J. Pincemall, C. Deby, Y. Lion, P. Braquet, P. Hans, K. Drieu and R. Goutier, Stud. Org. Chem., 23: 423–436 (1986).
8   M. E. Wall, M. C. Wani, G. Manikumar, P. Abraham, H. Taylor, T. J. Hughes, J. Warner and R. McGivney, J. Nat. Prod., 51: 1084–1091 (1988).
9   E. Middleton, Jr. and C. Kandaswami, Biochem. Pharmacol., 43: 1167–1179 (1992).
10   J. P. Brown and P. S. Dietrich, Mutat. Res., 66: 223–240 (1979).
11   S. Ogawa, T. Hirayama, Y. Sumida, M. Tokuda, K. Hirai and S. Fukui, Mutat. Res., 190: 107–112 (1987).
12   N. Kaneda, J. M. Pezzuto, D. D. Soejarto, A. D. Kinghorn and N. R. Farnsworth, J. Nat. Prod., 54: 196–206 (1991).
13   S. D. Varma, A. Mizuno and J. H. Kinoshita, Science, 195: 205–206 (1977).
14   D. J. Bauer, J. W. T. Selway, J. F. Batchelor, M. Tisdale, I. C. Caldwell and D. A. B. Young, Nature 292, 369–370 (1981).
15   G. Spedding, A. Ratty and E. Middleton, Jr., Antiviral Res., 12: 99–110 (1989).

16   L. F. Bjeldanes and G. W. Chang, Science, 197: 577–578 (1977).
17   J. T. McGregor and L. Jurd, Mutat. Res., 54: 297–309 (1978).
18   C. A. Elliger, P. R. Henika and J. T. McGregor, Mutat. Res., 135: 77–86 (1984).
19   K. A. Rashid, C. A. Mullin and R. O. Mumma, Mutat. Res., 169: 71–79 (1986).
20   H. Czeczot, B. Tudek, J. Kusztelak, T. Szymczyk, B. Dobrowolska, G. Glinkowska, J. Malinowski and H. Strzelecka, Mutat. Res., 240: 209–216 (1990).
21   J. Jurado, E. Alejandre-Duran, A. A. Moraga and C. Pueyo, Mutagenesis, 6: 289–295 (1991).
22   M. Nagao, N. Morita, T. Yahagi, M. Shimizu, M. Kuroyanagi, M. Fukuoka, K. Yoshihira, S. Natori, T. Fujino and T. Sugimura, Environ. Mutagen., 3: 401–419 (1981).
23   J. H. Carver, A. V. Carrano and J. T. McGregor, Mutat. Res., 113: 45–60 (1983).
24   S. Suzuki, T. Takada, Y. Sugawara, T. Muto and R. Kominami, Jpn. J. Cancer Res., 82: 1061–1064 (1991).
25   B. N. Ames, J. McCann and E. Yamasaki, Mutat. Res., 31: 347–364 (1975).
26   A. A. Hardigree and J. L. Epler, Mutat. Res., 58: 231–239 (1978).
27   L. E. Sacks and J. T. McGregor, Mutat. Res., 95: 191–202 (1982).
28   W. A. F. Watson, Mutat. Res., 103: 145–147 (1982).
29   J. T. McGregor, C. M. Wehr, G. D. Manners, L. Jurd, J. L. Minkler and A. V. Carrano, Mutat. Res., 124: 255–270 (1983).
30   R. K. Sahu, R. Basu and A. Sharma, Mutat Res., 89: 69–74 (1981).
31   W. D. Pennie and M. S. Campo, Virology, 190: 861–865 (1992).
32   A. M. Ambrose, D. J. Robbins and F. DeEds, J. Am. Pharm. Assoc. Sci. Ed., 41: 119–122 (1952).
33   D. Saito, A. Shirai, T. Matsushima, T. Sugimura and I. Hirono, Teratogen. Carcinogen. Mutagen., 1: 213–221 (1980).
34   A. M. Pamucku, S. Yalciner, J. F. Hatcher and G. T. Bryan, Cancer Res., 40: 3468–3472 (1980).
35   S. Hosaka and I. Hirono, Gann., 72: 327–328 (1981).
36   I. Hirono, I. Ueno, S. Hosaka, H. Takanashi, T. Matsushima, T. Sugimura and S. Natori, Cancer Lett., 13: 15–21 (1981).
37   K. Morino, N. Matsukura, T. Kawachi, H. Ohgaki, T. Sugimura and I. Hirono, Carcinogenesis, 3: 93–97 (1982).
38   M. Hirose, S. Fukushima, T. Sakata, M. Inui and N. Ito, Cancer lett. 21, 23–27 (1983).
39   A. Sakai, K. Sasaki, H. Mizusawa and M. Ishidate Jr., Teratogen. Carcinogen. Mutagen., 10: 333–340 (1990).
40   NTP Technical Report (No. 409) on the Toxicology and Carcinogenesis Studies of Quercetin in F344/N Rats. NIH Publication No. 91–3140 (1991). US Department of Health and Human Services, Public Health Service, National Toxicology Program, Research Triangle Park, N. C.
41   N. Ito, Jpn. J. Cancer Res., 83: 312–313 (1992).
42   I. Hirono, Jpn. J. Cancer Res., 83: 313–314 (1992).
43   M. T. Huang, A. W. Wood, H. L. Newmark, J. M. Sayer, H. Yagi, D. M. Jerina and A. H. Conney, Carcinogenesis, 4: 1631–1637 (1983).
44   T. Torigoe, M. Arisawa, S. Itoh, M. Fujio and H. B. Maruyama, Biochem. Biophys. Res. Comm., 112: 833–842 (1983).
45   G. M. Shah and R. K. Bhattacharya, Chem. Biol. Interact., 59: 1–15 (1986).
46   Y. H. Chae, S. L. Coffing, V. M. Cook, D. K. Ho, J. M. Cassady and W. M. Baird, Carcinogenesis, 12: 2001–2006 (1991).
47   Y. H. Chae, C. B. Marcus, D. K. Ho, J. M. Cassady and W. M. Baird, Cancer Lett., 60: 15–24 (1991).

48 J. E. Nixon, J. D. Hendricks, N. E. Pawlowski, C. B. Pereira, R. O. Sinn-huber and G. S. Bailey, Carcinogenesis, 5: 615–619 (1984).
49 K. Yasukawa, M. Takido, M. Takeuchi, Y. Sato, K. Nitta and S. Naka-gawa, Chem. Pharm. Bull., 38: 774–776 (1990).
50 E. E. Deschner, J. Ruperto, G. Wong and H. L. Newmark, Carcinogenesis, 12: 1193–1196 (1991).
51 L. Liu and A. Castonguay, Carcinogenesis, 12: 1203–1208 (1991).
52 H. Nishino, E. Naito, A. Iwashima, K. Tanaka, T. Matsuura, H. Fujiki and T. Sugimura, Gann., 74: 311–316 (1984).
53 T. Horiuchi, H. Fujiki, H. Hakii, M. Suganuma, K. Yamashita and T. Sugimura, Jpn. J. Cancer Res. (Gann.), 77: 526–531 (1986).
54 E. M. Bickoff, A. L. Livingston and A. N. Booth, Arch. Biochem. Biophys., 88: 262–266 (1960).
55 D. A. Shutt and R. I. Cox, Endocrinology, 52: 299–304 (1980).
56 B. Y. Tang and N. R. Adams, J. Endocr., 85: 291–296 (1980).
57 B. M. Markaverich, R. R. Roberts, M. A. Alejandro, G. A. Johnson, B. S. Middleditch and J. H. Clark, J. Steroid Biochem., 30: 71–78 (1988).
58 L. M. Larocca, M. Piantelli, G. Leone, S. Sica, L. Teofili, P. Benedetti Panici, G. Scambia, S. Mancuso, A. Capelli and F. O. Ranelletti, Br. J. Haematol., 75: 489–495 (1990).
59 G. Scambia, F. O. Ranelletti, P. Benedetti-Panici, M. Piantelli, C. Rumi, F. Battaglia, L. M. Larocca, A. Capelli and S. Mancuso, Int. J. Cancer, 46: 1112–1116 (1990).
60 G. Scambia, F. O. Ranelletti, P. Benedetti-Panici, M. Piantelli, G. Bo-nanno, R. De Vincenzo, G. Ferrandina, L. Pierelli, A. Capelli and S. Man-cuso, Cancer Chemother. Pharmacol., 28: 255–258 (1991).
61 M. E. Baker, J. Steroid Biochem. Molec. Biol., 41: 301–308 (1992).
62 Chiang Su New Medical College: Chon Yao Da Tze Dian, Shanghai Science Technology Publisher, 1979.
63 H. Y. Hsu, Y. P. Chou and M. Hong, The Chemical constituents of Oriental herbs, OHAI, Long Beach (1982).

Progress in Drug Research, Vol. 42
Edited by Ernst Jucker
© 1994 Birkhäuser Verlag Basel (Switzerland)

Serenics

Berend Olivier[1,2], Jan Mos[1], Maikel Raghoebar[3],
Paul de Koning[4] and Marianne Mak[4]

[1]CNS-Research, Drug Discovery Section, Solvay Duphar b.v., P.O.Box 900, 1380 DA Weesp, The Netherlands; [2]Dept. of Psychopharmacology, Faculty of Pharmacy, University of Utrecht, Utrecht; [3]Project Management, Solvay Duphar b.v.; [4]Department of Clinical Research, Solvay Duphar b.v.

1   Introduction

The development of drugs, specifically aimed at reduction of pathological destructive behaviour in psychiatric patients, was started by
our company halfway through the seventies. It was conceived, and
this idea has been reinforced over the years, that pathologically
destructive behaviour, sometimes called "aggressive", "violent", "agitated" or "dysfunctional", presents a delicate problem in psychiatry.
Such behaviour, which is often a secondary complication of an
underlying organic disorder such as dementia, traumatic brain injury,
or profound mental retardation, is very often severely troublesome to
family care-givers and leads to their unwilling commitment of their
loved ones to institutional care. After these patients are institutionalized, their behaviour often continues to pose serious management
problems. In some cases various behavioural modification techniques
may facilitate functional integration within the institutional community. However, these techniques are labour intensive and not invariably successful. In most institutions, a residue of patients exhibiting
significant destructive behaviour remains. These individuals demand
a disproportionate measure of staff time, may require isolation and
even physical or chemical restraint to protect other patients, the staff
or themselves from undue risk of injury.
A striking variety of drugs has been tried in these patients (Tuinier,
1980), but historically, neuroleptics or hypnotics, used for their sedative properties, and benzodiazepines (BDZ) have been most commonly used. The sedatives, of course, in doses adequate to control
behaviour, often obliterate virtually all active behaviour, leading to a
semi-vegetative state and BDZ may even lead to paradoxical increases
in destructive behaviour (Azcarate, 1975; Bond and Lader, 1979;
DiMascio, 1973). More recently, lithium, beta-blockers and anticonvulsants have been tried. However, there are few well-controlled
studies and, indeed, the actual modes of treatment, essential characteristics of the treated patients, or clear outcome measures are often
missing in published reports. In any event, the drugs used have no
specific effects upon behaviour (e.g., the neuroleptics) or are associated with significant adverse effects (e.g., neuroleptics and tardive
dyskinesia, beta-blockers and hypotension; lithium and renal problems), or both. Therefore, we recognized at the end of the 1970's that
there was a real need for compounds which might specifically inhibit

destructive behaviour without other significant behavioural, psychiatric or somatic side effects. However, when addressing ourselves to the problems of synthesis, qualification and development of such compounds, we were immediately faced with limitations of the pharmacological models many of which (if not most) had been developed empirically based upon the activity of known psychotropics.

To progress beyond the state-of-the-art at the time, therefore, we had to develop a set of functionally animal models which could be feasible applied to a large number of candidate drugs; which might define the pharmacologic characteristics of classes of compounds yet unknown; and which could provide a credible basis for evential trials in man. Section 2 has been devoted to a description of the animal models used. In the remainder of this volume, the results of that effort are outlined and the characteristics of the series of such compounds called "serenics", which answer to a pharmacologic profile apparently unique in specific inhibition of offensive aggression, are described (section 2). Moreover, the putative mechanism of action is described (section 3). In section 4 the pharmacokinetic profile of eltoprazine in various species is examined. The final section discusses some of the therapeutical implications and results and existing pharmacotherapeutic options.

1.1   Animal models

Through the sixties and seventies, psychopharmacology laboratories often used simple and somewhat unnatural models involving agonistic behaviours (generically, if somewhat nonspecifically termed aggressive behaviours) in animals to detect putative psychoactivity of newly synthesized compounds. Generally, these models were focused upon a single response variable, such as isolation-induced fighting among male mice, to indicate psychoactivity essentially unrelated to the observed behaviour, in this case to indicate neuroleptic activity (Janssen et al., 1959). While such models are functionally simple to run and score and, therefore, suitable for screening, they do not reveal the mechanism of action and, therefore, can predict little of anything about the specificity of the observed effect and, excepting relative potency, nothing which might distinguish the compound under test from existing neuroleptics.

The aforementioned "isolation-induced aggression" in male mice was used as a primary screening model to determine a simple and straightforward effective dose (ED_{50}-value in mg/kg orally) for the reduction of aggression. This measure, the dose of a drug which reduces aggression by 50%, is not informative as to how a drug reduces aggression and is consequently not predictive about the specificity of its behavioural effect. To describe the behavioural profile of a drug, we developed an ethological screening procedure, social interaction in mice, which is based on extensive ethological observation and recording of the ongoing behavioural items (Olivier and van Dalen, 1982). For this purpose we divided the behaviour into several elements which have been described before in detail (Grant and Mackintosh, 1963). These elements adequately describe the diverse aspects in the behaviour of an isolated male mouse as offense, defence, social interest, flight, exploration and self care. By carefully observing and recording the ongoing behaviour, often assisted by slow-motion video-analysis, it appeared possible to differentiate the behavioural profile of several drugs (Olivier and Van Dalen, 1982; Olivier et al., 1984; Olivier et al., 1986; Olivier et al., 1987). Using this animal model it appeared possible to distinguish specific anti-aggressive drugs from non-, or less-specific drugs.

In several publications (Olivier and Van Dalen 1982; Olivier et al., 1986), we have shown that inhibition of aggression can be accompanied by inhibition of other behaviours (social interest, exploration) leading to a nonspecific profile (e.g. neuroleptics), but it also shows the profile in which social behaviour and exploration remain intact (e.g. fluprazine, eltoprazine). This latter, highly specific anti-aggressive profile has been depicted by us as the SERENIC profile (Olivier et al., 1986).

This profile has been elaborated in other animal models describing the anti-aggressive profile of drugs, e.g., in rats.

In our laboratory we have tested new putative serenic compounds in what we call a behavioural cascade (Fig. I-1).

After a first screening of all newly synthesized compounds in aggressive mice for anti-aggressive activity, in which the only criterion is a certain ED_{50}-value, any compound which has better activity than the preset ED_{50}-value is tested in the Social Interaction test in mice. Compounds are tested in a dose range comprising the ED_{50}-value to 25 times higher than the ED_{50}-value for inhibition of aggression.

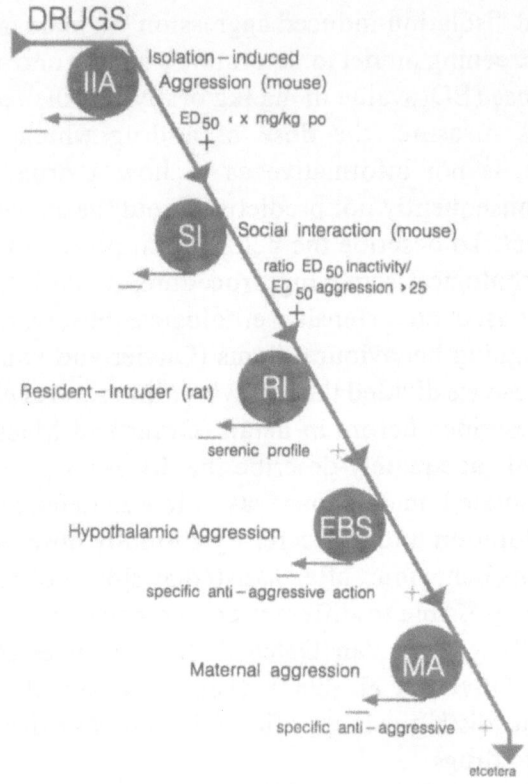

Fig. I-1

Behavioural cascade to detect serenics. The primary test is isolation-induced aggression in mice. When a certain ED_{50}-value (mg/kg p.o.) is found, a social interaction test in mice is performed. When a large ratio (25) between the ED_{50}-value for enhancement of inactivity (sedation) and the ED_{50}-value for inhibition of aggression is found, the drug proceeds to the resident-intruder paradigm in rats where a specific anti-aggressive profile is needed before continuation occurs along the cascade towards hypothalamic aggression and maternal aggression.

A compound will only proceed through the cascade if the ratio ED_{50}-value inactivity/ED_{50}-value aggression is larger than 25, which means that we want at least a factor of 25 between anti-aggressive and non-specific effects like sedation, muscle relaxation, etc. A drug with such a profile will consecutively be tested in the Resident-Intruder, the Hypothalamic Aggression and Maternal Aggression paradigms in rats, in order to judge whether it exerts a behaviourally specific, i.e. serenic, profile. The extensive description of all the models used is given in section 2.

1.2   Chemistry

In a combined lead-finding and screening operation in the mid-seventies, about 2,000 chemical structures, selected from different chemical classes, were screened for potential anti-aggressive activity in the isolation-induced aggression test in mice. In 1975 we detected some phenylpiperazine-analogues (e.g. DU 24527) which fulfilled our primary pharmacological criteria for an anti-aggressive structure. These compounds were the starting point for further chemical optimalisation (see fig. I-2).

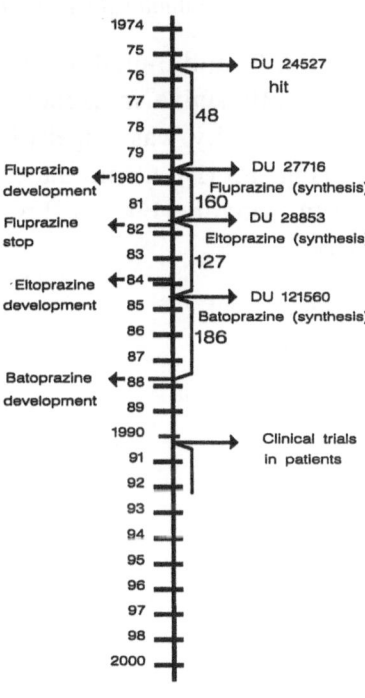

Development Serenics

Fig. I-2
Time frame for the development of serenics. To the left of the timebar the important events in the development of serenics are depicted. To the right the chemical synthesis of antiaggressive drugs within the serenic project is shown. From 1990 on eltoprazine has been tested in patients.

During the following exploration and optimalisation period, about 50 new phenylpiperazine analogues were synthesized (Hartog et al., 1986). In 1980, one of them (DU 27716, fluprazine) was, based on its promising anti-aggressive and pharmacological profile, selected for further development. This development was stopped in 1982 because of toxicity problems in animals. Mean while, the optimalisation strategy, directed by increasing knowledge of the structure-activity relationship of this chemical class, shifted to a new class of up to then unknown bicyclic-heteroaryl-piperazines.

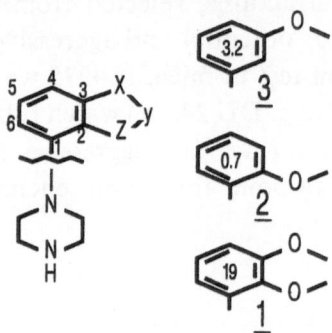

Fig. I-3
Structure-activity relation of serenics. The mother molecule basic to several modifications has been depicted on the left. The figures in the phenylring show the oral ED_{50}-value to inhibit aggression in mice.

This was based on our findings that 2- and 3-methoxy-phenylpipe-razines (Fig. I-3 (**2** and **3**)) were both active in isolation-induced aggression, whereas anti-aggressive activity was largely lost in the 2,3-dimethoxyphenyl compound (Fig. I-3 (**1**)). Combination of these two substituents into a benzodioxan structure (Fig. I-4-1) resulted in a remarkable anti-aggressive activity.

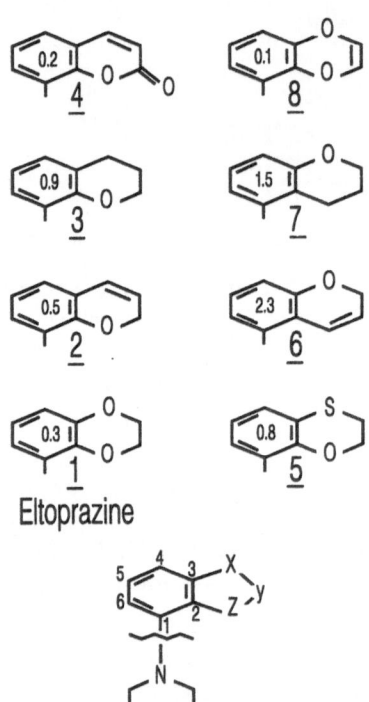

Eltoprazine

Fig. I-4
Structure-activity relation of serenics. The mother molecule basic to several modifications has been depicted at the bottom. The figures in the phenylring show the oral ED_{50}-value to inhibit aggression in mice.

This finding was further explored by designing an extensive series of analogues, using structure-activity relation studies (SAR). All these compounds were tested for anti-aggressive activity in the isolation-induced aggression test. This resulted in the selection of a number of interesting compounds, of which, in 1984, after the withdrawal of fluprazine, a new serenic (eltoprazine, Fig. I-4-1) was selected for further investigation. Based on the information that it was allowed to combine the substituents on position 2 and 3 in the phenyl ring, a series of bicyclic compounds were designed with the general structure shown in all the figures I-3 to I-9, containing one or more atoms from the group of carbon, oxygen, sulphur or nitrogen in the annelated ring. These new heterobicyclic structures were screened for anti-aggressive activity, resulting in additional information about the relation between the chemical structure and anti-aggressive activity in mice. It appeared that annelation of a heterocyclic ring was allowed and that there were neither large differences in potency between the compounds with the annelated 5-, 6- or 7-hetero ring analogues, nor between oxygen, sulphur and/or nitrogen containing rings, as illustrated in Figs. I-4, I-5 and I-6.

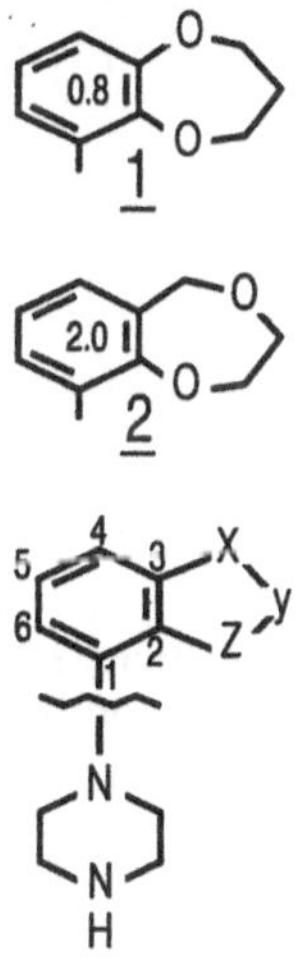

Fig. I-5
Structure-activity relation of serenics. The mother molecule basic to several modifications has been depicted at the bottom. The figures in the phenyl-ring show the oral ED_{50}-value to inhibit aggression in mice.

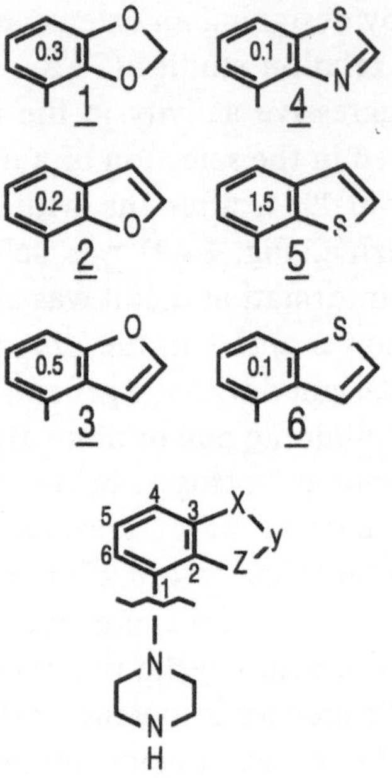

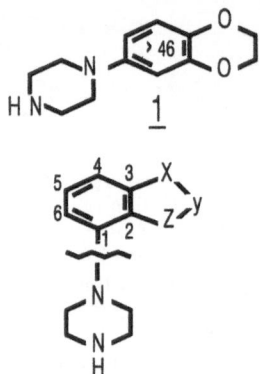

Fig. I-6

Structure-activity relation of serenics. The mother molecule basic to several modifications has been depicted at the bottom. The figures in the phenyl-ring show the oral ED_{50}-value to inhibit aggression in mice.

Moving the piperazine ring from the 1-position to the 6-position (Fig. I-7) of the phenyl ring resulted in a complete loss of the anti-aggressive activity, indicating that substitution of the para-position (opposite to the piperazine nitrogen) is not allowed.

Fig. I-7

Structure-activity relation of serenics. The mother molecule basic to several modifications has been depicted at the bottom. The figures in the phenyl-ring show the oral ED_{50}-value to inhibit aggression in mice.

This may be explained by alterations in physical-chemical properties and/or steric factors. Additional substitution in the phenyl ring, for instance by chlorine or fluorine (as illustrated in Fig. I-8, 1-5), resulted in a strong decrease of anti-aggressive activity when compared to the unsubstituted compound (eltoprazine).

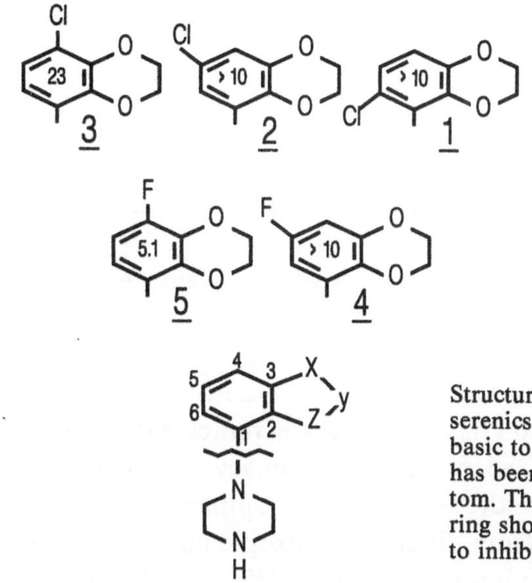

Fig. I-8
Structure-activity relation of
serenics. The mother molecule
basic to several modifications
has been depicted at the bottom. The figures in the phenyl-
ring show the oral ED_{50}-value
to inhibit aggression in mice.

Relatively small variations in the piperazine ring, or insertion of a
carbonyl- or methylene function between the phenyl and the piperazine ring (Fig. I-9, 1-5) also strongly diminished the anti-aggressive
potency compared to the parent compound.
Besides an ED_{50}-value for inhibition of isolation-induced aggression,

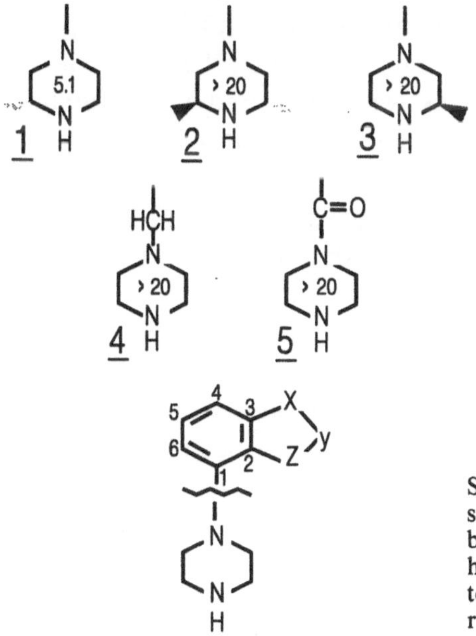

Fig. I-9
Structure-activity relation of
serenics. The mother molecule
basic to several modifications
has been depicted at the bottom. The figures in the phenyl-
ring show the oral ED_{50}-value
to inhibit aggression in mice.

all compounds were also screened for in vitro serotonergic (5-HT$_1$) receptor affinity.

High affinities for serotonin receptors were found for all derivatives with anti-aggressive properties. Correlation of the latter with serotonin 1A, 1B or 1C receptor affinity strongly suggested that the anti-aggressive activity is mediated by a 5-HT$_1$-like activity.

2   Behavioural pharmacology of the serenic, eltoprazine
2.1   Introduction

An overview of the general rationale underlying the animal models used to discover and characterise the serenics has been given in the introduction. Here we present a summary of the main results of experiments in which the serenics were compared and contrasted with a number of drugs from other psychotropic classes using the modelling techniques of ethopharmacology. We believe that these results support the contention that the serenics have a unique activity profile which differentiates them from other classes of compounds. In particular, they inhibit the offensive components of agonistic behaviour in a variety of animal models without motor or CNS retardation, social inhibition, or other such effects. To our knowledge, their specificity in this regard is unparalleled by other compounds notwithstanding some apparent similarities, for example, of receptor binding profiles.

In these studies eltoprazine and fluprazine, the most widely studied representatives of the serenics, were compared with a number of other putative anti-aggressive compounds or drugs used clinically in an attempt to ameliorate aggressive behaviour of patients. Although a number of compounds have been used clinically (Itil and Mukhopadhyay, 1978; Gunn, 1979), no drug with a specific anti-aggressive profile is available.

Depending on the underlying disorder, such as schizophrenic syndromes, epileptic disorders, acute brain syndromes, chronic organic brain syndromes, mental retardation, behavioural disturbances or personality disorders, various drugs have been used (Itil and Mukhopadhyay, 1978; Itil, 1981; Sheard, 1983, 1984, 1987). Among these are neuroleptics, tranquillizers, lithium and some newer compounds assumed to be anti-aggressive. In the course of the present investigation, compounds belonging to these pharmacological categories were used for comparison.

Some of the comparators used are: the neuroleptics chlorpromazine and haloperidol, the tranquillizer chlordiazepoxide, putative anti-aggressives Sch 12679 and YG-19-256 (Itil and Mukhopadhyay, 1978; Bell and Brown, 1979), alcohol and some other drugs chosen because of their pharmacological profile in comparison to eltoprazine.

2.2 Offensive aggression paradigms

Social isolation has long been known to induce offensive behaviour in mice (Scott and Fredericson, 1951), and this led to development by Yen et al. (1959) of a laboratory model in which such behaviour was consistently induced. They were also the first to report the effects of selected pharmacological agents on isolation-induced aggression in mice.

This model has been extensively used in assessing the effects of drugs (Malick, 1979; Miczek and Barry, 1976; Miczek and Krsiak, 1979). The model clearly measures offensive aggression because the behaviour exhibited by these isolated male mice is highly offensive (Miczek and Krsiak, 1979; Blanchard et al., 1979), although defensive properties may still be present in (some of) these animals (Krsiak, 1975, 1979).

Because the complete behavioural repertoire is manifested in isolated male mice (Miczek and Krsiak, 1979; Krsiak, 1979; Poshivalov, 1987), the isolation-induced aggression model is also attractive for assessing the effects of drugs on total behaviour using ethological methods. This variant of the model is presented here as "social interaction" (Olivier and Van Dalen, 1982) and, as in the less elaborated form, reflects predominantly the offensive qualities of agonistic behaviour.

Isolation-induced aggression in mice

The detailed methodology is given in Olivier et al. (1989). Short male mice were isolated for four weeks and selected for aggressive behaviour. Drugs were given intraperitoneally or orally, 30, 60 or 240 mins before testing, which lasted three minutes. The results shown in Table II-1 demonstrate that eltoprazine has a marked anti-aggressive effect 30 minutes after an intraperitoneal and one hour after an oral dose when tested in isolation-induced aggression. Four hours after oral dosing, it still had an anti-aggressive action, although its duration of action seems to be shorter (ratio 7.5) than fluprazine, another serenic, which was also active after both i.p. and oral administration. Chlordiazepoxide, diazepam, fluvoxamine, alcohol and Sch 12679 have a weak or no anti-aggressive action, whilst chlorpromazine, d-amphetamine, YG-19-256, and haloperidol are quite potent.

Social interaction in male mice – acute treatment

Male albino (DAP) mice (16-19 g) were kept singly in macrolon cages (13x17.5x11.5 cm) for 3 weeks. To measure social interactions, such an isolated mouse was placed for 5 min in a neutral observation cage (21x30x30 cm) of which the floor was covered with sawdust. Then a male group-housed opponent was introduced and for 5 minutes the behaviour of the "isolated" mouse was scored according to a previously described ethogram (Olivier et al., 1989; Grant and Mackintosh, 1963). Drugs were given orally (except 8-OH-DPAT-s.c.) 60 min before testing. Each dose group included 13 animals and on one testing day 5 groups were tested, using a randomized design.

Table II-1

Effect of various psychoactive drugs on isolation-induced aggression in male mice

Drug	Route	n	30 min	60 min	n	240 min
				Mean ED_{50}-values ($\pm$ SEM)*		
				injection-test interval		
Eltoprazine	po	4		0.4±0.06		
	po	2			2	2.9
	ip	1	0.1			
Fluprazine	ip	2	0.7			
	po	7		1.2±0.1	2	0.8
Chlordiazepoxide	po	8		73±13		
Diazepam	po	2		12		
Sch 12679	po	5		37±9		
YG-19-256	po	3		1.0±0.2		
Chlorpromazine	po	2		4.7		
Haloperidol	po	2		0.8		
d-Amphetamine	po	2		4		
Fluvoxamine	po	2		70		
Alcohol	po	1		>3 g/kg		

* Mean ED_{50}-values ($\pm$ SEM) calculated from ED_{50}-values of separate experiments; n = number of experiments (5 groups of 5 animals per experiment.)

Figure II-1 shows the effects of a dose range (0.5 – 20 mg/kg p.o.) of eltoprazine after acute administration on social interaction. Eltopra-

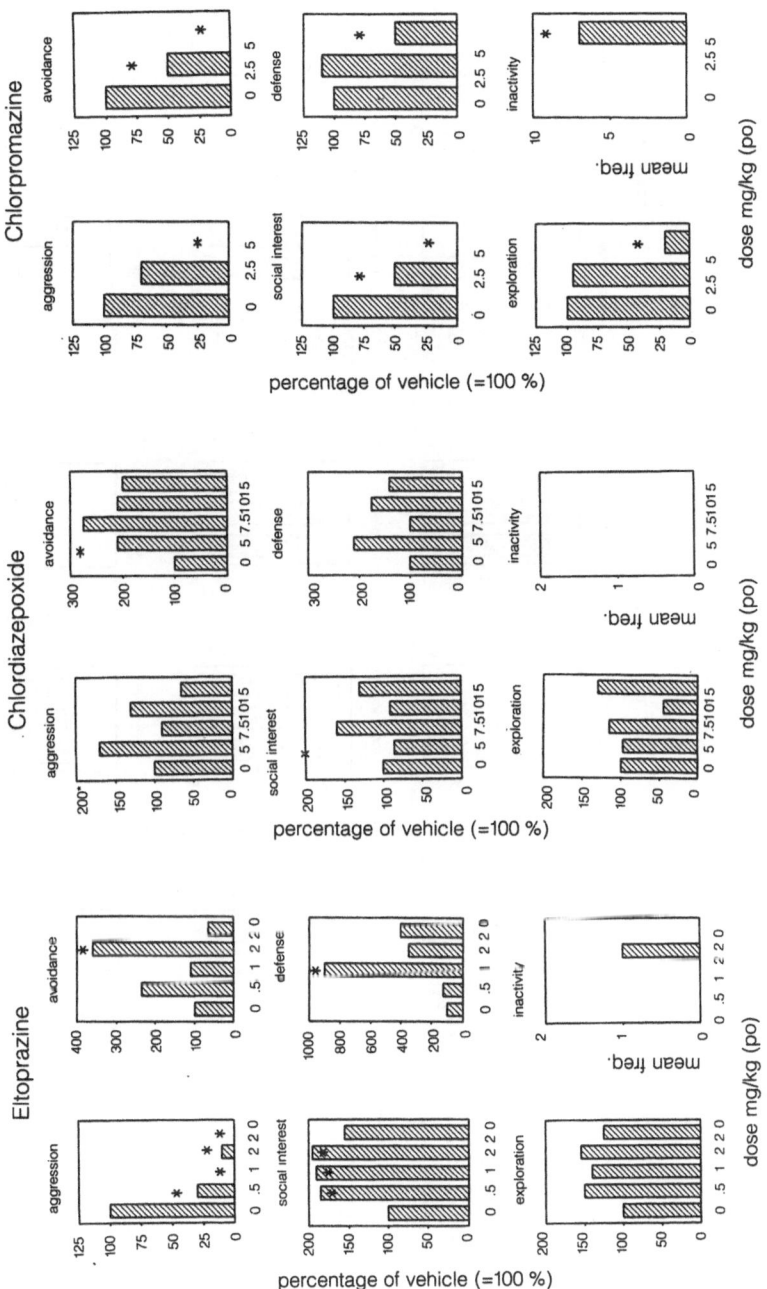

Fig. II-1

Effects of eltoprazine (0.5–20 mg/kg p.o.), chlordiazepoxide (5–15 mg/kg p.o.) and chlorpromazine (2.5–5 mg/kg p.o.) on the frequency of occurrence of 6 behavioural categories in intermale aggression in mice. For inactivity the mean frequency has been depicted, for the other categories the frequency is shown as % of 0 mg/kg.

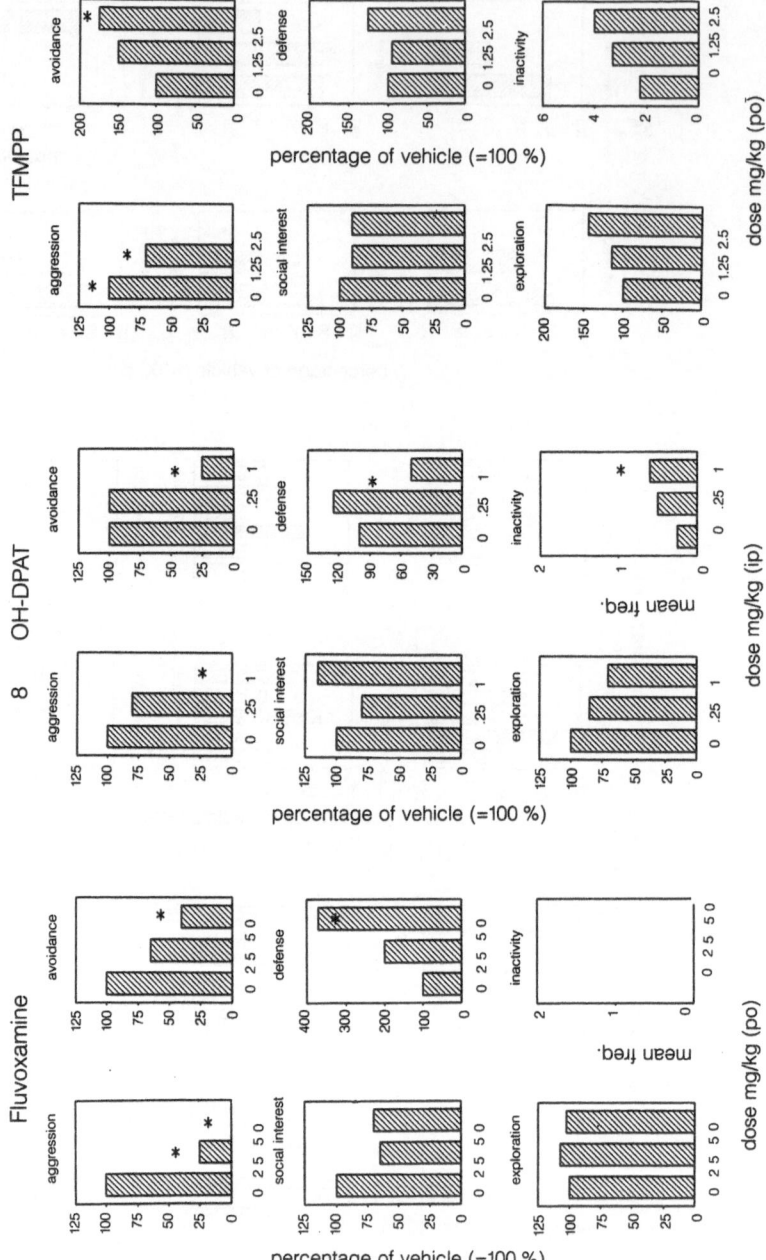

Fig. II-2

Effects of fluvoxamine (25–50 mg/kg p.o.), 8-OH-DPAT (0.25–1 mg/kg s.c.) and TFMPP (1.25–2.5 mg/kg p.o.) on the frequency of occurrence of 6 behavioural categories in intermale aggression in mice. For inactivity the mean frequency has been depicted, for the other categories the frequency is shown as % of 0 mg/kg.

zine dose-dependently inhibits aggression, both in introductory aggressive elements, aggression and tail rattling. Concomitantly, social activities, except "crawling under", increased, but not in a dose-dependent way, up to a certain level (approx. 100% increase). No effects were found in exploration and inactivity, whereas avoidance and defence were somewhat enhanced (particularly at 1 and 2 mg/kg). It should be noted that at 20 mg/kg p.o., which is roughly 50 times the ED_{50}-value for aggression, aggression was completely gone. No sedation, myorelaxant or psycho-stimulant activities were induced by eltoprazine, illustrating the very specific anti-aggressive (serenic) activity of this kind of drug.

Figures II-1 and II-2 also show the results for a number of reference compounds, viz. chlordiazepoxide, chlorpromazine, TFMPP (trifluoromethylphenyl piperazine), fluvoxamine and 8-OH-DPAT (8-hydro-2-di-n-propylaminotetralin). Chlordiazepoxide was tested in two separate experiments (5 and 10 mg/kg; 7.5 and 15 mg/kg). As can be seen from the figure, the effects of the different doses in the two experiments are not entirely consistent. The differences between the two experiments may be due to the high level of aggression and low level of social activity measured in the control group of the second experiment, which can clearly influence the effects of psychoactive drugs on behaviour (Miczek and Krsiak, 1979). However, it is clear that chlordiazepoxide does not have anti-aggressive activity. At low doses it even enhances aggression, thereby confirming the pro-aggressive activity of low doses of benzodiazepine agonists (Mos and Olivier, 1987, 1989).

While chlorpromazine significantly inhibited aggressive activities at a dose of 5 mg/kg, both social and non-social activities were also strongly suppressed and must be considered non-specific. At 2.5 mg/kg aggressive components were only slightly influenced. Fluprazine, a prototype serenic (Olivier et al., 1986), shows a behavioural profile generally comparable to that of eltoprazine.

For reference purposes, a number of serotonergic drugs has also been tested in intermale aggression in mice. TFMPP, a rather specific 5-HT_{1B}-agonist (Asarch et al., 1985; Glennon, 1986; Olivier et al., 1987) and an important metabolite of fluprazine, has a more or less similar behavioural profile as eltoprazine, whereas fluvoxamine, a specific 5-HT-reuptake blocker (Claassen et al., 1979), also inhibits aggression, but in a less specific way because it is accompanied by a decrease in social interest and an increase in defence. A specific 5-HT$_{1A}$-agonist, 8-OH-DPAT (Middlemiss and Fozard, 1983), also reduced aggression, but it decreased non-social activities somewhat and reduced defence (at 1 mg/kg) and avoidance.

It can be concluded that serenics, the class to which eltoprazine belongs, have a very specific behavioural profile in this intermale aggression paradigm in mice. This profile is unrivalled by any other drug tested so far (Olivier and Van Dalen, 1982; Olivier et al., 1984a,b 1986, 1987).

We also performed an experiment to judge whether eltoprazine keeps its anti-aggressive properties when given subchronically to isolated aggressive mice.

Social interaction in male mice – subchronic treatment

Fifteen groups of male mice (N = 13/group) were used. Each male was isolated for four weeks and received during the last 7 days vehicle (1% glucose) or eltoprazine (3, 5 or 10 mg/kg/day) via their drinking water. Three experiments were run in parallel; each experiment consisted of 2 vehicle groups and 3 groups receiving eltoprazine. After this 7-day treatment one wash-out day was given and then the pre-treated mice were acutely dosed with vehicle or eltoprazine (0.5, 1.0 and 2.0 mg/kg) orally, one hour before a 5-min intermale aggression test, which was otherwise similarly performed as described before.

Although the whole behavioural repertoire was measured, we only present data on social interaction and aggression (fig. II-3).

Figure 3 shows the results after pretreatment aimed at, respectively, 0, 3, 5 and 10 mg/kg/day in the drinking water. The actual eltoprazine intake measured was 0, 3.0, 6.5 and 14.0 mg/kg/day for the respective groups.

In general, eltoprazine has similar effects after subchronic dosing than after acute dosing. Both the enhancing effects on social behaviour and the dose-dependent decreases in aggressive behaviour remain after subchronic pretreatment. This indicates the absence of any tolerance or rebound phenomena after subchronic treatment.

Resident-intruder aggression in rats – acute treatment

Although resident-intruder aggression somewhat resembles the intermale aggression situation in mice described above, there are some attractive differences. Because rats are social animals (Barnett, 1975;

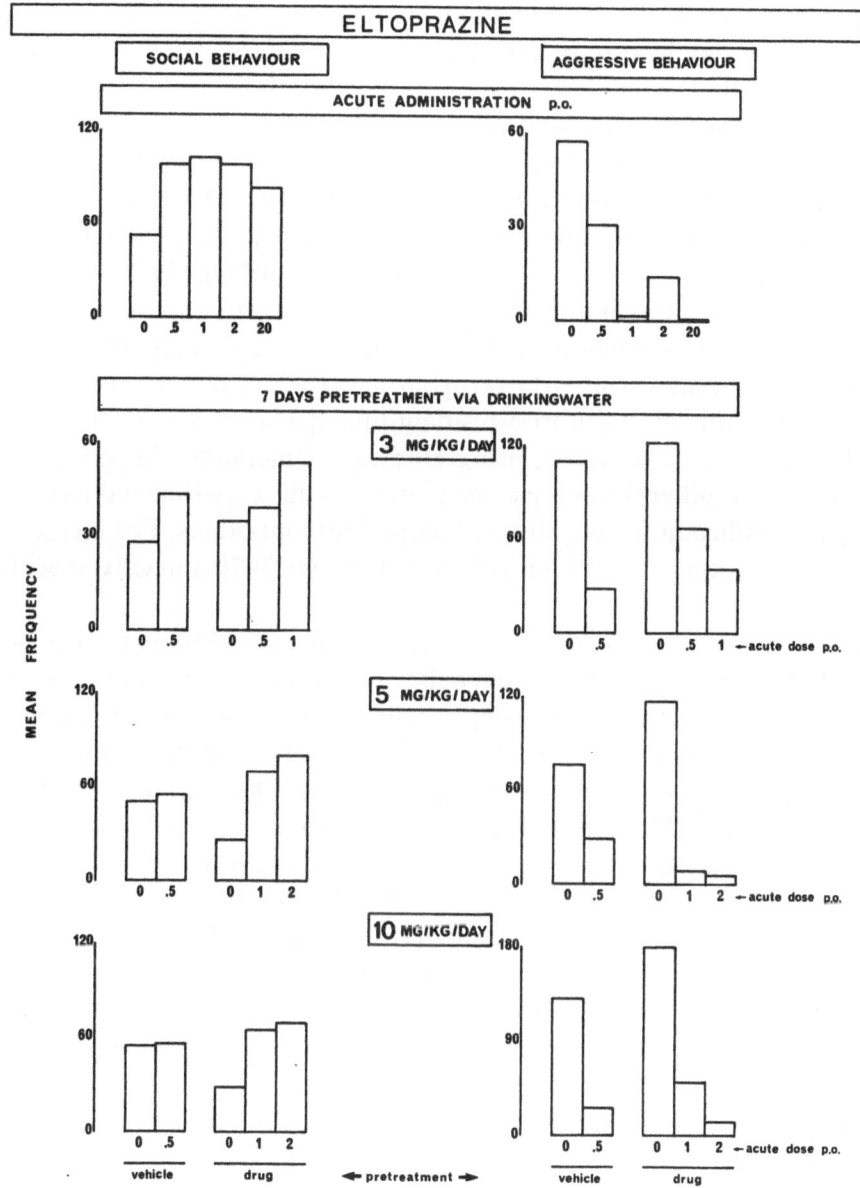

Fig. II-3

The effect of acute doses of eltoprazine after subchronic-treatment with vehicle, 3, 5 or 10 mg/kg/day eltoprazine p.o. for 7 days on the frequency of occurrence of aggression and social behaviour in intermale aggression in mice. For comparison the acute experiment has been included. (Note that scales are different.)

Timmermans, 1978), the isolation involved in the social interaction paradigm may lead to behavioural disturbances (Valzelli, 1973; Valzelli and Bernasconi, 1980).

Moreover, male rats are territorial (Barnett, 1975) and the test set-up as used in the resident-intruder paradigm seems a reasonable natural condition to induce territorial aggression (Adams, 1976; Olivier, 1977). According to several authors (Miczek and Krsiak, 1979; Olivier, 1977; Blanchard and Blanchard, 1977; Lehman and Adams, 1977; Miczek, 1979), introduction of a strange male in such a (semi-natural) territory evokes an almost complete pattern of aggression, strongly resembling the natural patterns of wild rats (Barnett, 1975; Timmermans, 1978). Therefore, in this territorial resident-intruder model, the effects of eltoprazine were assessed, using ethological methods. For comparison, several other drugs have been tested in this experimental model; e.g. d-amphetamine, buspirone, haloperidol and others. For methodological aspects the reader is referred to Olivier (1981) and Olivier et al. (1984).

Figures II-4, II-5 and II-6 summarize the effects of different drugs on five categories of the resident's behaviour towards a male opponent. Eltoprazine exerted a dose-dependent decrease in offence (aggression). This coincided with a slight increase in social interest and an increase in exploration. Avoidance was somewhat enhanced at 1.25 and 2.5 mg/kg but this had returned to normal at 5 mg/kg, whereas inactivity was somewhat enhanced at the highest dose.

This profile is specific for serenics. In this paradigm no other drug tested so far (which, apart from those presented here, comprise a considerable number of drugs from different drug classes) exerted such a specific serenic profile. This is illustrated here by haloperidol (fig. II-4), which is a very non-specific anti-aggressive drug; by oxazepam (fig. II-4), which enhances aggression concomitant with increases in social interest and decreases in exploration and avoidance behaviour, and by d-amphetamine (fig. II-6), which exerts anti-aggressive activity together with reduced social interest, increased exploration (stereotypy) and (at lower doses) increased avoidance behaviour and decreased inactivity.

For comparative reasons we also studied some serotonergic drugs in the resident-intruder paradigm, viz. 8-OH-DPAT (fig. II-5), buspirone (fig. II-6), ipsapirone (fig. II-5; specific 5-HT_{1A}-agonists) and RU24969 (fig. II-5; a nonspecific 5-HT_1-agonist).

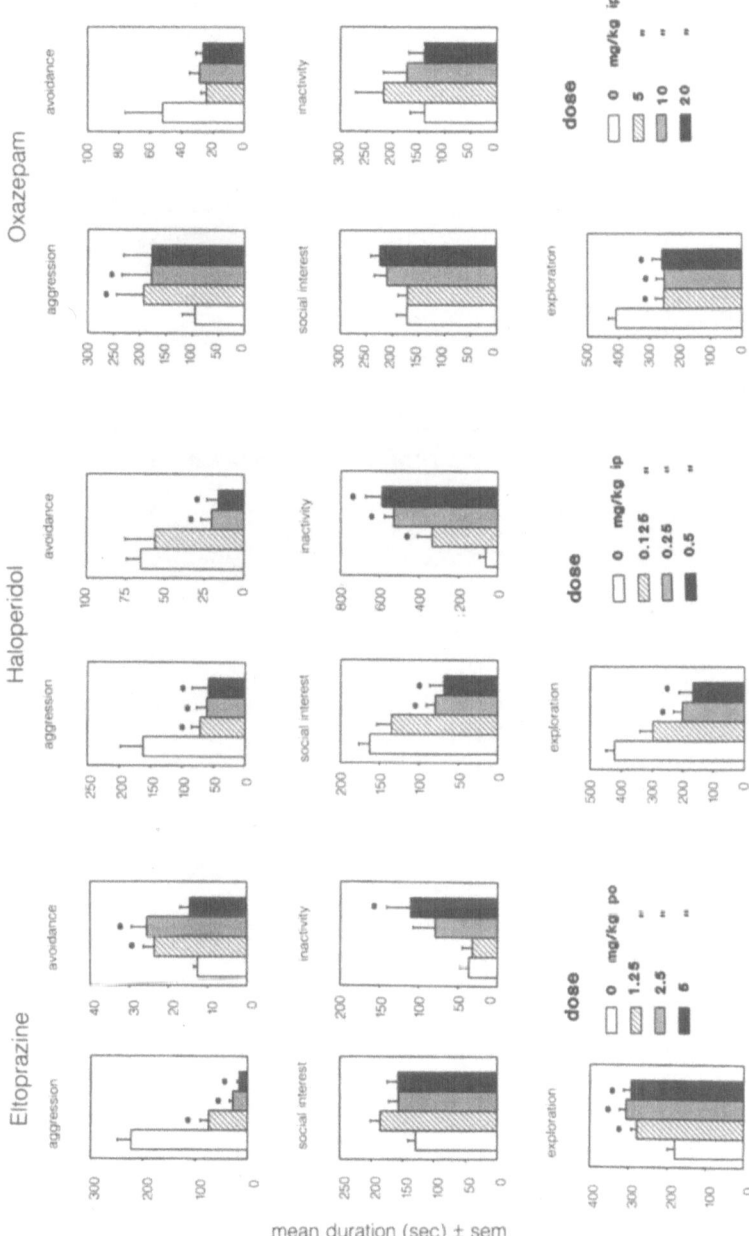

Fig. II-4

The effects of eltoprazine (1.25–5 mg/kg p.o.), haloperidol (0.125–0.5 mg/kg i.p.) and oxazepam (5–20 mg/kg i.p.) are shown on the mean duration of 5 representative behavioural categories in resident-intruder (territorial) aggression in male rats. Doses were given intraperitoneally and subcutaneously 30 min before testing and orally 60 min before testing. Each drug was tested in 12 rats.

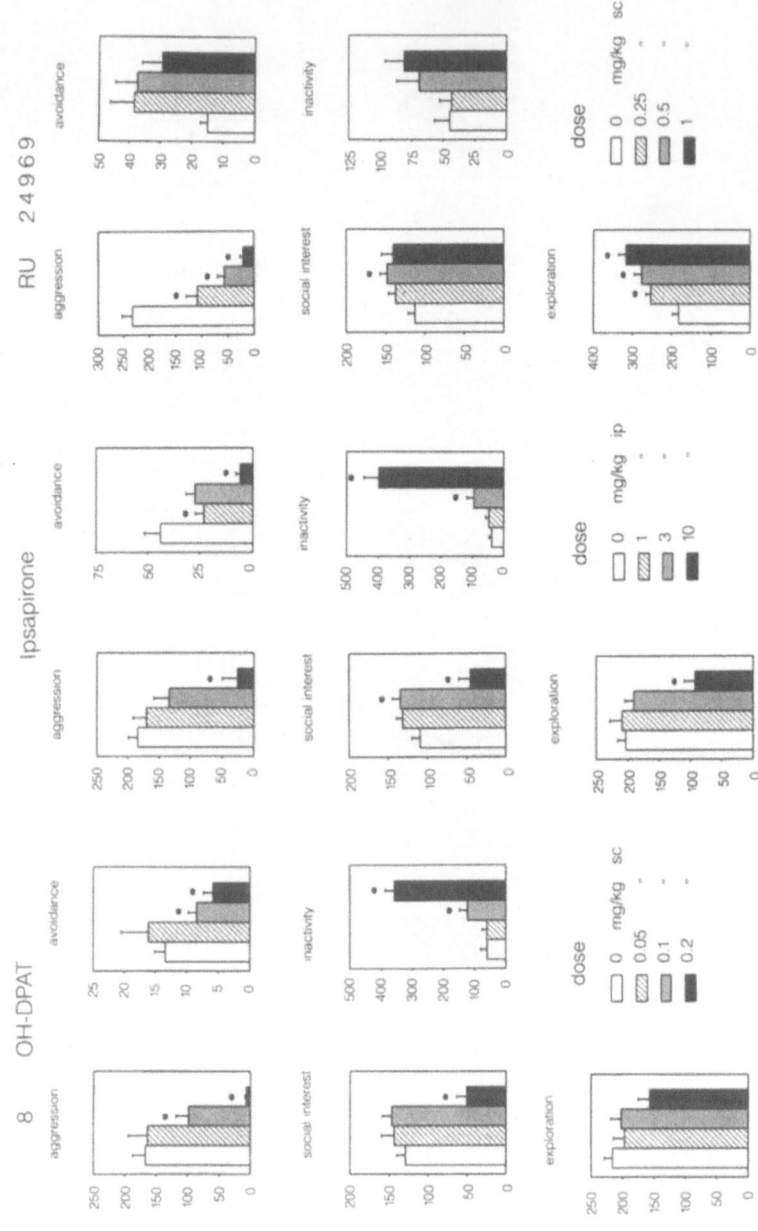

mean duration (sec) ± sem

Fig. II-5

The effects of 8-OH-DPAT (0.05–0.2 mg/kg s.c.), ipsapirone (1–10 mg/kg i.p.) and RU 24969 (0.25–1 mg/kg s.c.) are shown on the mean duration of 5 representative behavioural categories in resident-intruder (territorial) aggression in male rats. Doses were given intraperitoneally and subcutaneously 30 min before testing and orally 60 min before testing. Each drug was tested in 12 rats.

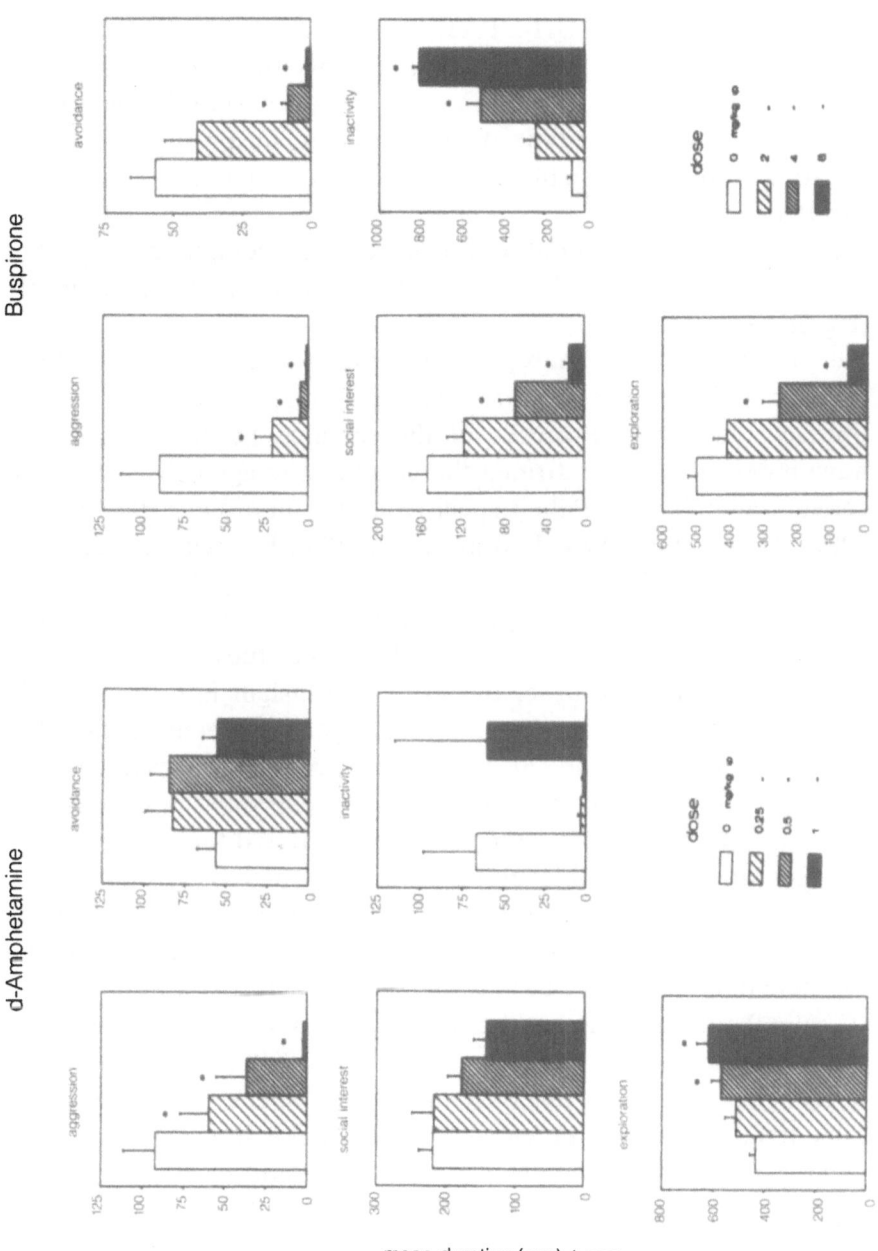

Fig. II-6
The effects of d-amphetamine (0.25–1 mg/kg i.p.) and buspirone (2–8 mg/kg i.p.) are shown on the mean duration of 5 representative behavioural categories in resident-intruder (territorial) aggression in male rats. Doses were given intraperitoneally 30 min before testing. Each drug was tested in 12 rats.

The 5-HT$_{1A}$-agonists, 8-OH-DPAT, buspirone and ipsapirone, all decreased aggressive behaviour but in a non-specific manner; simultaneously social interest, exploration and avoidance were decreased and inactivity enhanced (sedation). In particular, buspirone had a very sedative profile, presumably also caused by its dopamine-antagonistic properties.

RU24969 has a behavioural profile more or less comparable to that of eltoprazine, although it has a more pronounced stimulatory profile (e.g. in exploration).

Detailed behavioural analysis using sequence- and cluster-analyses (Olivier, 1981; Olivier and Mos, 1986 a, b) supports the view of the unique anti-aggressive profile of the serenics. Several laboratories have independently confirmed the specific anti-aggressive action of serenics and also stress their specific effects on offence (Poshivalov, 1987; Benton et al., 1984; Dijkstra et al., 1984; Flannelly et al., 1985).

Resident-intruder aggression in rats – subchronic treatment

We also performed a preliminary subchronic study in the resident-intruder paradigm, in order to have some insight into the possible development of tolerance for eltoprazine's anti-aggressive action. We administered eltoprazine (20 mg/kg/day) or saline for seven days via Alzet® osmotic minipumps. After 7 days, one day's wash-out was given and thereafter each resident male was tested for 15 minutes, 30 minutes after an acute injection of saline or 10 mg/kg i.p. eltoprazine. Figure II-7 shows an overall picture in which the individual elements have been grouped according to categories and the effects of the different treatments have been expressed as a percentage of the (saline + saline) treatment. It can be seen that 7 days pre-treatment with saline does not affect the acute effectiveness of 10 mg/kg eltoprazine in reducing offence; at this dose no offensive behaviour occurs. The same treatment somewhat enhances exploration and slightly reduces social interest. Avoidance is clearly reduced and inactivity strongly enhanced (especially the duration).

Acute treatment with saline, after 7 days pre-treatment with 20 mg/kg/day eltoprazine, indicates that the inhibitory effects of eltoprazine have still not completely waned. Compared to the (saline + saline) level, offence is reduced to 30% (frequency) or 40% (duration). This indication is supported by a similar pattern in the categories of exploration, social interest, avoidance and inactivity compared with acute treatment.

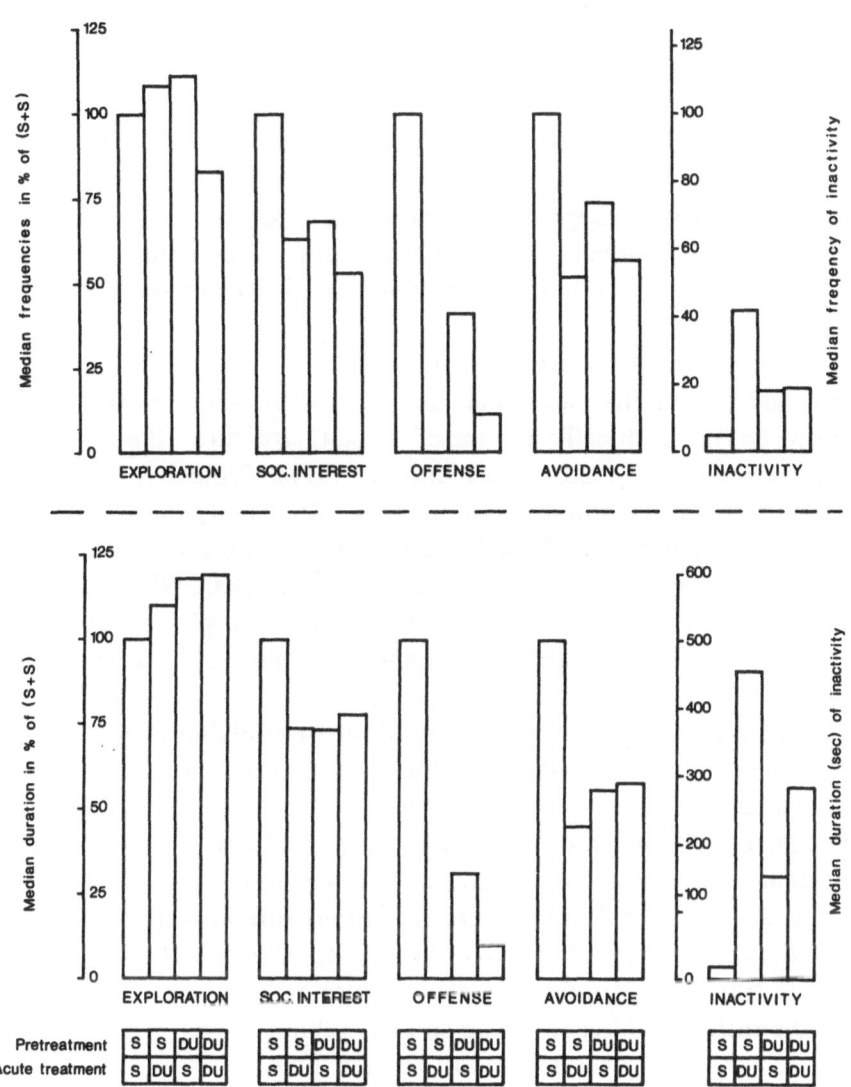

Fig. II-7
After seven days pre-treatment with saline (S) or eltoprazine, 20 mg/kg/day (DU) via minipump, the acute behavioural effects of saline (S) or eltoprazine, 10 mg/kg i.p. (DU) are measured in a resident-intruder paradigm. The top panel reflects the frequencies, the bottom panel the duration of 5 behavioural categories.

Acute treatment on day 8 of the 7-day pretreated eltoprazine group shows that eltoprazine is still able to exert its anti-aggressive action, whereas the whole behavioural profile also suggests that the drug in these eltoprazine-pretreated animals is still active. The difference observed in offence between acute eltoprazine treatment in saline or eltoprazine pre-treated animals may suggest that some tolerance occurs after 7 days pre-treatment with 20 mg/kg eltoprazine administered via minipumps (subcutaneous). A clear disadvantage of the present experiment was that the minipumps were not removed, so that the exact time of stopping of delivery of eltoprazine was not known. However, the removal of such a pump 1 day before behavioural tests would heavily interfere with the behavioural performance.

Colony-aggression in rats

Rats are socially living animals and groups of male and female rats show an hierarchically organized social structure (Barnett, 1975; Timmermans, 1978; Lore and Flannelly, 1977). Typically, a dominant (or α-male) emerges and maintains that role usually for an extended period (Blanchard and Blanchard, 1981, 1984; Blanchard et al., 1977). The remaining males are subordinates (Dijkstra et al., 1984; Mos et al., 1984) which, like females, do not ordinarily take part in attacks on strange male intruders (Blanchard and Blanchard, 1977; Blanchard et al., 1977).

The attractiveness of a colony situation for studying drug effects is that one can treat all males, only the α-male or only the subordinates, or one can remove several members (e.g. the α-male) and then see what happens when a strange intruder is placed into the colony. In the present experimental paradigm, a limited colony consisting of two males and one female is used. During colony formation the emergence of a dominant male is verified by weekly intruder tests. Typically, after two to three weeks, one male (the α-male) makes most of the attacks on the intruder. After reaching such a stable hierarchy, drug experiments were performed (Mos and Olivier, 1988).

Two male (400–500 g) and one female (250–275 g) TMD-S3 rats were placed in a colony ($65 \times 50 \times 50$ cm) in which two small Macrolon cages ($15 \times 20 \times 20$ cm) were situated and coupled via a tube in such a way that a kind of burrowing system was created. Food and water were always available. During weekly 15-min intruder tests (male Wistar intruders of 300–350 g) the emergence of an α-male was noted. After 3–5 weeks practically each colony (a total of 24 colonies were used) has a stable hierarchy.

Experiments were performed on these stable colonies. Sixty minutes
before testing the female and the two macrolon cages were removed
from the colony, both males received the drug or vehicle orally and
were replaced in the colony. Both members of a colony received a
similar treatment, either vehicle (tragacanth 1%) or one dose of a drug.

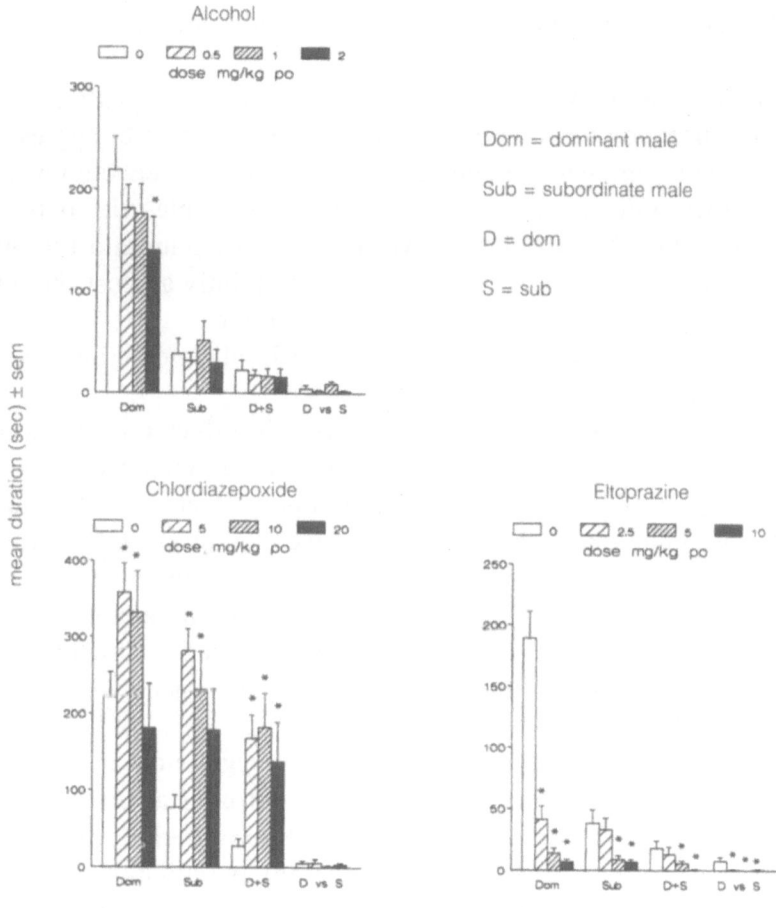

Fig. II-8
Effects of eltoprazine (2.5, 5 and 10 mg/kg p.o.), chlordiazepoxide (5, 10 and 20 mg/kg
p.o.) and ethyl alcohol (0.5, 1 and 2 g/kg p.o.) on dominant and subordinate male rats
in a colony situation when a strange intruder was present. * : p<0.05 significant
difference from 0 mg/kg.

An experiment lasted two weeks and each colony was tested on Monday and Thursday of each week. Treatments were randomized according to a latin square design. Sixty minutes after administration of vehicle or drug, an intruder was placed into the colony and for the following 15-min the ongoing behaviour was videotaped and recorded directly via the computer system described before. For the present purpose only the time spent on aggression, both for the α-male and the subordinate, was recorded.

As reference compounds, chlordiazepoxide and ethyl alcohol were used.

Figure II-8 shows the results of acute treatment with eltoprazine, chlordiazepoxide and ethyl alcohol on the duration of aggression (all summed aggression elements) during a 15-min encounter with an intruder. Four kinds of interaction are possible, viz. between the α-male and the intruder, between the subordinate and the intruder, between the α-male and the subordinate jointly against the intruder, and between the α-male and the subordinate.

Eltoprazine clearly reduced aggression in all interactions in a dose-dependent way.

Chlordiazepoxide (CDP) had a biphasic effect on aggression, increasing it at 5 and 10 mg/kg (except in the dominant vs. subordinate interaction). Moreover, CDP differentially affected the dominant and subordinate male. The pro-aggressive action of CDP was more marked in the subordinate than in the dominant male (around 300% in the subordinate and approx. 150% in the dominant male). This pro-aggressive action of CDP has been described before (Olivier et al., 1986 a, b; Mos and Olivier, 1986) in several aggression paradigms (Mos et al., 1987).

Ethyl alcohol had no clear effects of aggression in any type of interaction, except in the dominant vs. intruder at the highest dose, where aggression was reduced. The failure of high doses (2 g/kg) of alcohol to affect aggression in this colony paradigm confirms earlier data obtained in resident-intruder aggression, maternal aggression and in hypothalamically-induced aggression. For reviews of alcohol effects see Winslow et al. (1987), Blanchard et al. (1987) and Olivier and Mos (1986). Under specific conditions alcohol may lead to pro-aggressive actions (Winslow et al., 1987), but neither we (Olivier and Mos, 1986) nor others (Blanchard and Blanchard, 1987; Brain, 1986) were able to detect such pro-aggressive actions.

Hypothalamically-induced behaviour in rats

Electrical stimulation in the hypothalamus of rats (Koolhaas, 1978; Kruk et al., 1979) in the presence of an appropriate goal object, typically a conspecific, will induce behaviour very similar to normal offensive aggression (Kruk et al., 1979; Kruk and Van der Poel, 1980). Hypothalamic aggression in male rats is sensitive to manipulations of androgen levels (Bermond et al., 1982). Moreover, it can be induced in an area (Kruk et al., 1983) roughly coinciding with the areas where levels of circulating sex hormones are regulated (Orsini et al., 1985). In female rats aggression can also be elicited in this same area (Kruk et al., 1984; Mos et al., 1987). This behaviour is readily reproduced under controlled circumstances, thereby meeting an important requirement for a model to study aggression. In this model the effects of eltoprazine were assessed and compared to a number of reference compounds. Previous studies have shown that serenics (Olivier et al., 1986; Olivier and Mos, 1986; Kruk et al., 1984; Van der Poel et al., 1982) exert a very specific profile in this hypothalamically-induced aggression paradigm in both males and females.

In addition to aggressive behaviour, this stimulation in the hypothalamus also induces locomotion and teeth-chattering (Kruk et al., 1984; Van der Poel et al., 1982). The effects of drugs are measured by the changes in the current thresholds required to evoke the respective behaviours (Van der Poel et al., 1982). Comparison of the effects on the different thresholds gives information about the specificity of the drug effect. A specific anti-aggressive effect is present when only the thresholds for aggression and teeth-chattering are enhanced and locomotion is unaffected.

Threshold Determinations – Adult male rats of the Wezob, Wistar or TMD-S3 strains were used as experimental subjects. They were equipped with two bipolar electrodes aimed at a certain site in the hypothalamus (Kruk et al., 1979). Threshold current intensities for attack, teeth-chattering, locomotion and switch-off were determined according to an up-and-down method. During the experiments the current was on for 10 sec and off for 50 sec periodically. The current was increased in fixed steps till the desired response was induced, then decreased until the response was lost, etc. The threshold of a behaviour, i.e. the current intensity inducing that behaviour in 50% of the stimulation trials, was calculated from six subsequent response changes. Aggression (with a male partner) and teeth-chattering (without a partner) were tested in a plexiglass cylinder (35 cm; height 45 cm). Prior to drug testing at least 5 thresholds were obtained for all behaviours. Locomotion was tested in a large cage ($60 \times 50 \times 100$ cm) with a floor area covered with an absorbent material, which was divided into 8 squares of 25×25 cm. The number of squares crossed during 10 sec stimulation trials was counted. A trial was scored as positive if at least 6 crossings were obtained. Each animal received saline, or one of three doses of a drug according to a randomized block-design. Each dose was given twice, separated by at least one day of rest; the first dose was followed after 30 minutes by a threshold determination of aggression followed by a locomotion test; the second dose was followed after 30 minutes by a test for teeth-chattering. The mean threshold current levels of the last three pre-drug determinations were used as initial current levels in the drug test.

Figure II-9 shows the changes in thresholds (%) for aggression, teeth-chattering and locomotion after treatment with eltoprazine, fluprazine, chlordiazepoxide, haloperidol, 8-OH-DPAT and fluvoxamine.

Eltoprazine clearly enhanced the threshold for aggression and teeth-chattering (slightly), whereas the threshold for locomotion was even decreased, indicating the specificity of action on aggression. Fluprazine had a comparable effect on aggression but did not influence locomotion (Van der Poel et al., 1982), whereas haloperidol enhanced aggression, teeth-chattering (slightly) and locomotion-thresholds (which could not even be measured) at the same time, indicating its non-specific effects.

Chlordiazepoxide had no effect on aggression and teeth-chattering thresholds at lower doses and enhanced the thresholds for both aggression and locomotion only at the highest dose, presumably indicating the muscle relaxant properties at that dose.

8-OH-DPAT had no influence on thresholds for aggression and teeth-chattering, whereas fluvoxamine had a somewhat specific anti-aggressive profile.

Recent evident (Kruk et al., 1987) showed that this electrical brain stimulation (EBS)-induced behaviour paradigm in rats shows a quite specific profile for serenics: enhancement of thresholds for aggression and teeth-chattering, no effect of even a decrease on locomotion thresholds and no effect on switch-off behaviour, a measure for the interference of a drug with the aversive qualities also resulting from

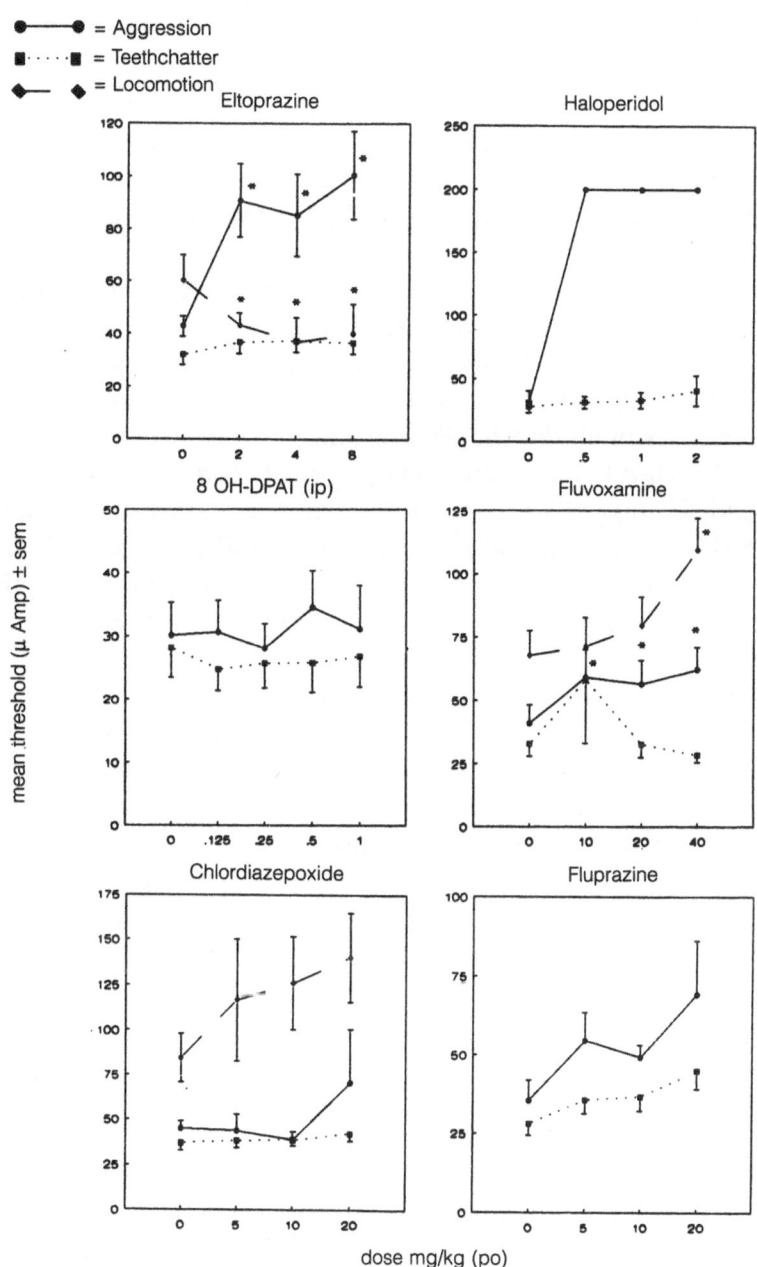

Fig. II-9

The mean thresholds (±SEM) in μA are given for three behaviours evoked by electrical stimulation from the hypothalamus of male rats: aggression, teeth-chatter and locomotion. The effects of eltoprazine, haloperidol, 8-OH-DPAT, fluvoxamine, chlordiazepoxide and fluprazine are given on these thresholds. Significant difference (* : p<0.05) from 0 mg/kg is depicted.

the electrical brain stimulation. d-Amphetamine (0.5 – 2 mg/kg i.p.) had no effect on aggression, teeth-chattering and switch-off behaviour, but decreased the locomotion threshold, illustrating its stimulatory action. Scopolamine, a (muscarinic) anticholinergic drug, had (at 0.25 – 1.0 mg/kg i.p.) no effect on aggression and teeth-chattering, but decreased locomotory thresholds and also decreased switch-off thresholds.

Alcohol, up to a dose of 2 g/kg orally, had no effect on any parameter, which was also observed after naloxone (0.1 – 10 mg/kg, i.p.), an opiate antagonist. Quipazine, a non-specific 5-HT_1-agonist and potent 5-HT_3 antagonist, had a quite non-specific action in EBS behaviours: increases in all thresholds, indicating its behavioural non-specificity. 8-OH-DPAT, a specific 5-HT_{1A}-agonist, had, at doses between 0.05 and 0.2 mg/kg i.p., no effects, whereas TFMPP, a rather specific 5-$HT_{1B/1C}$-agonist, and a putative metabolite of fluprazine, exerts a specific effect at 0.5 – 2 mg/kg i.p. on aggression (and teeth-chattering) without interference with locomotion. Interestingly, TFMPP enhanced switch-off thresholds, indicating at least that the anti-aggressive action is not caused by fear-induction. dl-Propranolol, a β-adrenergic blocker (at 5 – 20 mg/kg i.p.) also has a specific anti-aggressive profile; it inhibited aggression and teeth-chattering, but had no influence on locomotion and switch-off.

Summarizing, serenics, like eltoprazine and fluprazine, have a specific profile in this hypothalamically-induced behavioural model; enhancement of aggression-related behaviours, without disturbing side effects like sedation or muscle relaxation, nor fear-enhancing effects as revealed by enhancement of stimulation-escape (switch-off behaviour).

Maternal aggression (MA) in the rat

The majority of studies on animal aggression deals with interactions between males (Moyer, 1968). However, females can be quite aggressive under certain conditions, as, for instance, in hypothalamically-induced aggression in rats (Kruk et al., 1984; Mos et al., 1987), aggression in non-oestrus hamsters (Floody and Pfaff, 1977; Payne and Swanson, 1970) and maternal aggression in several rodent species (mice, voles, rats, hamsters; cf. (Floody, 1983; Svare and Mann, 1983)). In a female analogue of the resident-intruder paradigm, female rats display appreciable levels of aggression versus female intruders but to a lesser extent against male intruders. In general, however, attack frequencies in female aggression are lower than in males (Blanchard and Blanchard, 1981, 1987; Van der Poel et al., 1982). The use of a female aggression paradigm for psychopharmacological purposes has been uncommon and, only the last decade, the development of models has been undertaken using maternal aggression in female rats (Olivier and Mos, 1986; Olivier et al., 1985; Van der Poel et al., 1984) and mice (Yoshimura, 1987).

Maternal aggression is restricted to the postpartum period (Erskine et al., 1978 a,b; 1980; Haney et al., 1989; Svare and Gandelman, 1974) during which the lactating female is highly aggressive towards strange intruders, particularly males (Wise, 1974; Svare, 1977; Takahashi and Lore, 1982).

Aggression, at least in mice, has been reported to be dependent upon stimuli from the litter, especially suckling (Svare et al., 1980). Although suckling and growth of the nipples are necessary conditions for the display of maternal aggression, the associated changes in prolactin levels are not a necessary requirement (Svare, 1981).

Maternal aggression seems very purposeful, viz. protection of the offspring, and occurs universally throughout the animal kingdom including humans (Archer, 1988).

The effects of eltoprazine and a number of reference compounds were studied in a maternal aggression paradigm, specifically developed in our laboratory to test psychoactive drugs (Olivier and Mos, 1986; Olivier et al., 1985, 1986; Van der Poel et al., 1984; Mos et al., 1989). Female rats of approximately 250–350 g (4–9 months old) were used as experimental animals. Females of the Tryon Maze Dull (S3) and the Wistar strains were used. All strains were derived from CPB-TNO at Zeist, The Netherlands. The females were placed together with a breeding male in their Makrolon® cage ($30 \times 20 \times 15$ cm). The male was left for two weeks with the female, after which she was placed in the observation cage ($40 \times 30 \times 30$ cm) where she stayed for the rest of the experiment. This cage was provided with nesting material and food and water were always available. These cages were situated in the observation room, with a reversed day-night rhythm (12L/12D), night starting at 07.00 h. The day of birth was regarded as postpartum day 0. In the experiments parturient females were tested on alternate days from day 3 to 11 against a naive male Wistar intruder, which had a lower bodyweight (by ca. 25 g) than the female. Pups were present during tests.

Tests were performed in the first part of the dark period (from 08.30 –12.30 h) under red light conditions. A male intruder was placed in the female's home cage for 5 min. The ongoing behaviour was videotaped and analysed later. Each intruder was used once and was sacrificed immediately after the morning sessions with an i.p. overdose of pentobarbital. Drugs were given intraperitoneally 30 min before testing. Animals were tested on days 3, 5, 7, 9 and 11. Each animal was its own control. Drugs and vehicle were completely randomized over days.

All statistical analyses were performed using non-parametric statistics since the variability or the structure of the data did not always warrant a normal or a symmetrical distribution. A modified Friedman analysis was used to detect overall differences between the test days, and was followed by the contrast method for specific comparisons (Klotz, 1980), or the matched pair Wilcoxon test (Siegel, 1956). From the behaviour of females we always recorded directly the number of attacks and the latency to the first attack.

The full behavioural repertoire was scored according to the methodology described in Olivier et al. (1985). In fig. II-10 the effects of eltoprazine on maternal aggression are shown, measured in a 5-min confrontation between a lactating mother and a strange male intruder. Eltoprazine reduced aggression in a dose-dependent way, but also had an effect on several other categories, e.g. decrease in social interest (ISB), exploration and body-care, whereas inactivity and pup care, two closely related categories in this paradigm, were enhanced.

Typically, eltoprazine had a similar effect on this maternal behaviour as had fluprazine but a different one from both haloperidol and chlordiazepoxide.

To illustrate the efficacy of eltoprazine in inhibiting aggression in this model, the effects on the mean number of attacks, the attack latencies and the mean number of wounds are shown in figure II-11. The mean number of attacks is dose-dependently decreased after both eltoprazine and fluprazine, whereas chlordiazepoxide showed no decrease, but an aggression-enhancing effect in this model, at least at low doses. Haloperidol reduced attacks only at the highest dose, presumably caused by severe sedative effects at that dose. d-Amphetamine reduces the number of attacks in a dose-dependent manner, whereas even high doses of alcohol (up to 2 g/kg) have no apparent effect (fig. II-11). Eltoprazine, fluprazine and haloperidol enhance the attack latencies

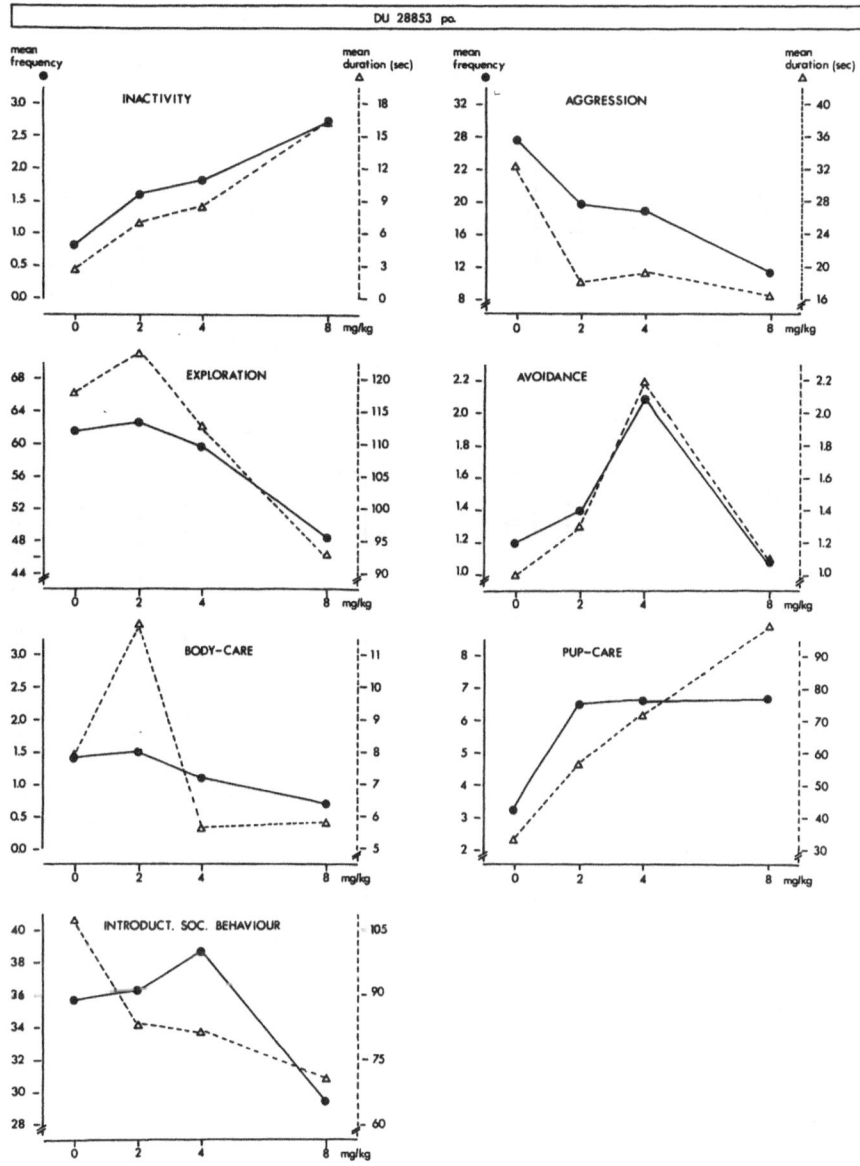

Fig. II-10
Effects of eltoprazine (DU 28853) on 7 behavioural categories of maternal aggression of lactating female rats (note the different scales in the figures).

only at the highest dose used, whereas chlordiazepoxide (at least at low dosages) shortens it.

In summary, eltoprazine has a good anti-aggressive action in maternal aggression. Although the behavioural effects after eltoprazine are

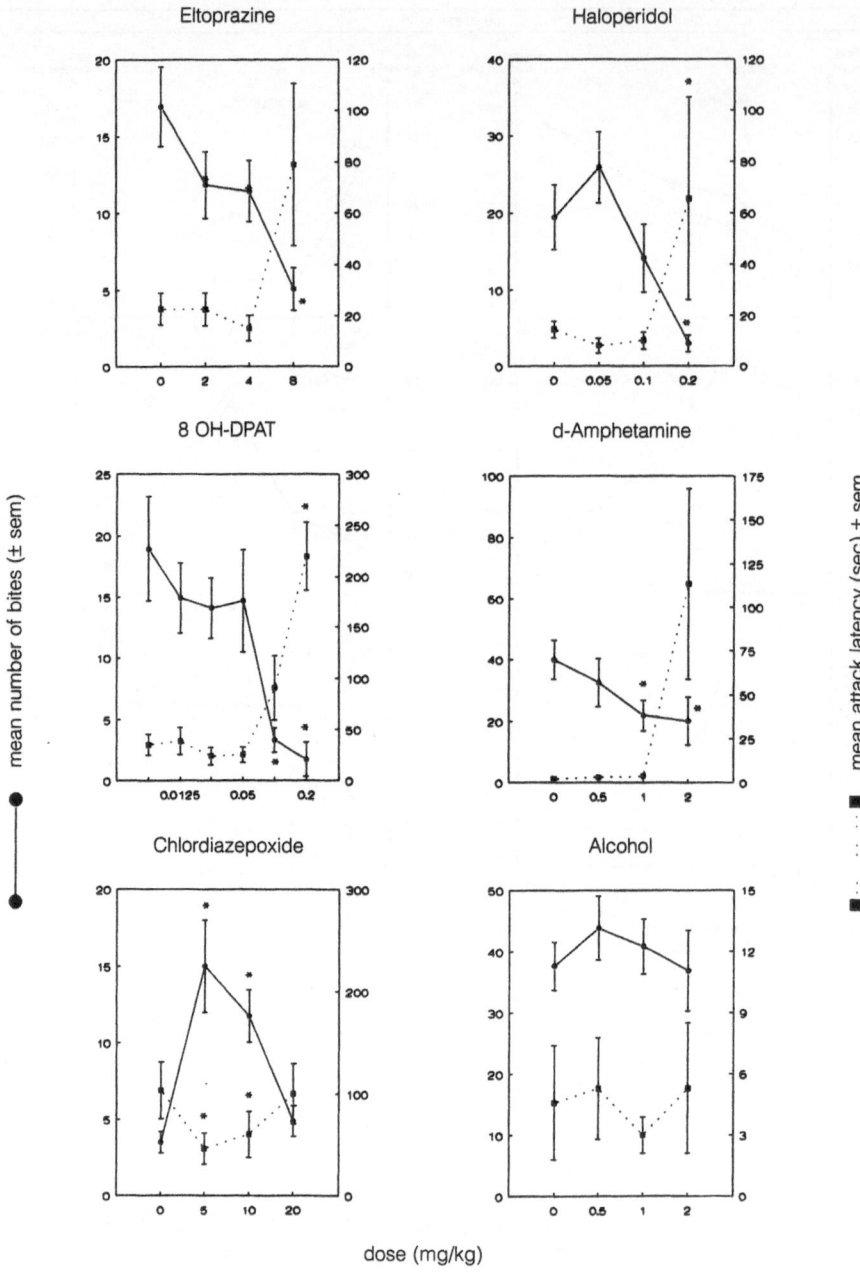

Fig. II-11

Effects of eltoprazine (p.o.), 8-OH-DPAT (i.p.), chlordiazepoxide (p.o.), haloperidol (i.p.), d-amphetamine (i.p.) and alcohol (g/kg p.o.) on the mean number of bites and the latency of the first attack within a maternal aggression test against a naive male intruder. * : $p < 0.05$ denotes a significant difference from vehicle-treatment (0 mg/kg). Note that the alcohol treatment is in g/kg instead of mg/kg.

quite different from those observed in male aggression paradigms, the behavioural structure indicates that interference with aggression in such a female paradigm may lead to several strategies for the female. One such, displayed e.g. by haloperidol or 8-OH-DPAT treated females, leads to interference with pup care; another one, spending more time on pup care (and consequently on inactivity) is shown after serenics (eltoprazine; fluprazine) and some other serotonergic drugs (TFMPP).

Play-fighting in juvenile rats

It has been suggested (Panksepp et al., 1987) that play can be considered a fundamental neuro-behavioural category found in a wide variety of mammalian species, including man. One of the functions of mammalian play behaviour may be to gain experience for later social and agonistic interactions (Hinde, 1974). Play-fighting can be readily observed in juvenile rats (Panksepp, 1981) when such animals are socially deprived for some time (Panksepp and Beatty, 1980) and when a "paired-encounter" technique is used, in which two animals can interact in a neutral arena (Panksepp et al., 1987). When young rats are observed in a neutral arena, after some exploration they begin vigorous play and play-fighting. They solicit play by pouncing on each other, ofter followed by a chase, until they end up in a brief "wrestling bout". These bouts are generally short and end with a "pin" in which one animal is lying on its back and the other standing on it (Panksepp et al., 1984, 1987). By measuring the number of pins and the activity of the animals we tried to get a picture of the effects of eltoprazine on this juvenile agonistic behaviour model. As a reference compound chlordiazepoxide was used.

There have been quite a few psychopharmacological studies on play-fighting (cf. Panksepp et al., 1987 for a review).

After weaning at 21 days old, male juvenile rats were isolated in small cages (13 × 17.5 × 11.5 cm) for a couple of weeks. In the first experiment 100 juveniles were used. At the moment of testing the mean body-weight ± SEM was 52.6±0.9 g. Test animals were matched by weight in pairs and both animals of a pair obtained the same treatment. During testing the latency to the first pin and the frequency of pinning were scored, and also the general activity was counted by measuring the number of crossings over a vertical line dividing the cage into two equal parts (via video recordings). Animals were injected intraperitoneally 30 minutes before testing. Testing occurred in a rather large cage ($30 \times 40 \times 20$ cm) and lasted 5 minutes. In the first experiment eltoprazine was tested in doses of 0 (vehicle = saline), 0.5, 1, 2 and 4 mg/kg. Each dose was given to 10 pairs.

In the second experiment 100 juvenile rats (82.9 ± 1.4 g bodyweight) were used. Animals obtained 0 (gelatin-mannitol microsuspension as vehicle), 1.25, 2.5, 5 and 10 mg/kg i.p. chlordiazepoxide 30 minutes before testing.

All treatments were randomized over animals and time. Figure II-12 shows the effects of different doses of eltoprazine on the pinning frequency and pinning latency. Eltoprazine reduced pinning in a dose-dependent manner. At the same time, it had a stimulatory action on activity, at least at doses from 0.5–2 mg/kg i.p., indicating that pinning was not reduced due to sedation or other non-specific behavioural effects.

Chlordiazepoxide enhanced the number of pinnings at 5 mg/kg, but had no significant effects on the general activity, although it certainly did not reduce it. The reduction in pinning after eltoprazine and the enhancement after chlordiazepoxide parallel findings observed in maternal aggression (Olivier et al., 1985) and resident-intruder aggression (Mos and Olivier, 1987; Mos et al., 1987; Olivier and Mos, 1989) and support the evidence that pinning (and play-fighting) are juvenile correlates of later adult agonistic behaviours.

Agonistic behaviour in pigs

When young pigs from different litters are first housed together, e.g. at weaning, intense fighting can occur (Dantzer and Mormède, 1979; McGlone et al., 1981) which may lead to severe wounds or even death. Often, agonistic interactions continue till a clear hierarchy has been established, a process which may last for 48 hours (McGlone, 1985). Fraser (1974) recognized two distinct patterns of aggressive behaviour during these agonistic interactions. One involved biting while the other, less intense, involved butting and pushing.

In fatstock farms, the neuroleptic azaperone is often used to reduce the undesired aggression observed after mixing unfamiliar pigs (Symoens and Van den Brande, 1969). Azaperone is a strong sedative (Porter and Slusser, 1985) and acts only by shifting the hierarchy fights forward in time: after the sedative effects wane, these fights still occur. Treatment of pigs with a specific anti-aggressive drug, which does not

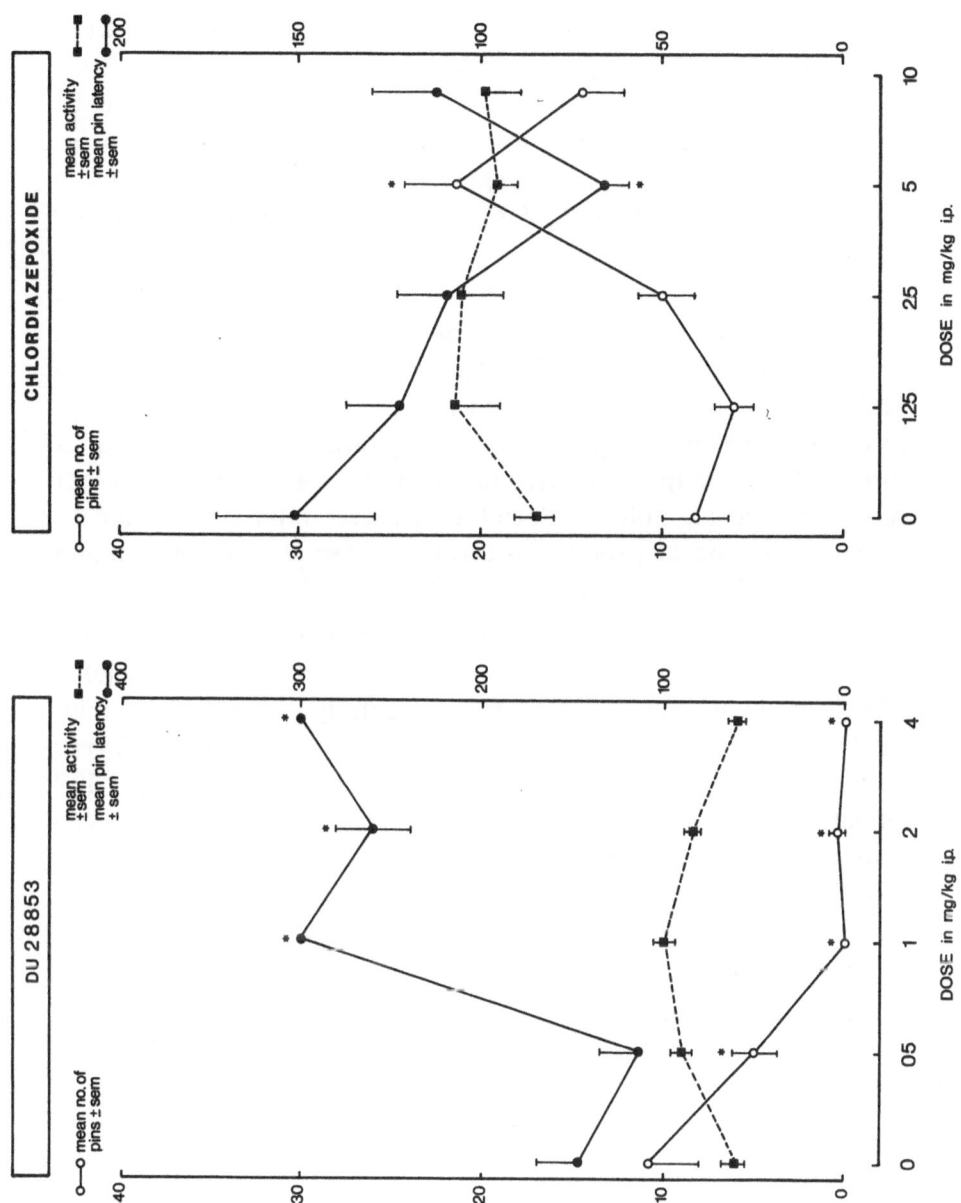

Fig. II-12
The effects of eltoprazine (mg/kg, i.p.) and chlordiazepoxide (mg/kg, i.p.) on the
frequency of pinning, the latency of the first pin and the mean activity of the pair after
eltoprazine or chlordiazepoxide treatment. * : p<0.05 compared to 0 mg/kg.

sedate the animals nor interfere with the communication between them, may have the advantage that the treated pigs are able to interact and to familiarize with each other. This might allow a hierarchy to be settled without the heavy fighting normally observed. Therefore, we tested eltoprazine in a porcine aggression paradigm, which includes mixing of unfamiliar piglets. For comparison, azaperone (Stresnil®) was also tested.

Three litters of female and castrated male piglets, about 10–14 weeks old and 15 to 40 kg bodyweight at the beginning of the experiment, were used. Animals within a litter (11 per litter) were familiar to each other, but unfamiliar to animals of the other litters. The three groups were housed in one of the piggeries at the farm of Solvay Duphar at Muiden. Each group was housed in a pen of 3×4 m. Food and water were available ad libitum. Social encounters took place after an adaptation period of 1 week. Observations started between 8.30 and 10.00 a.m. and lasted 4 hours.

Social encounters were arranged in a neutral pen (3×3 m). Of each litter, 3 animals were introduced, resulting in a mixed group of 9 animals. Animals were injected intramuscularly in the neck, 15 minutes before encounters, with saline, eltoprazine (2.5 and 10 mg/kg) or azaperone (1.5 mg/kg) in a volume of 1 ml/20 kg bodyweight. All 9 animals of a mixed group received the same treatment. The experiments were conducted in such a way that animals of the three litters were always unknown to each other.

Each animal had an identification number on its back to facilitate behavioural observations. The observation and registration took place by video-recording and direct observations by three observers who recorded: a) the piglet taking initiative to a fight and the piglets who suffered the attack and b) the duration of the interaction. For a description of the social ethogram of pigs we refer to McGlone (1985) and Schouten (1986). Shortly, agonistic interactions consisted of bites (bites at the ears, neck, shoulder and face), pushes, head under push, head up push, head-jumps, body turns and flight. When one or more of these elements occurred it was scored as aggression.

In fig. II-13 the results of treatment with saline, eltoprazine (2.5 and 10 mg/kg, i.m.) and azaperone (1.5 mg/kg, i.m.) are summarized on three aspects of agonistic behaviour: i.e., the number of agonistic interactions/15 minutes; the percentage of total time spent on agonistic

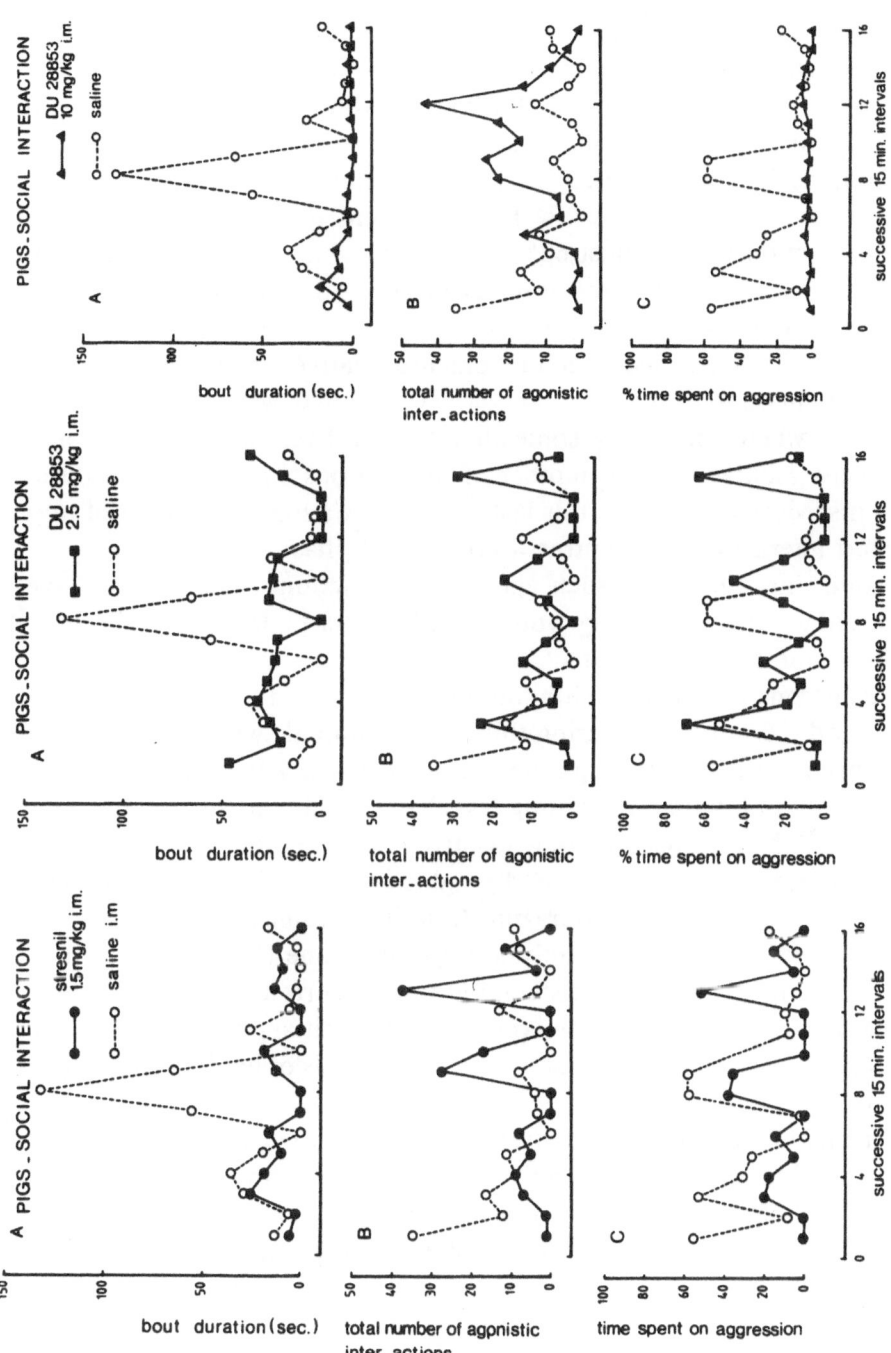

Fig. II-13

The effects of azaperone (Stresnil®; left column) and eltoprazine (DU 28853) 2.5 (middle column) and 1 0 (right column) mg/kg in social interactions in pigs are shown on the bout duration (panels A), the total number of agonistic interactions (panels B) and the time spent on aggression (panels C). All items are expressed per 15 mins observation time. The total observation time was 4 hours.

behaviour (per 15 minutes); and the bout duration of agonistic interactions, that is, the mean time spent on one such interaction.

In each of the columns of the figure, saline-treatment is shown in order to facilitate the comparison with the respective drug treatments. Under saline conditions, agonistic interactions start immediately after mixing the pigs (latency < 1 minute) and during the first 15 min observation time, almost 60% of total time was spent on aggression (Fig. II-13C). The greatest number of agonistic interactions occurred during this time and included almost all individual piglets (Fig. II-13B). Typically most interactions are relatively short-lasting.

After this initial period, aggression waxes and wanes for about 2.5 hours, when, apparently, some hierarchy has been settled, as indicated by the relatively small number of interactions and short bout durations. Moreover, during this last phase, only a limited number of pigs start interactions, in contrast to the initial phase.

Following 4 hours of such agonistic interactions, most piglets have sustained many bleeding wounds and scratches, mainly on the ears, head and behind the ears.

Azaperone (left column) inhibits aggression only for a relatively short period (30 minutes). During this period, animals were lying flat and sedated, dispersed through the observation pen. After this, aggression appeared (although remaining less than in saline-treated animals for about 2 h). Intense fighting occurred after 3 hours, probably indicating that the usual hierarchy fights have simply been postponed.

The lowest dose of eltoprazine (middle column; 2.5 mg/kg, i.m.) inhibited aggression for only a very short time (30 min). After this period, intense and persistent fighting occurred, leading to many wounds and scratches. However, during the initial phase of inhibition, animals were not sedated and showed all kinds of exploratory behaviour.

The higher dose of eltoprazine (right column; 10 mg/kg, i.m.) reduced aggression almost completely during the four-hour confrontation. Very limited time (less than 6%) was spent on aggression in any period. Moreover, the nature of interaction was dramatically shifted from intense fighting and severe injury among the saline-treated animals to subtle and non-damaging interactions among the eltoprazine-treated (10 mg/kg, i.m.) animals. Furthermore, eltoprazine-treated pigs were neither sedated nor showed any other debilitating effects which might have interfered with their ability to engage in agonistic behaviour. Instead, animals showed high levels of social (introductory agonistic) interactions, especially in the second part of the four-hour observation period. This may indicate that no serious fighting would follow and that possibly a hierarchy has already been settled.

2.3   Defensive aggression paradigms

Those forms of agonistic behaviour in which elements of initiative and approach prevail belong to the offensive repertoire, which is characterized by initiative, attack, and similar pro-active behaviours. This contrasts with the defensive repertoire, which is characterised by submission, flight and similar reactive behaviours. Fighting, when it occurs in a defensive animal, is merely a reaction to attack. Other defensive behaviours, such as flight or submission, are apparently intended to escape from or prevent further agonistic interactions (Dixon and Kaesermann, 1987). Some of the drugs known to suppress offensive behaviours effectively have highly undesirable effects on defensive ones. For example, neuroleptics inhibit all activities, including social interest and defensive reactions.

It should also be pointed out that aggressive behaviour is, in evolutionary terms, a necessary component of the total behavioural repertoire. Therefore, drugs which may be useful in pathological behaviour should ideally inhibit offensive components, but should not inhibit initiative, as in social interaction, defensive and flight behaviours or other activities required for self-preservation. Consequently, we routinely test putative anti-aggressive agents for effects upon the defensive behavioural repertoire.

One of the most frequently used models in the psychopharmacology of aggression is foot-shock induced defence or pain-induced aggression in mice or rats (Sheard, 1981). Several recent studies have shown that this kind of aggression is primarily defensive (Blanchard et al., 1977; Rodgers, 1979; Scott, 1966). Although the defensive responses are readily evoked by electric foot-shock (Ulrich and Azrin, 1962) or drugs (Sbordone et al., 1981), there are a number of difficulties in this "defensive" model. It is difficult to dissociate non-specific motor effects from specific effects on defence, whereas alterations in pain reactivity may obscure effects on behaviour. Therefore one should be very cautious in interpreting drug effects in this "defensive" model (Miczek, 1987).

A more natural model of defensive behaviour uses one of the resident-intruder paradigms described above, but focussing upon the intruder who must defend himself effectively against attack by a resident male or a lactating female (Olivier and Mos, 1986; Miczek and Krsiak, 1981; Mos et al., 1987; Rodgers, 1981). In this situation, a defending rat displays all behavioural elements occurring in natural situations: e.g., defensive upright postures, freeze-crouch postures, full submissive posture, fleeing and vocalisations (sonic and ultrasonic). This model offers an opportunity to record the effects of psychotropic agents on the complete defensive behavioural repertoire.

Foot-shock induced defence in mice

Effects upon defence activity were determined according to a modification of the test method described by Tedeschi et al. (1959). Five selected pairs of male albino mice were used for each dose of the test compound. The test compounds were orally administered to the pairs of mice in a range of doses, and the mice were tested for fighting episodes and paralysis 60 minutes later. Pairs of mice showing three or more fighting episodes within three minutes were considered as not being protected by the test compound. Lack of paralysis was assessed by the ability of mice, hanging by their forelimbs from a thin bar, to bring their hind limbs on to the bar within 3 seconds. The ED_{50}-value for anti-aggressive activity or paralysis (being the dose preventing fighting episodes in half the pairs of mice, or causing paralysis), were calculated according to the method of Horn (1956). To indicate the specificity of the anti-defence effect, the ratio paralysis/defence is given; high values indicate specific anti-defence effects, whereas low values suggest strong interfering effects from, e.g., muscle relaxation. As can be seen from Table II-2, eltoprazine has no activity in this paradigm either on defence or on muscle tone.

Fluprazine, on the other hand, shows marked activity against foot-shock induced fighting, at doses which do not influence muscle tone, which may suggest analgesic effects. Sch 12679 is far less active in this test and had only a marginal specificity, while the activity of chlordiazepoxide, diazepam, YG-19-256, chlorpromazine, amitriptyline, imipramine, desmethylimipramine and chlorimipramine were found to be non-specific. Chlordiazepoxide and diazepam (benzodiazepines) nicely illustrate their well-known muscle relaxing effects.

Table II-2
Effect on foot-shock induced defence (D) and paralysis (P) in male mice

Compound	n	Oral ED_{50}-value $\pm$ SEM (mg/kg p·o)		
		defense	paralysis	ratio P/D
Eltoprazine	1	>46.4	>46.4	n. d.
Fluprazine	3	2.4±0.6	>40	>20
Diazepam	2	6.8	2.5	0.4
Chlordiazepoxide	9	15.4±1.6	11.7±1.8	0.76
Fluvoxamine	3	>215	>215	n. d.
Sch 12679	3	32.9±3.0	64.3±18.3	1.96
YG- 19-256	1	27.1	31.0	1.14
Chlorpromazine	2	8.2	7.3	0.91
Imipramine	1	108	190	1.7
Desmethylimipramine	1	215	>215	n.d.
Chlorimipramine	1	147	176	1.2
Amitriptyline	1	27	50	1.8

Mean ED_{50}-value $\pm$ SEM of repeated experiments; n = number of experiments; n.d. = not determinable.

Defensive behaviour in rats

Those forms of agonistic behaviour in which elements of initiative and approach prevail belong to offensive aggression. This offence contrasts with defence, in which fighting is merely a response to being attacked, without initiative and essentially "reactive". Flight and submission is behaviour aimed at escaping or preventing further agonistic interactions (Dixon and Kaesermann, 1987). Some of the drugs known to suppress aggression effectively have highly undesirable effects; e.g., neuroleptics decrease activity, including social interest, whereas low doses of benzodiazepines may even increase aggression (Mos and Olivier, 1987; Mos et al., 1987). However, aggression is not always detrimental and often badly needed, e.g. in cases of being attacked (Blanchard and Blanchard, 1988).

Therefore, ideally, drugs should inhibit aggression but leave animals competent to deal with situations that require initiative and adequate defence and flight in response to threat and danger. To test the effects of drugs on this aspect of defensive/flight behaviour, we tested drug-treated male intruders in an aggression paradigm, where they will be attacked by lactating females and are strongly dependent on their own defensive capabilities to minimize injury.

For the details of the experimental set-up see the methodology described in the section on maternal aggression. In this case, not the females, but the male intruders were treated. Male intruders of the Wistar strain (CPB-TNO) were used which were approx. 25 g lower in weight than the females. All intruders were naive and used only once. Animals were treated with vehicle or drug intraperitoneally or orally, 30 min or 60 min, respectively, before testing.

Drugs and vehicles were randomized over testing days. The behaviour was recorded on video and analyzed later. Although the intruder was treated, the behaviour of both the lactating females and of the intruder was observed. In the former case only the number of attacks on the intruders was noted, whereas in the latter case the complete behavioural repertoire was scored. Always 12 intruders per dose were used. As acute treatment, eltoprazine (0, 2, 4 and 8 mg/kg, orally), haloperidol (0, 0.5, 1 and 2 mg/kg, i.p.), d-amphetamine (0, 1, 2 and 4 mg/kg, i.p.), fluprazine (0, 5, 10 and 20 mg/kg, i.p.), chlordiazepoxide (0, 5, 10 and 20 mg/kg, orally) and naloxone (0, 0.1, 1 and 10 mg/kg, i.p.) were used. Acute tests lasted 5 minutes. Eltoprazine was also tested after 7 days pre-treatment. During 7 days, and two times a day (8.00 a.m. and 8.00 p.m.) male intruder rats were treated with vehicle (0), 5, 10 or 20 mg/kg orally. Approximately 12–14 hours after the last drug administration, animals were tested for 5 min in the cage of an untreated lactating female. Tests were performed in a similar way to normal maternal aggression tests.

Figure II-14 shows the effect of acute oral treatment of eltoprazine of the intruders on the attack behaviour of the untreated females. No significant effects were noted on the frequency of bite attacks or the attack latency, although at 2 mg/kg there was a trend toward a decreased number of attacks on these intruders. This "Indirect" drug effect indicates that the qualities of eltoprazine-treated intruders to evoke aggression from the lactating females are apparently unchanged. Table II-3 shows the effects of acute oral treatment of eltoprazine on the defensive/flight behaviour of the intruders. In the defence/flight categories there is some shift from active forms of defence/flight to more passive forms; upright posture is decreased at higher doses where on back (inactive) is enhanced.

The absence of effect upon exploration (except the decrease in rearing

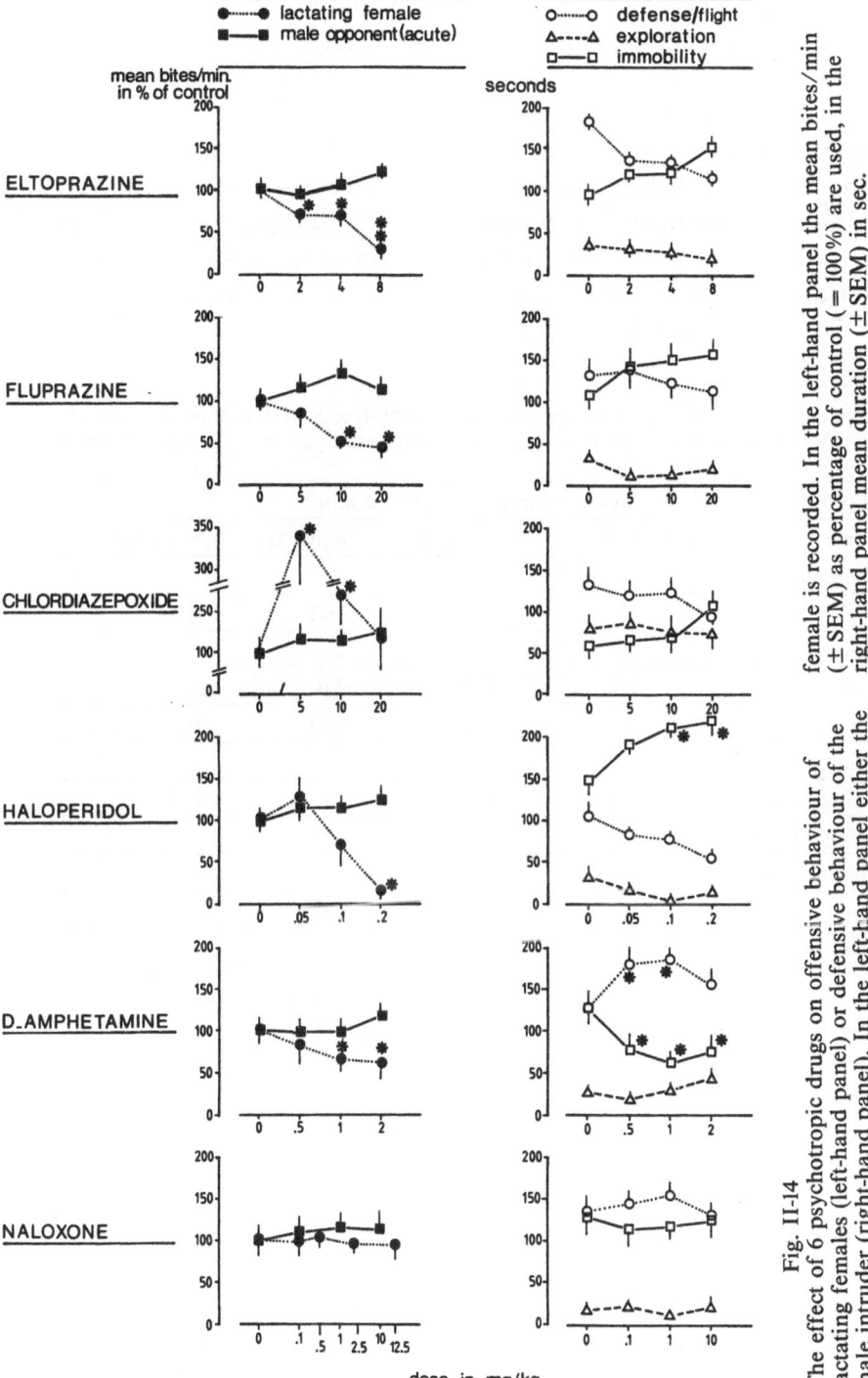

Fig. II-14

The effect of 6 psychotropic drugs on offensive behaviour of lactating females (left-hand panel) or defensive behaviour of the male intruder (right-hand panel). In the left-hand panel either the lactating female is treated (direct drug effects) or the male opponent (indirect drug effect), but in both cases the behaviour of the female is recorded. In the left-hand panel the mean bites/min (±SEM) as percentage of control (=100%) are used, in the right-hand panel mean duration (±SEM) in sec.
* : (p<0.05) denotes significant difference from vehicle (0 mg/kg).

at 8 mg/kg) and social interest, together with the lack of effect upon
flight and avoidance capabilities, suggests that the increase of inactive
behaviours after eltoprazine has not been caused by muscle relaxation
or other debilitating drug effects.

After 7 days pre-treatment with eltoprazine (0, 5, 10 and 20 mg/kg
orally b.i.d.), the behaviour of intruders, measured 12–14 hours after
the last drug administration, was not altered by this pretreatment. This
can be deduced from the indirect drug effects (Fig. II-14) which show
no effects upon the attack behaviour of the lactating females and from
the direct behavioural effects (Table II-4).

Table II-3
Effects of acute vehicle or eltoprazine treatment (p.o.) of the intruders on the
behaviour of intruders in the maternal aggression-paradigm. N = 12 animals/dose.

Behavioural Categories	Median duration (sec) / 10 min			
	0 mg/kg	2 mg/kg	4 mg/kg	8 mg/kg
Exploration				
Sniffing	13.4	8.3	14.1	6.9
Rearing	4.3	1.2	2.2	0.6*
Locomotion	6.8	8.4	7.0	8.5
Attention	6.1	2.4	0.01*	0.6
Social Interest				
Moving towards	0.0	0.0	0.0	0.0
Sniffing intruder	1.3	2.1	0.9	0.4
Defense/flight				
Flight (escape)	5.5	2.6	2.9	0.7
Avoid (evade)	2.7	4.0	2.7	2.9
On back (keep off)	147.5	93.3	95.4	106.9
Upright posture (active)	35.7	31.1	8.8*	6.7*
Crouching	22.9	19.6	24.1	31.9
On back (inactive)	1.1	80.6*	100.0*	104.8*

* significant difference from 0 mg/kg (p<0.05, t.t.)

Only a small increase in rearing at the highest dose was noted. This
may indicate that chronic pre-treatment of eltoprazine does not
induce rebound effects on defence/flight behaviour.

Figure II-14 summarises the effects of several compounds (eltoprazine, fluprazine, chlordiazepoxide (CDP), haloperidol, d-ampheta-

Table II-4

Effects on the behaviour of intruders after 7 days (2x/day) oral treatment with eltoprazine. The defensive behaviour was measured 12–14 hours after the last drug administration in the maternal aggression paradigm. N = 12 animals/dose.

Behavioral Categories	Median duration (sec) / 5 min			
	0 mg/kg	2 mg/kg	4 mg/kg	8 mg/kg
Exploration				
Sniffing	28.1	28.9	24.9	50.9
Rearing	7.8	19.8	23.5	22.9*
Locomotion	7.5	5.7	4.3	0.8
Attention	8.7	7.1	1.3	5.0
Social Interest				
Moving towards	0.0	0.0	0.0	0.0
Sniffing intruder	0.4	1.1	0.0	0.0
Defense/flight				
Flight (escape)	0.0	0.6	0.4	1.4
Avoid (evade)	2.8	3.0	2.4	2.9
On back (keep off)	34.4	37.7	57.5	64.4
Upright posture (active)	8.0	31.9	24.7	34.1
Crouching	70.7	45.1	44.0	68.3
On back (inactive)	22.8	12.7	16.4	0.0

* significant difference from 0 mg/kg (p<0.05, t.t.)

mine and naloxone) both upon the behaviour of the treated (direct drug effects) and untreated lactating female (indirect drug effects) and on the behaviour of the treated male intruders (direct drug effects). In the latter case three categories have been used to describe the behaviour: immobility, reflecting all inactive defence behaviours like inactive on back, crouching, inactive upright posture, sitting and lying; defence, reflecting all active defensive/flight elements including active upright posture, active on back (keep off lying), avoid and flight; and exploration, e.g., rearing, locomotion, attention and sniffing. Serenics (eltoprazine and fluprazine) clearly reduce the attacks of the lactating female when she is treated, but have no significant effects upon the (untreated) female when only the intruders are treated. Results of exploration, defensive behaviour and immobility of male intruder rats against lactating females are summarized in the right-hand panel of Fig. II-14. The categories attention, social interest and flight comprise only a very small proportion of total time. Moreover, no major effects were noted in these categories after drug treatment and they are therefore not shown.

The average duration of the behavioural categories shows considerable variation, which arises both from individual reactions of intruders and from variations in the intensity of offensive behaviour exhibited by individual, lactating females. Due to this variability, exploration was never significantly changed by drug treatment of the intruder.

Although d-amphetamine treatment increased exploration somewhat, most of the time was spent on defence. Haloperidol tended to decrease exploration, in accordance with the known sedative action of this drug. Fluprazine, CDP and naloxone did not affect exploration. Fluprazine, although effectively reducing Offensive aggression, does not decrease the defensive capacities of male intruders. At the highest dose, a non-significant decrease in defence is seen following CDP treatment of the intruders. Naloxone has no influence on defence, whereas defence is increased by d-amphetamine. Haloperidol reduces the time spent on defence in a dose-dependent manner, although this did not quite reach statistical significance at the 5% level. As expected, immobility increased after haloperidol and decreased after amphetamine. The other drugs, including fluprazine, did not significantly affect immobility.

In summary, drugs of various classes differentially influenced offence and defence in the maternal aggression paradigm. CDP increased aggression at lower doses but left defence intact. Haloperidol decreased both offensive and defensive behaviour. d-amphetamine suppressed offensive behaviours in the lactating females, and increased defensive behaviours of the male intruders.

Naloxone, an opiate antagonist, changed neither offence nor defensive behaviours in this maternal aggression paradigm. The probable antagonism of defeat-induced analgesia (Miczek et al., 1984) apparently does not modify the behaviour of the attacked opponent. Fluprazine and eltoprazine markedly inhibited offensive behaviours in maternal rats, but had no effect on adequate defence and flight.

These findings, although in agreement with expectations derived from the literature (Flannelly et al., 1985; Blanchard et al., 1985), suffer in part from the high levels of aggression displayed by the females in the defence experiments. This leaves little opportunity for the male intruders to display social behaviour or exploration. The clear-cut dominance of the females suppresses the extent to which social interactions may develop during the test period, and may thus mask some more subtle drug effects, notably the pro-aggressive effects claimed for amphetamine and CDP when given to the opponent (Miczek, 1974). Nevertheless, the data obtained strengthen the unique profile of the serenics in the field of aggression, defence and social stress. Since aggression usually results in wounding the opponent (Mos et al., 1984), effective control of aggressive behaviour may be very beneficial, especially for the victims. The decrease in aggression, concomitant with maintaining the integrity of social interest and defence, implies that serenics are good candidates for the effective amelioration of maladaptive social behaviour.

2.4   Predatory behaviour

Mouse killing (muricide) by rats occurs spontaneously in a proportion of rats, but not all, confronted with a mouse (Karli, 1956). There has been a lot of dispute about the nature of muricide, resulting in describing it as inter-species aggression (Karli et al., 1969), predatory aggression (Moyer, 1976; Potegal, 1979) or simply predatory behaviour (Adamec and Himes, 1978; Baenninger, 1978; O'Boyle, 1974; Rossi, 1975). The nature of this muricidal response depends on one's definition of aggression. Following Huntingford (1976), three categories of aggression can be defined according to the three main situations in which they occur: viz., social aggression between members of the same species; predatory aggression, which includes hunting, stalking and preycapturing shown by the predator towards the prey; and anti-predator aggression, which includes a prey attacking its predator. By this definition, predatory behaviour is aggressive in nature, although this aggression differs on neurophysiological, endocrinological and topographical grounds from "social" or "intraspecific" aggression (Moyer, 1976; O'Boyle, 1974). The neurophysiology of aggressive behaviour indicates that different neural substrates in the CNS are involved in different types of aggressive behaviour (Moyer, 1976; Karli, 1981). This suggests, in turn, that different experimental manipulations may have diverse results when comparing their effects on different types of aggression. The outcome of studies on muricide, therefore, cannot be used to predict general effects on aggression, but such results should be evaluated against the background of that particular type of aggression, i.e. predation.

Muricidal behaviour in rats

Adult male (400–500 g) and adult female (300–350 g) TMD-S3 rats were used. All were experienced mouse-killers, which means that they kill with a latency of less than 1 min after intrusion of a mouse. They were individually housed in macrolon cages ($30 \times 20 \times 15$ cm). Day-night rhythm was reversed (day 19.00 to 7.00 hrs). The observations were facilitated by dim light during the experiments. An experiment started with intraperitoneal injection (30 minutes before testing) of the S3-animal with saline or the test compound(s). Thirty minutes after injection, a mouse (female DAP) was placed in the cage of the S3-rat and the time (in minutes) when the mouse was killed was noted for the following 30 or 120 minutes. Afterwards the mouse was removed.

For oral administration the same procedure was used, except that drugs were given 60 minutes before testing using 1% tragacanth as vehicle.

Rats treated with placebo (saline) all killed the mouse within one minute of its intrusion into the cage. The i.p. effects of drugs are shown in Table II-5 (left columns) giving the LEDs for each drug. Eltoprazine inhibited muricide in both males and females, although to a lesser extent in the latter. A considerable number of drugs with diverse mechanisms of action may exert inhibitory effects on muricide.

TFMPP, a rather specific 5-HT$_{1B}$-agonist, quite potently inhibited this behaviour. Several other serotonergic drugs (5-HT-reuptake blocker (fluvoxamine), 5MeODMT (agonist), RU24969 (agonist), fenfluramine (release), fluprazine (weak agonist), quipazine (agonist), inhibited muricidal behaviour, while others, such as chlorpromazine, scopolamine, d-amphetamine, haloperidol and dl-propranolol, did so also, suggesting that inhibition of muricidal behaviour merely represents a measure of psychoactivity of drugs. However, some drugs, like 8-OH-DPAT (a 5-HT$_{1A}$-agonist), naloxone (opiate-antagonist), ipsapirone (and to a lesser extent buspirone), methysergide and chlordiazepoxide, do not affect muricidal behaviour.

In general, drugs (excepting TFMPP) are less potent (on a mg/kg basis) in females than in males.

Table II-5 (right column) shows the lowest effective doses (LED) after oral drug treatment. Eltoprazine inhibits muricide at 20 mg/kg p.o. Fluprazine inhibits muricide at 32 mg/kg orally and TFMPP at 3 mg/kg p.o. Chlordiazepoxide and diazepam, both benzodiazepines, have no influence up to 32 and 20 mg/kg orally respectively. Haloperidol (8 mg/kg) also inhibits muricidal behaviour, whereas chlorpromazine could not be determined, due to toxic side-effects.

Compared with the i.p. route, oral treatment of compounds in this muricidal model in S3-male rats seems very ineffective, as indicated by ratios of oral/i.p. of 3 to 80.

Table II-5
Inhibition of muricidal behaviour 30 min (i.p.) or 60 min (p.o.) after drug administration is expressed as the Lowest Effective Dose (LED) which significantly inhibits mouse killing.

	Lowest Effective Dose (mg/kg)			
Route of administration	intraperitoneal		oral	
Drug	in males	in females	in males	Ratio oral / i.p. in males
Eltoprazine	5	1.5	20	4
TFMPP	1	0.5	~3	3
Fluprazine	8	3	32	4
Naloxone	>10	n.t.	n.t.	–
5-Me-0-DMT	1	~5	n.t.	
Quipazine	4	4	n.t.	–
Chlorpromazine	5	n.t.	>20*	>4
Scopolamine	0.5	>2	n.t.	
d-Amphetamine	0.5	1.5	n.t.	
Ipsapirone	>10	n.t.	n.t.	
Buspirone	~20	~20	n.t.	–
Fluvoxamine	~20	~10	>50	>2.5
RU24969	1	2	n.t.	–
8-OH-DPAT (s.c.)	>5	>0.2	n.t.	
Fenfluramine	~2	~4	n.t.	–
Haloperidol	0.1	1	8	80
dl-propranolol	~10	n.t.	n.t.	–
Methysergide	>20	>30	n.t.	
Chlordiazepoxide	>20	n.t.	>32	n.d.
Diazepam	>20	n.t.	>20	n.d.

n.t. = not tested; n.d. = not determinable.
* indicates that at that dose toxic symptoms precluded higher dosing.

2.5   Discussion

Table II-6 compares the effects of eltoprazine with several psycho-tropics from a variety of drug classes in several paradigms involving both offensive and defensive components of agonistic behaviour and in a model of predatory behaviour. In general, eltoprazine exemplifies the very specific inhibition of the offensive components of agonistic interactions without material effects upon flight, defensive and social capabilities (Olivier et al., 1986). In models involving spontaneous offensive behaviour in male mice and rats (viz. isolation-induced aggression in mice, intermale aggression in mice and rats, resident-intruder aggression in rats, colony aggression in rats), eltoprazine typically reduces the offensive components of agonistic behaviour concomitant with enhanced social interest. Defensive behaviour in these paradigms is not directly affected and sedation, muscle relaxa-tion or motor/sensory impairment is not found at doses which clearly inhibit offensive behaviour. In this profile, eltoprazine is comparable to other serenics like DU 27725, TFMPP, fluprazine or DU 28412 (Olivier and Van Dalen 1982; Olivier et al., 1986, 1984a,b; Olivier, 1981; Bradford et al., 1984).

This very specific "serenic" profile has not been found in any other drug tested so far (table II-6). Other drugs claimed to have specific anti-aggressive activity such as YG-19256 (Owen, 1980; Roubicek et al., 1972) and Sch-12679 (Itil and Mukhopadhyay, 1978) have very non-specific profiles in these naturalistic animal paradigms (Olivier and van Dalen, 1982; Olivier et al., 1986; Olivier et al., 1984a,b). Moreover, other drugs, among them some which have been used clinically to attempt management of aggressive behaviours (Sheard 1983, 1984), have no apparent anti-aggressive activity (e.g., anxiolytics) or also have non-specific activity (typically sedation) which inhibits aggressive or agitated behaviour only at the cost of generalized depression of all behaviours.

Another paradigm, EBS or hypothalamically-induced aggression, has supported the specificity of the serenics, including eltoprazine. This EBS-model is a very potent offence paradigm in which aggression can be evoked directly by stimulation of the neural structures involved in aggression (Kruk and van der Poel, 1980; Mos et al., 1987). In this model, the serenics inhibit only aggressive elements (including teeth-chattering), while other drugs have no effect or quite non-specific effects in this paradigm. In addition, both eltoprazine (unpublished) and fluprazine inhibit aggression in both males and females in a comparable way (Kruk et al., 1984). This gender-independent effect of serenics suggests that their behavioural effects are apparently independent of androgens. Although the predictive value of these models will finally be determined only when there has been adequate clinical work, it is tempting to speculate that such an EBS paradigm may prove to be one of the most valid for identifying drugs intended for the treatment of pathological forms of aggressive or hostile behaviours in man.

Finally, eltoprazine (as well as fluprazine and TFMPP) has potent anti-aggressive effects in a model of female aggression: maternal aggression in lactating rats. Not only is the behavioural profile in this model different from that found in models of spontaneous male aggression, but this model also detects unique differences in the pharmacological profiles of drugs. Anxiolytics (e.g., chlordiazepoxide), at least at low doses, increased aggression in this paradigm (Olivier et al., 1985; Mos and Olivier, 1986; Mos et al., 1987 a, b; Olivier and Mos, 1989), but such aggression-enhancing doses of CDP did not antagonize the dose-dependent decrease after fluprazine (Olivier et al., 1986). Currently, about 50 different drugs from different classes have been tested in maternal aggression but none (excepting perhaps RU24969) showed a clear serenic profile (Olivier et al., 1986, 1987; Olivier and Mos, 1986).

Eltoprazine was active in a model of agonistic behaviour in juvenile rats, i.e., play-fighting, again without unwanted side-effects.

On the other hand, chlordiazepoxide increased play-fighting. These data show that young and adult animals react in a similar way to drugs which suggests that serenics may also influence juvenile forms of aggressive or hostile behaviours in humans.

Eltoprazine was, unlike fluprazine, very active in a porcine aggression model without disturbing side-effects, especially without sedation, and quite different in this respect from a much used sedative neuroleptic, azaperone.

As would be expected of a drug with specific anti-offensive effects, eltoprazine was not active in shock-induced fighting, a model of defensive aggression. However, when eltoprazine was given acutely to intruders who were subsequently attacked by lactating females, the defensive strategy of the treated intruders was somewhat altered,

Table II-6

Summary of effects in agonistic paradigms. ↑ = increase; alcohol (g/kg). ED_{50} = dose that gives 50% suppression of ↓ = decrease; ∅ = no effect; – = not tested; sp = specific effect; aggression. LED = Lowest Effective Dose. nsp = nonspecific effect. Doses are given in mg/kg, except for

Paradigms	Elto prazine	Flupra zine	Chlordia zepoxide	Halo peridol	Chlor promazine	d-Amphet amine	Alcohol	TFMPP	Fluvox amine	RU24969	8OH-DPAT	Buspirone
Offense												
Isolation-induced aggr. in mice(ED_{50})	↓0.39 po / ↓0.1 ip	↓1.2 po / ↓0.7 ip	↓73 po	↓<1 po	↓4.7 po	↓4 po	>3 g/kg po	↓0.2 po	↓70 po	↓0.7 po	↓0.3 ip	>20 po
Social Interaction in mice (LED)	<0.5 po ↓sp	<1.25 po ↓sp	>15 po ↓nsp	<1 po ↓nsp	3 po ↓nsp	–	–	<1.25 po ↓sp	<25 po ↓nsp	<1 po ↓nsp	<1 ip ↓nsp	1.0 ip ↓nsp
Resident-intruder aggr. in rats (LED)	<1.25 po ↓sp	5 po ↓sp	5–10 po ↑↓ >20 po	0.1 ip ↓nsp	–	0.5 ip ↓nsp	∅(>3 g/kg) po	1 ip ↓sp	5 ip ↓nsp	0.25 sc ↓sp	0.1 sc ↓nsp	2 ip ↓nsp
Colony aggression in male rats (LED)	<2.5 po ↓sp	<16 po ↓sp	5–10 po ↑↓ 20 po	–	–	–	∅-62 g/kg po	–	–	–	–	–
Hypothalamic-ind. aggr. in rats (LED)	<2 po ↓sp	4 po ↓sp	∅>20po nsp	<0.5 ip ↓nsp	–	∅(<2 ip) po	∅(2 g/kg) ↓sp	0.5 ip ↓nsp	10 ip	–	∅(>1.0 ip) –	–
Maternal aggression in female rats (LED)	2 po ↓sp	5 ip ↓sp	5–10 po ↑↓ >20 po	0.1 ip ↓nsp	–	1 ip ↓nsp	∅(>2 g/kg) po	0.5 ip ↓sp	20 ip ↓nsp	0.5 ip ↓sp	0.1 ip ↓nsp	2.0 ip ↓
Play fighting in juvenile rats (LED)	<2 po ↓sp	–	5–10 ip ↑↓ >20 ip	–	–	–	–	–	–	–	–	–
Aggression in pigs	↓2.5 im / ↓10 im sp	>30 im	–	–	–	–	–	–	–	–	–	–
Defense												
Shock-induced defense in mice (ED_{50})	>46.4 po	↓2.4 po sp	↓15.4 po nsp	–	↓8.2 po nsp	–	–	–	–	–	–	–
Defensive/flight of intruder	∅ unchanged strategy	∅ unchanged strategy	∅ changed strategy	→ changed strategy	–	→ changed strategy	–	–	–	–	–	–
Predation												
mouse killing in rats (LED)	↓5 ip / ↓20 po sp	↓8 ip / ↓32 po sp	∅>20 ip / ∅>32 po	↓0.1 ip / ↓8 po nsp	↓5 ip / ↓>20 po nsp	↓0.5 ip nsp	–	↓1.0 ip / ↓3 po sp	↓20 ip / ∅>50 po	↓1 ip sp / sp	∅>5 ip	∅20 ip –

although the animals were fully capable of all behavioural elements in the defensive repertoire. That is, there were no signs of motor deficit or other debilitating effects. In contrast, for example, haloperidol or d-amphetamine showed a number of such non-specific effects.

When intruders were treated for seven days with eltoprazine, no behavioural effects were noted when these animals were subsequently tested as intruders against attackers. Finally, eltoprazine, like a number of drugs from other drug classes, inhibited predatory aggression, viz. muricidal behaviour in male and female rats.

Eltoprazine was, after a 7-day pre-treatment in intermale aggression in mice, able to inhibit aggression without significant tolerance, while also no rebound effects were noted. In male rat aggression paradigms, there were some indications of (mild) tolerance.

While there are similarities between eltoprazine (and other serenics) and other drugs in one or another of the animal models, there is no other drug which, to our knowledge, shows such a consistent inhibition of offensive behaviour across several disparate models without concomitant suppression of other major components of physical or behavioural function. It is to describe this very specific behavioural profile that we have suggested this class of compounds should carry the cognomen "serenics".

While the effects of these drugs in animal models do not, in themselves, prove that similar (or similarly specific) effects will be found if these compounds are administered to man, there are several factors to suggest such similarities.

However, we would contend, regardless of what similarities of effects may or may not be found, that the very specificity of these drugs in disparate animal models strongly supports two very positive speculations:

1. The development of new animal models in ethopharmacology can lead in turn to the discovery and characterisation of compounds with novel psychotropic activity. In this way, psychopharmacology can move beyond the constraints of "me-too" models and drugs.

2. Drugs with an activity affecting only specific components of complex behavioural systems are feasible. Although the serenics, even in the animal models, may not yet be the "magic bullet", they are rather more rifle than shotgun. This encourages belief that drugs with effects significantly more specific than many in common use can be anticipated when better modelling techniques are perfected.

3   **Mechanism of action of serenics**

This section focusses on the presumed mechanism of action of
serenics as exemplified by a number of representative drugs. Most
studies have been performed on eltoprazine as a representative compound of the class. However, the behavioural profile of TFMPP, RU
24969 and fluprazine is to a large extent comparable to eltoprazine,
thus these compounds will be used to show the generality of the
principles of the mechanism of action. Since these compounds have
received less thorough attention, some caution is needed in the
extrapolation of the data of eltoprazine to general principles underlying a serenic action. Moreover, the mechanistic studies have largely
used rodent species which further limits possible generalizations. First
we will describe the results of receptor binding studies, followed by
autoradiographic studies narrowing the scope to serotonergic receptors. Neurochemical properties will then be presented. At the behavioural level drug discrimination experiments shed light on the relative
contribution of different serotonergic receptor subtypes involved in
the action of eltoprazine. Finally the site of action of serenics in the
CNS has been investigated.

3.1   Receptor binding

In the early days of the search for specific anti-aggressive compounds,
a behavioural screening was used extensively. In the 80's the rapid
development of receptor binding techniques and the discovery of
subtypes for various neurotransmitters began to play an important
role in unravelling the mode of action of drugs. The most prominent
feature of serenic compounds appeared to be their affinity for the
serotonin receptor. Later developments have subsequently shown that
a considerable number of receptors exist, ranging from $5\text{-}HT_1$ to 5-HT.
Within this division various subtypes exist. In table 3.1 the affinities of
eltoprazine, RU 24969, TFMPP and serotonin are presented for a
number of receptors. It is clear that eltoprazine is a mixed $5\text{-}HT_1$
ligand, similar to TFMPP. Compared to the natural agonist serotonin
the affinity is somewhat lower. The $5\text{-}HT_2$ affinity is too far away from
the other affinities to play an important role, but the $5\text{-}HT_3$ affinity is
rather potent.
Unpublished observations have suggested that eltoprazine is a weak

5-HT$_3$ antagonist compared to for example ondansetron and other established 5-HT$_3$ antagonists (Olivier et al., 1992). Since the 5-HT$_3$ antagonists MDL 72222 and ondansetron have no anti-aggressive properties whatsoever (Mos et al., 1990), it seems unlikely that the affinity of serenics for the 5-HT$_3$ receptor is crucial for their anti-aggressive action.

Of the other significant affinities, the β-receptor affinity deserves special attention. Since for example ($\pm$)-propranolol and ($\pm$)-pindolol have been found anti-aggressive in animal aggression models (Olivier et al., 1993; Da Vanzo, 1988) as well as clinically this affinity might be responsible for the anti-aggressive actions. Several arguments can be used to refute this idea. First it should be noted that propranolol as well as pindolol have significant 5-HT$_{1B}$ affinity, which could explain their anti-aggressive actions as well. Second, we (Olivier et al., 1993) found (-)-timolol, a β-adrenergic antagonist without 5-HT affinity, without any effect on aggression. In drug-discrimination studies (see later) both pindolol and propranolol substitute for eltoprazine, but again timolol did not generalize to the eltoprazine cue (Ybema et al., 1992). In mice (Da Vanzo, 1988; Yoshimura et al., 1987) the differential activity of β-blockers in suppressing aggression has also been noted. In summary, the evidence points to modulation of the 5-HT$_{1B}$ receptor as the responsible mechanism, rather than a β-adrenergic mechanism. Other affinities that possibly play a role in modulating the activity of eltoprazine are those for the α_1 and α_2 receptor. Functional in vivo studies only have suggested weak partial agonism and it seems unlikely that these actions explain the anti-aggressive actions.

3.2   Autoradiographic studies

Autoradiography can be elegantly used to compare the binding of eltoprazine with the natural agonist serotonin.

Sijbesma et al. (1990) have performed detailed autoradiographic studies using [^{3}H]-eltoprazine, [^{3}H]-serotonin and the selective 5-HT$_{1A}$ agonist [^{3}]H-8-OH-DPAT. In vitro autoradiographic studies with [^{3}H]-eltoprazine demonstrate a widespread but heterogenous distribution throughout the rat brain (fig. III-1).

Nearly all the binding is to grey matter areas with non-significant levels present in white matter tracts such as the corpus callosum. The nonspecific binding, obtained either in the presence of 1 μM 5-HT or

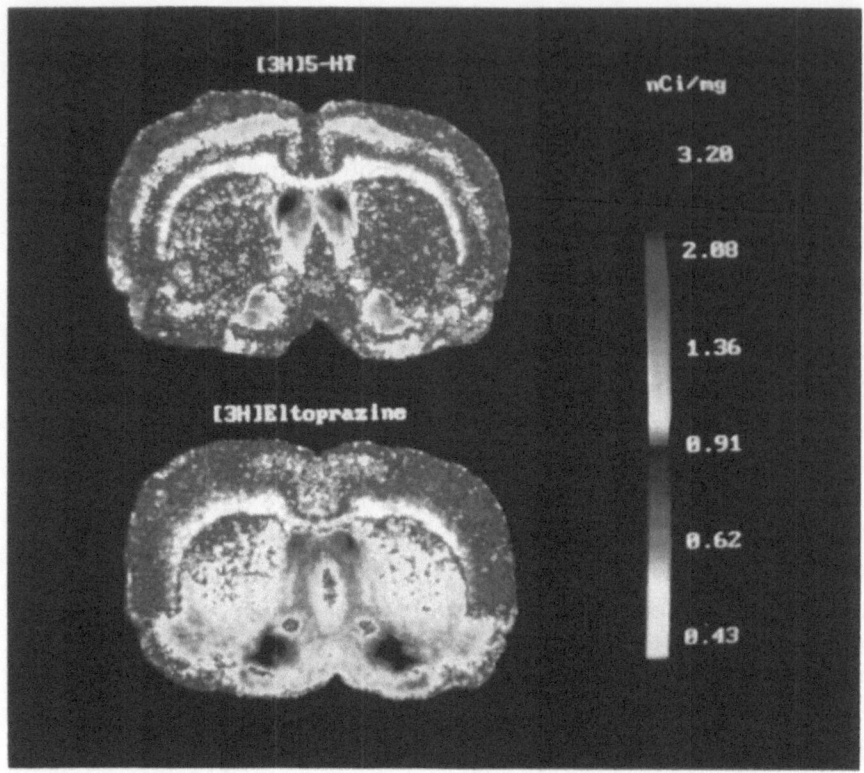

Fig. III-1

Comparison between [³H]-5-HT and [³H]-eltoprazine binding sites in coronal sections of rat brain. The images are bright-field photographs of digitized and colour-coded autoradiograms generated from adjacent coronal brain sections (20 μm) incubated with either 1.8 nM [³H]-5-HT or 12 nM [³H]-eltoprazine.

1 μM eltoprazine, results in virtually blank images. The highest specific [³H]-eltoprazine binding is found in substantia nigra, dorsal subiculum and basal ganglia (ventral pallidum and globus pallidus). Relatively high specific binding is also present in limbic structures, such as the dentate gyrus and CA_1-CA_2 region of the hippocampus, as well as in entorhinal cortex, lateral septum, central grey and dorsal raphe nucleus.

Table III-1
Receptor Binding Profiles
>:>10,000 nM

Compound: Receptor	Serotonin K_i(nM)	Eltopraz. K_i(nM)	RU-24969 K_i(nM)	TFMPP K_i(nM)
α_1-adrenergic	>	790	1,200	1,300
α_2-adrenergic	>	3,100	2,800	1,700
$\beta_{1,2}$-adrenergic	>	420	680	950
dopamine-D_1	3,800	>	>	>
dopamine-D_2	>	1,100	1,300	810
dopamine-D_3	>	>	>	620
5-HT$_{1A}$	4.2	40	8.7	200
5-HT$_{1B}$	3.6	52	5.9	49
5-HT$_{1C}$	4.3	81	48	13
5-HT$_{1D}$	3.4	390	42	690
5-HT$_2$	1,300	1,700	1,700	780
5-HT$_3$	360	25	1,500	240
5-HT$_{uptake}$	890	>	280	1,300
tryptamine	1,600	>	>	>
histamine-H_1	>	3,900	>	2,500
muscarine-M_1	>	>	1,500	5,800
muscarine-M_2	>	>	>	>
muscarine-M_3	>	>	>	>
μ-opiate	1,400	>	6,300	>
κ-opiate	>	>	>	>
δ-opiate	>	>	>	>
Ca^{++}$_{chan}$-(DHP)	>	>	>	>
Ca^{++}$_{chan}$-(VER)	>	>	3,100	510
Na$^+$$_{chan}$-(BTX)	>	>	9,800	10,000
benzodiazepine	>	>	>	>
GABA$_A$	>	>	>	>
glycine	>	>	>	>
TRH	>	>	>	>
sigma (σ)	9,300	9,300	2,300	300
LTD$_4$	>	>	>	>
CCK(CNS)	>	>	>	>
CCK(pancreas)	>	>	>	>
Substance P	>	>	>	>
NMDA	>	>	>	>

Areas containing moderate levels of [^{3}H]eltoprazine binding sites include the amygdala, the hypothalamus, the caudate putamen, the superior colliculus and the medial raphe nucleus. The cerebral cortex, thalamic nuclei and the cerebellum expressed only low densities of binding sites.

superior colliculus and the medial raphe nucleus. The cerebral cortex, thalamic nuclei and the cerebellum expressed only low densities of binding sites.

The overall distribution of [³H]eltoprazine binding sites bears a strong resemblance to the location of 5-HT binding sites labelled by [³H]5-HT. Furthermore, [³H]eltoprazine binding is reduced to levels of nonspecific binding by low concentrations (0.1 μM) of unlabelled 5-HT. Brain areas containing high amounts of 5-HT$_{1B}$ sites (e.g. ventral pallidum and caudate putamen) exhibit relatively more [³H]eltoprazine binding as compared to [³H]5-HT binding, while relatively dense [³H]5-HT binding is present in areas enriched in 5-HT$_{1A}$ sites such as lateral septum, and the internal layers of the cerebral cortex (fig. III-1). Also, the choroid plexus of ventricles, which mainly contains 5-HT$_{1C}$ sites, shows higher levels of [³H]5-HT than of [³H]eltoprazine binding. Saturation analyses with [³H]eltoprazine and [³H]5-HT demonstrate high affinity binding of both ligands in many brain regions. Their apparent dissociation constants (K_D) and maximal binding capacities (B_{max}) in a few selected frontal brain areas are presented in table III-2. [³H]-5-HT has almost equal affinity for the various anatomical regions, whereas the K_D values of [³H]eltoprazine are consistently higher in 5-HT$_{1A}$ as compared to 5-HT$_{1B}$ receptor dense areas.

Table III-2
Saturation analysis of [³H]5-HT and [³H]eltoprazine binding in coronal rat brain sections as determined by quantitative autoradiography

Brain areas	[³H]5-HT		[³H]eltoprazine	
	K_D (nM)	B_{max} (fmol/mg)	K_D (nM)	B_{max} (fmol/mg)
5-HT$_{1A}$ regions				
Parietal cortex lamina IV-VI	1.3±0.24	57±1.8	9.1±0.99	55±3.9
Septal nuclei	1.5±0.26	319±11.9	9.5±0.73	278±5.9
5-HT$_{1B}$ regions				
Ventral pallidum	1.4±0.31	298±22.8	4.3±0.42	337 ±6.7
Caudate putamen	1.9±0.28	72±3.8	5.8±0.65	79±4.1

The autoradiographic studies were performed in rats and guinea pigs because these species differ with respect to the 5-HT$_{1B/D}$ receptor. The rat brain contains 5-HT$_{1B}$ receptors which are closely related to the more ubiquitous occurring 5-HT$_{1D}$ receptor which also occurs in humans. Molecular biological studies have confirmed that these receptors belong to the same family, but functional studies have shown important species differences. In the rat the distribution of eltoprazine followed the distribution of 5-HT$_{1B}$ receptors more closely than that of 5-HT$_{1A}$ receptors. This confirms the significant 5-HT$_{1B}$ and 5-HT$_{1A}$ affinity of eltoprazine, but also suggest that in rats the 5-HT$_{1B}$ plays an important functional role in the mechanism of action. In guinea pigs however, the distribution of [^{3}H]-eltoprazine binding sites showed a good correlation with that of the 5-HT$_{1A}$ sites (Sijbesma et al., 1991), thereby confirming the absence of 5-HT$_{1B}$ sites in guinea pig brain. Notwithstanding the apparent absence of 5-HT$_{1B}$ mediated activity of eltoprazine in the guinea pig, eltoprazine exerts anti-aggressive actions in this species (Mak et al., 1993).

The binding of [^{3}H]-eltoprazine has also been studied, although in less detail, in postmortem brain tissue of monkey and human. In these species, we found, similar to the guinea pig, a preferential binding of [^{3}H]-eltoprazine to brain regions containing high levels of 5-HT$_{1A}$ recognition sites (e.g. hippocampus, dorsal raphe and entorhinal cortex), which could be displaced by unlabelled 8-OH-DPAT. In addition, significant levels of [^{3}H]-eltoprazine binding sites were observed in the choroid plexus, which mainly comprises 5-HT$_{1C}$ receptor sites. Specific [^{3}H]-eltoprazine binding was virtually absent in brain regions predominantly containing 5-HT$_{1D}$ recognition sites (e.g. putamen and substantia nigra). Interestingly, eltoprazine has been shown to inhibit offensive aggression in both pigs (Olivier et al., 1987) and vervet monkeys (McGuire and Raleigh, unpublished results) without causing sedation.

3.3   Neurochemistry

As a representative of the serenics, we will present data on the neurochemical effects of eltoprazine, in comparison to reference compounds. By and large TFMPP and fluprazine have similar effects, but RU 24969 has additional effects on dopaminergic neurotransmission. The neurochemical experiments were mainly aimed at the establishment of the serotonergic properties of eltoprazine since receptor binding and autoradiography had already shown the importance of serotonin in the serenic activity of those drugs.

The functional 5-HT$_{1A}$ activity of eltoprazine was assessed in a model using the forskolin-stimulated c-AMP production in rat hippocampal slices. The selective 5-HT$_{1A}$ agonist 8-OH-DPAT induces a concentration-dependent inhibition of forskolin stimulated adenylate cyclase activity (for details see Schipper et al., 1990).

Under those conditions is the maximal inhibition $23\pm3\%$, whereas 50% inhibition of the maximal effect (IC_{50}-value) occurs at 4 nM. The selective 5-HT_{1A} agonist flesinoxan induced an inhibition of adenylate cyclase activity comparable to 8-OH-DPAT. The maximal inhibition of flesinoxan was $24\pm2\%$ and the IC_{50}-value value 3 nM. In this functional model for 5-HT_{1A} receptor activity, eltoprazine inhibited adenylate cyclase activity, reaching significance only at the highest concentration tested (1 μM). The maximal response, however, is $16\pm5\%$, which is 70% of the maximal effect obtained by 8-OH-DPAT. Thus eltoprazine behaves as a partial 5-HT_{1A} agonist and is considerably less potent than the prototypical 5-HT_{1A} agonists 8-OH-DPAT and flesinoxan.

5-HT_{1B} receptors occur both presynaptically at the nerve terminal (autoreceptor) and postsynaptically. 5-HT release from the terminal is under influence of the 5-HT_{1B} autoreceptor. Agonists inhibit the release of 5-HT after K^+ stimulation. The effects of eltoprazine and TFMPP on the 5-HT_{1B} autoreceptor in rats were determined, using 5-HT as the natural ligand.

The K^+ stimulated release of [^3H]-5-HT from cortex slices is inhibited by exogenous 5-HT. As illustrated in fig. III-2, 5-HT induced a dose-dependent inhibition, which resulted in a maximal inhibition of about 70% of the control values. Based on these dose response curves, the pD_2 value of 5-HT was estimated at 7.7 ± 0.1 in 10 independent experiments. Eltoprazine also inhibited the K^+ stimulated 5-HT release, but the maximal inhibition is much lower than that of 5-HT. The pD_2 value of eltoprazine was estimated at 7.8 ± 0.1 with an intrinsic activity (α) of 0.5 ± 0.1 based on 4 independent experiments. 8-OH-DPAT up to concentrations of 1 μM was inactive (see fig. III-2). TFMPP inhibited the K^+ stimulated 5-HT release, with a similar affinity ($pD_2 = 7.5\pm0.1$) as eltoprazine, but with a slightly higher intrinsic value ($\alpha = 0.7\pm0.1$).

In summary, the mixed 5-HT_1 compounds eltoprazine and TFMPP act as partial agonists at the 5-HT_{1B} autoreceptor. The potencies are high enough to expect a significant in vivo effect on 5-HT_{1B} receptors, in contrast to 8-OH-DPAT.

Besides the 5-$HT_{1A/1B}$ affinity, eltoprazine possesses significant 5-HT_{1C} affinity. A functional model to test eltoprazine's activity is the choroid

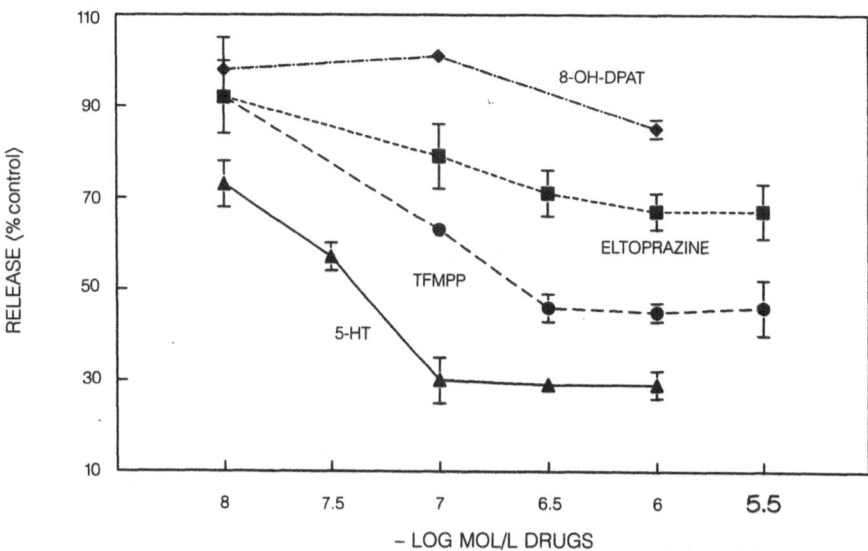

Fig. III-2

Concentration curves of eltoprazine, 5-HT, TFMPP, and 8-OH-DPAT on K⁺-stimula-
ted release of [³H]-5-HT from neocortical rat slices. Data are means ± SEM of values
from four measurements and are expressed as % of control (= 100%).

plexus of the pig which contains a high density of 5-HT_{1C} receptors.
These receptors are functionally linked to the phosphoinositol pathway. Stimulation of the 5-HT_{1C} receptors results in an increased PI
turnover as measured by the inositol phosphate accumulation in the
presence of lithium (Conn et al., 1986). In our experiments, 5-HT
induced a 7-fold increase in the inositol phosphate accumulation in
the choroid plexus as illustrated in fig. III-3. In this functional 5-HT_{1C}
model, eltoprazine and 8-OH-DPAT have no stimulatory effects on
the PI turnover as shown in fig. III-3. This is in contrast to TFMPP
which increased PI turnover about fourfold, suggesting (partial)
agonistic properties in this model.

To evaluate the antagonistic properties on 5-HT_{1C} receptors, the
effects of compounds were studied in the presence of 1 μM 5-HT. The
5-HT_{1C} antagonist mianserine reduced the 5-HT induced increase of
PI turnover (see fig. III-4), with an IC_{50} of 0.05 μM. Spiperone, a
compound with high affinity for the 5-HT_2 receptor, did not inhibit the
5-HT induced effects on PI turnover in concentrations up to 1 μM.
Eltoprazine was able to inhibit the 5-HT induced stimulation of PI
turnover (see fig. III-4), but these antagonist properties occur at rather
high concentrations (IC_{50} is 7 μM).

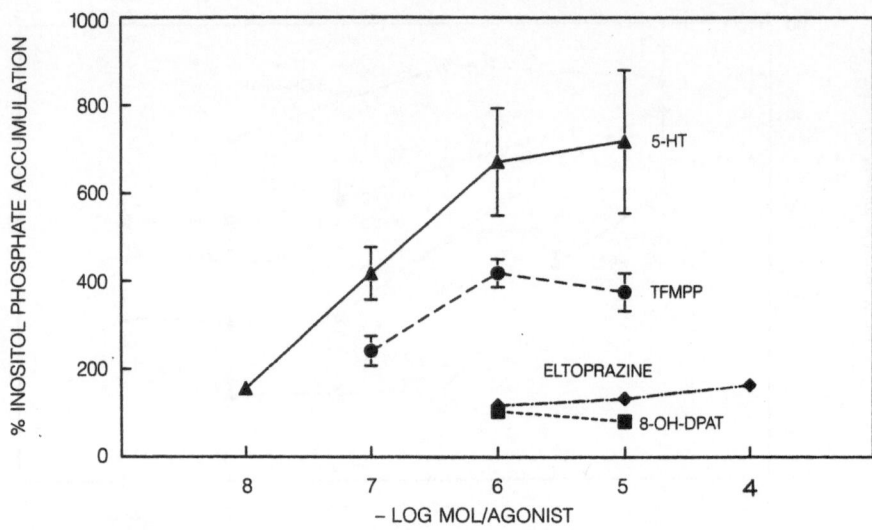

Fig. III-3

Concentration curves of eltoprazine, 5-HT, TFMPP and 8-OH-DPAT on phosphatidyl inositol turnover in pig choroid plexus. Each point is the mean ± SEM of 6 determinations and the data are presented as % stimulation above basal (= 100%).

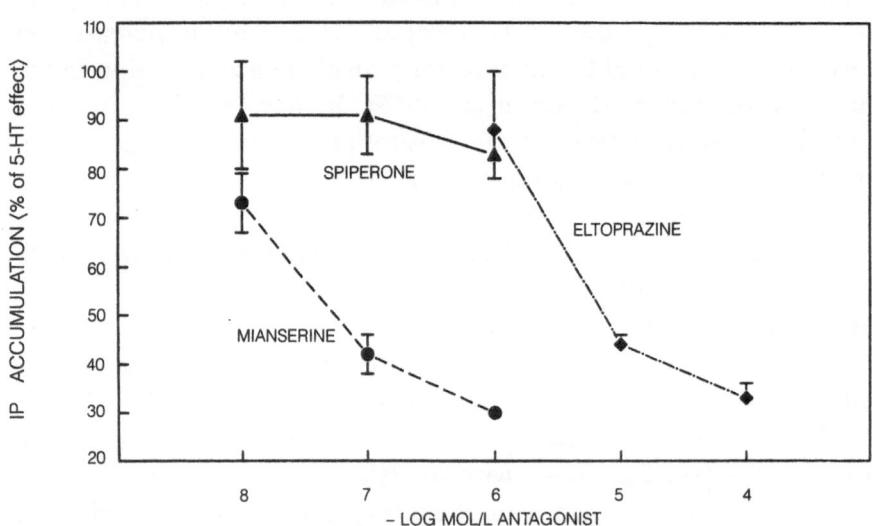

Fig. III-4

Concentration curves of eltoprazine, mianserine and spiperone on 5-HT stimulated phosphatidyl inositol turnover in pig choroid plexus. The data are presented as % of the maximal response occurring without antagonist added. Each point is the mean ± SEM of 6 determinations.

In summary, the in vitro functional tests suggest a mixed $5\text{-HT}_{1A/1B}$ agonistic profile of eltoprazine and TFMPP, but the 5-HT_{1C} actions of eltoprazine and TFMPP are opposite. To further evaluate the role of eltoprazine in vivo, several other experiments were performed.

Eltoprazine did not affect 5-HT levels in the striatum of the rat (table III-3), but levels of its major metabolite 5-hydroxy indole acetic acid (5-HIAA) were decreased at doses of 10 mg/kg p.o. and higher. The decreased 5-HIAA levels without a change in 5-HT levels are generally found with 5-HT agonists and excludes MAO inhibiting or 5-HT releasing properties. At doses of 3 and 10 mg/kg, which are effective in inhibiting aggressive behaviour, eltoprazine has no significant effects on the DA system. At high doses of 30 mg/kg p.o. eltoprazine shows no effect on DA levels, but a small increase in its major metabolites, 3,4-dihydroxyphenylacetic acid (DOPAC) and homovanillic acid (HVA), is observed.

Table III-3
Effects of eltoprazine on dopamine, serotonin and their metabolites in rat striatum

Dose (mg/kg po)	% of control (mean ± SEM)				
	DOPAC	HVA	DA	5-HT	5-HIAA
Eltoprazine 0	100±5	100±3	100±3	100±4	100±8
3	100±10	97±9	101±10	107±7	91±7
10	129±13	112±9	88±6	102±4	74±8*
30	166±18*	138±16	88±9	97±4	82±7*

* $p<0.05$, Student t-test (2-tailed); the levels (ng/g tissue) in vehicle treated animals were for DOPAC: 464±21; HVA: 756±38; DA: 10444±277; 5-HT: 378±32; 5-HIAA: 260±11.

The effects of eltoprazine on 5-HT turnover were studied as well. After inhibition of the aromatic L-amino-acid decarboxylase by NSD 1015, 5-hydroxytryptophan (5-HTP) accumulates in brain regions containing 5-HT terminals. The rate of accumulation of 5-HTP has been used as an index of 5-HT turnover (Carlsson et al., 1972).

Eltoprazine decreased 5-HTP accumulation as shown in fig. III-5 at doses as low as 0.3 mg/kg p.o. Maximal inhibition of 60% of the 5-HTP accumulation was obtained at oral doses of 3 mg/kg of eltoprazine. 8-OH-DPAT is more potent than eltoprazine in inhibiting the 5-HTP accumulation (fig. III-5), whereas TFMPP is slightly less potent than eltoprazine.

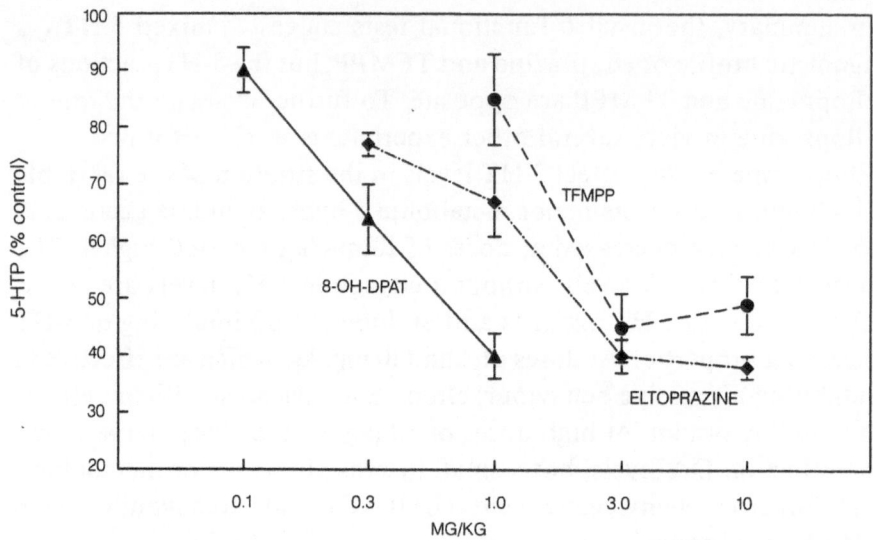

Fig. III-5

Effects of eltoprazine, TFMPP and 8-OH-DPAT on 5-HTP accumulation in the striatum of rats. All animals received the decarboxylase inhibitor NSD 1015 (100 mg/kg) 30 minutes before decapitation. 8-OH-DPAT was i.p. injected, the other drugs were given orally, all one hour before decapitation. Results are shown as % of control levels (100%). Data are means ± SEM of 6 observations in each group.

The collective data from receptor binding studies, autoradiography and neurochemistry strongly indicate the importance of mixed 5-HT$_1$ activity in the behavioural actions of eltoprazine. Probably the 5-HT$_{1A/1B}$ subtype are more involved than the 5-HT$_{1C}$ site which has been shown to differ between serenics (both agonists and antagonists are found). Several questions still remain unsettled, because 5-HT$_{1A}$ receptors occur both on the cell body of the serotonergic neuron as well as postsynaptically. The 5-HT$_{1B}$ receptor is also localized at two different sites, i.e. presynaptically as an autoreceptor as well as postsynaptically. Thus both the 5-HT$_{1A}$ and/or the 5-HT$_{1B}$ affinity may be important for the serenic activity, but in addition the site of action remains unclear. Two different sets of experiments have been carried out to elucidate these questions.

3.4   Drug discrimination studies

Methodological aspects

The drug discrimination paradigm is a very powerful and specific procedure for the 'in vivo' screening of (novel) compounds which takes a unique place within psychopharmacological research. This is because, in procedures designed to use discriminative stimulus properties of drugs, the distinctive physiological or interoceptive alterations (states, cues) induced by these psychoactive compounds are consequential, i.e. the animal must attend to ('discriminate') its own drug-induced altered internal milieu in order to escape from shock or to receive reward (food or water). No such 'attention' needs to occur in other, commonly used procedures in behavioural pharmacology.

In the drug discrimination procedure, experimental subjects (ranging from pigeons to humans, but usually rats) are trained to perform one response in the presence of a drug and another response when no drug or a different drug is present. Commonly, this consists of pressing either the left or the right lever in an operant chamber (Skinner box). Once trained, the animals are subjected to either generalization or antagonism tests. In generalization tests, the lever choice reflects the degree of similarity between the stimulus effects of the experiment ('test') and the training drug condition. In antagonism tests, the injection with the test drug is followed by an injection with the training compound in order to investigate whether the test drug can block the expression of the stimulus effect of the training compound. Drug discrimination procedures have been used successfully to distinguish different classes of drugs, for example benzodiazepines and barbiturates. With the development of selective ligands for different receptor (sub)types it is possible to further classify drugs within a single drug class, correlating the stimulus effects with affinities derived from binding studies. Rats trained to discriminate the 5-HT_{1A} selective agonist 8-OH-DPAT, also 'recognize' other specific 5-HT_{1A} agonists like ipsapirone and flesinoxan. However no generalization is found with mixed 5-HT_1 compounds. Similarly the cue of 8-OH-DPAT is blocked with 5-HT_{1A} antagonists, but not by specific 5-HT_2 or 5-HT_3 antagonist. Ybema et al. (1992) have published an extensive drug discrimination study on eltoprazine.

It was the aim of the experiment to determine whether eltoprazine can serve as a discriminative stimulus in rats, whether its stimulus effect is mediated by a 5-HT_1-based mechanism and to examine further possible distinctions between 5-HT_{1A}, 5-HT_{1B} and 5-HT_{1C} receptor involvement. Therefore, rats were trained to discriminate eltoprazine from saline in a 2-lever operant drug discrimination task. Thereafter, the animals were subjected to generalization and antagonism tests with a range of drugs having varying affinities for 5-HT$_1$ (i.e. 1A, 1B, 1C), 5-HT$_2$ and 5-HT$_3$ receptors, thus providing 'in vivo' evidence on the mechanism of action of eltoprazine, as far as its discriminative stimulus effects are concerned.

Table III-4

Effects of various drugs in drug-discrimination studies in rats trained to discriminate eltoprazine (0.5 mg/kg i.p.)

Compound	5-HT action	Generalization	Antagonism
Fluprazine	5-HT$_1$ mixed agonist	+	
TFMPP	5-HT$_1$ mixed agonist	+	
RU 24969	5-HT$_1$ mixed agonist	+	
8-OH-DPAT	5-HT$_{1A}$ agonist	+	
m-CPP	5-HT$_{1C/1B}$ agonist	±	
flesinoxan	5-HT$_{1A}$ agonist	±	
buspirone	5-HT$_{1A/D2}$ agonist	±	
DOI	5-HT$_{1C/2}$ agonist	−	
ketanserine	5-HT$_{1C/2}$ agonist	−	−
(±)pindolol	β antagonist 5-HT$_{1A/1B}$ agonist	+	−
(±)propranolol	β antagonist 5-HT$_{1A/1B}$ agonist	+	−
(−)timolol	β antagonist	−	−
mesulergine	mixed 5-HT$_{1/2}$ antag.	±	−
tropisetron	5-HT$_3$ antag.	−	−
methysergide	mixed 5-HT$_{1/2}$ antag.	−	

Fluprazine, TFMPP, RU24969 and 8-OH-DPAT substituted in a dose-related manner for the discriminative stimulus produced by 0.5 mg/kg of eltoprazine (Table III-4). Both flesinoxan and buspirone produced maximally 60% drug lever (DL) selection, m-CPP produced maximally 45.5% DL selection and less than 20% drug-lever selection was found after injections with DOI.

Finally, table III-4 also summarizes the results of substitution tests with the serotonergic antagonists ketanserin, mesulergine and tropisetron and the β-adrenergic antagonists (±)-pindolol, ±-propranolol and (−)-timolol. Ketanserin and tropisetron did not mimic the eltoprazine stimulus. Mesulergine partially substituted for eltoprazine, at doses (i.e. 2.0, 4.0 and 6.0 mg/kg) which reduced response rates. Both (±)-pindolol and (±)-propranolol completely mimicked eltoprazine.

The dose-response relationship of drugs showing maximally between 60 and 100% DL selection (i.e. eltoprazine, fluprazine, RU24969, TFMPP, 8-OH-DPAT, (±)-pindolol, flesinoxan and buspirone) are also presented in figure III-6. In this figure, DL selection is expressed as % animals that chose the drug lever. Eltoprazine, RU24969 and TFMPP had about the same ED_{50} (i.e. 0.09, 0.10 and 0.16 mg/kg, respectively), the ED_{50} of 8-OH-DPAT was 0.35 mg/kg, the ED_{50}s of (±)-pindolol, flesinoxan, fluprazine and buspirone were 1.78, 2.18, 4.84 and 4.92 mg/kg, respectively.

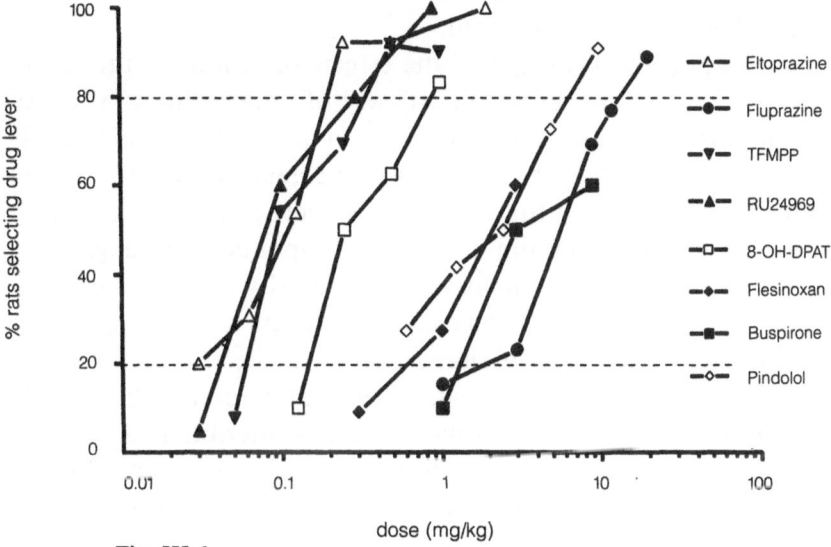

Fig. III-6
Drug-lever (DL) selection as % of animals choosing the drug lever. Generalization curves of eltoprazine, fluprazine, TFMPP, RU 24969, 8-OH-DPAT, flesinoxan, buspirone and (±)-pindolol are shown.

Antagonism tests

The results of antagonism studies with ketanserin, mesulergine, methysergide, tropisetron, (±)-pindolol and (±)-propranolol are also shown in table III-4. None of these antagonists blocked the eltoprazine stimulus.

Other studies (Ybema et al., in press) have revealed that non-serotonergic mechanisms are probably not involved in the stimulus properties of eltoprazine. In summary, the data suggest that the discriminative properties of eltoprazine are mediated through 5-HT_{1A} and 5-HT_{1B} receptors in the brain of rats. At present studies are underway to establish the stimulus properties of eltoprazine in a species lacking the 5-HT_{1B} receptor, e.g. the pigeon. Definitely the 5-HT_{1A} properties play a role, but not exclusively.

3.5   Site of action

Available evidence suggest the mixed $5\text{-HT}_{1A/1B}$ agonistic properties of eltoprazine to be responsible for its serenic activity. However, as previously noted, 5-HT_{1A} and 5-HT_{1B} receptors occur both pre- and postsynaptically. Eltoprazine might thus exert its anti-aggressive actions at different sites of the brain. Several studies were performed to evaluate this issue in more detail.

Sijbesma et al (1991) investigated the effects of lesions of the serotonergic system on the subsequent efficacy of eltoprazine to suppress aggression. Rats were tested for aggression and after lesioning of the major serotonergic nuclei by injection of the neurotoxic 5,7 DHT into the raphe nuclei retested for aggression. Severe lesions to the serotonin system had only minimal effects on spontaneous aggression, suggesting that even with the loss of the majority of the serotonergic innervation to the forebrain rats can still perform adequate aggressive behaviour. Administration of eltoprazine to the lesioned animals still reduced aggression significantly and even the hint of a slight potentiation of eltoprazine's anti-aggressive properties was obtained. Since 5,7 DHT injections destroy presynaptic 5-HT_{1A} and 5-HT_{1B} receptors, the remaining efficacy of eltoprazine to block aggression points to the importance of postsynaptic $5\text{-HT}_{1A/1B}$ receptors in controlling aggression. Even with major lesions of the presynaptic $5\text{-HT}_{1A/1B}$ receptors eltoprazine is effective. This does not rule out a role for the presynaptic 5-HT_{1A} and 5-HT_{1B} receptors in regulating aggression, but they are not absolute requirement for the action of serenics.

Another approach to study the site of action of serenics was followed by Mos et al. (1992). They equipped rats with canulas in the lateral ventricle, thus aiming to affect postsynaptic 5-HT receptors in parts of the forebrain. To unravel the contribution of postsynaptic 5-HT_{1A} and 5-HT_{1B} receptors in the control of aggression, different drugs were used. The specific 5-HT_{1A} receptor agonist 8-OH-DPAT (which after systemic injection results in a non-specific suppression of aggression,

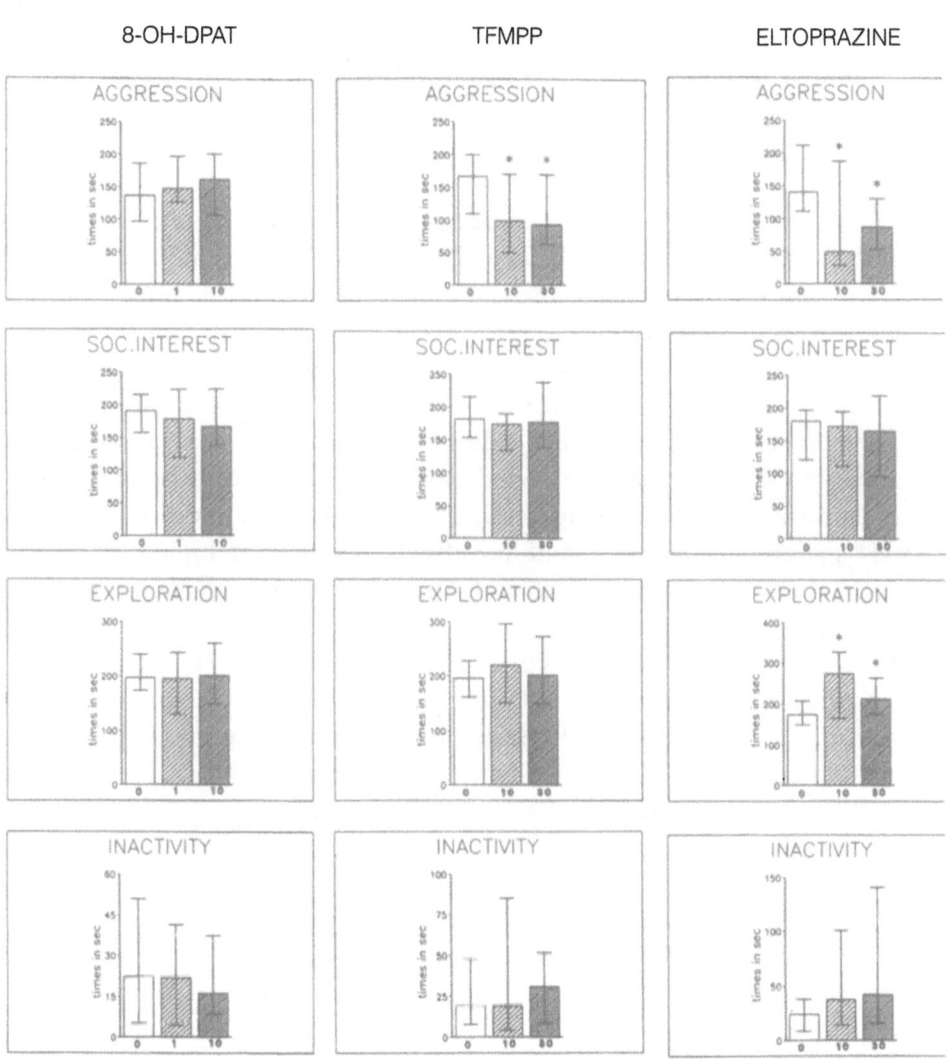

Fig. III-7
Median and interquartile values of the time spent (seconds) on four behavioural categories (aggression, social interest, exploration and inactivity) after intracerebroventricular administration of 8-OH-DPAT (N = 15), TFMPP (N = 14) and eltoprazine (N = 14). The abscissa shows the dose in μg, the ordinate time in seconds. * p$\leq$0.05.

see behavioural studies) did not induce any reduction in aggression. In contrast, the more specific 5-HT$_{1B/1C}$ receptor agonist TFMPP as well as eltoprazine exerted their serenic activity after intracerebroventricular injection in a similar way as after systemic administration (see figure III-7). These data virtually exclude a specific role of presynaptic 5-HT$_{1A}$ receptors in aggression. In combination with the previous study by Sijbesma et al. (1991) the present experiments reveal the importance of postsynaptic 5-HT$_{1B}$ receptors in the action of serenics to suppress aggression in rats. It should be remembered however, that in species lacking the 5-HT$_{1B}$ receptor similar studies have not been performed.

A final piece of evidence on the mechanism of action of eltoprazine stems from Mos et al. (1993). In a similar study as the one reported above, canulas were placed into the dorsal raphe nucleus, one of the major ascending serotonergic nuclei. The cell bodies of the serotonergic neurons contain 5-HT$_{1A}$ receptors which upon activation lead to a reduced serotonergic neurotransmission, i.e. these autoreceptors switch the serotonin neuron off. Administration of the 5-HT$_{1A}$ receptor agonist 8-OH-DPAT in the dorsal raphe led to a dose-dependent, non-specific reduction of aggression (fig. III-8). The more specific 5-HT$_{1B/1C}$ agonist TFMPP had no effects whereas at higher doses eltoprazine had similar effect as 8-OH-DPAT (Mos et al., unpublished).

This confirms the mixed 5-HT$_{1A/1B}$ properties of eltoprazine again. In summary, it appears that in rats the postsynaptic 5-HT$_{1B}$ receptor is particularly important for the specific reduction of aggression. The somatodendritic 5-HT$_{1A}$ autoreceptor is also involved in suppression of aggression, but sedative effects rapidly emerge.

4   **Pharmacokinetics of eltoprazine in mice, rats, dogs, hamsters, rabbits and humans**

4.1   Introduction

To produce a clinical response, a drug must achieve an effective concentration at its site of action, which must be maintained for an adequate length of time.

Pharmacokinetics is defined as the study of the kinetics of absorption, distribution, metabolism and excretion of compounds and their corresponding pharmacologic, therapeutic or toxic response in animals and man. To study the time course of concentrations of eltoprazine, a sensitive and specific analytical assay had to be developed for measurement of this compound in a biological fluid or tissue.

The application of pharmacokinetics is essential for the safety evaluation of drugs. The serenic compound eltoprazine has been eval-

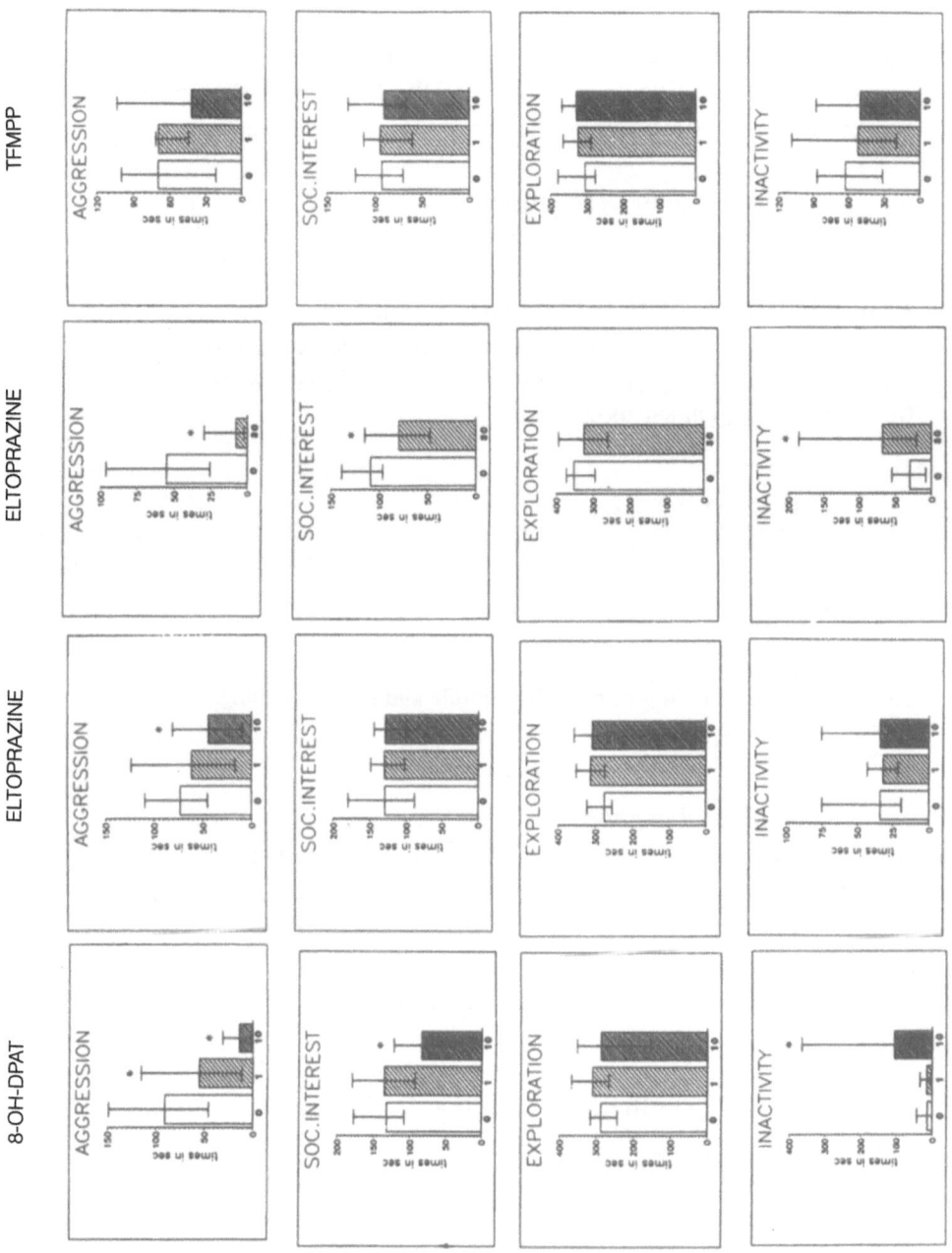

Fig. III-8
Median and interquartile values of the time spent (seconds) on four behavioural categories (aggression, social interest, exploration and inactivity) after administration of 8-OH-DPAT (N = 10), TFMPP (N = 9) and eltoprazine (N = 11) into the dorsal raphé nucleus. The abscissa shows the dose in μg, the ordinate the time spent in seconds. * p≤0.05.

for safety in human use by conducting studies in experimental animals. Qualitative comparisons of distribution and metabolite patterns, and quantitative comparisons of the kinetics of the compound, in both animals and humans, have been made and are reported here.

4.2   Experimental procedures

14C-labelled-eltoprazine

Eltoprazine (1-(2,3-dihydro-1,4-benzodioxin-5-yl) piperazine hydrochloride) was radiolabelled with ^{14}C in the piperazine moiety or with ^{14}C in the phenyl ring (Figure IV-1). Radiochemical purity as checked by HPLC was at least 98%.

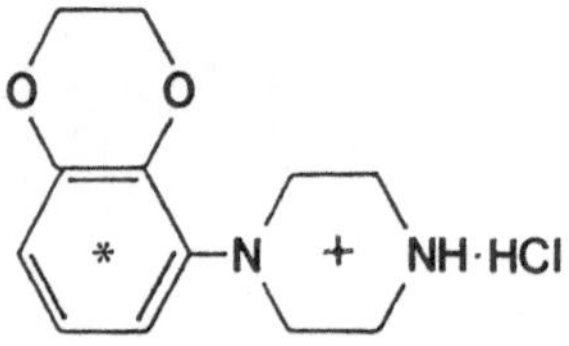

Fig. IV-1
Structural formula of eltoprazine hydrochloride and site of labelling.
* [U-phenyl-^{14}C] labelling.
# [U-piperazine-^{14}C] labelling.

Analytical methods

An HPLC assay was used for quantification of eltoprazine in biological fluids (Raghoebar et al., 1990). The determination limit was 1 ng·ml^{-1} plasma and 0.05 μg·ml^{-1} urine. The method was validated for linearity and reproducibility (CV = ± 8% in plasma and urine) at concentrations up to 100 ng·ml^{-1} in plasma and up to 1 μg·ml^{-1} in urine.

Radioactivity in plasma, urine, faeces, organs and tissues was measured by Liquid Scintillation Counting. Radioactivity in plasma and urine was determined directly, after mixing with Emulsifier Scintillator 299 (Packard) by Scintillation Counting. The counting results were automatically corrected for quenching by an external standard technique. Radioactivity in faeces and organs/tissues was determined after incineration of weighed samples in a Packard Combustion Analyser. The CO_2 formed was trapped in a mixture of Carbosorb and Perma Fluor (Packard) and radioactivity in the resulting solution was measured by Scintillation Counting. The results were corrected for incomplete recovery from combustion.

Eltoprazine metabolite patterns in animal and human urine were determined by HPLC on reverse-phase columns, using radioactivity detection (Koster et al., 1990). Metabolites are numbered in the order in which they are eluted from the HPLC system. Isolation, purification and characterisation of the metabolites is currently taking place.

Animal studies

Whole-body autoradiography studies were conducted both orally and intravenously at a level of 5 mg·kg^{-1} in male Sprague Dawley (SIV) rats and in male blackhooded rats of the BDE-strain. Rats were sacrificed by inhalation of an overdose of ether at selected time and frozen promptly in aqueous solution of carboxymethylcellulose and subsequently immersed in a mixture of isopropanol and dry ice for cryotomy. Sagittal sections (30 μm) were taken at several levels using a PMV 450 Cryomicrotome and dried at $-20°$C. The dried sections were put in contact with sheets of LKB [^{3}H]-Ultrafilm for 1 week. The films were then developed using standard techniques.

For kinetic and mass balance studies in rats, male and female Sprague-Dawley rats were used weighing about 200 g. Dog studies were performed on male and female Beagles weighing approximately 12 kg. Mass balance studies were performed in male and female New-Zealand white rabbits (1.7–2.7 kg) and Syrian BlOFID hamsters (110-130 g). The mice studies were performed in male and female CD-1 Swiss mice (18-25 g).

Human studies

Healthy male subjects, aged between 18 and 40 years, weighing between 56 and 95 kg, participated in three single-dose studies (radioactive excretion study, IV/PO study, dose-proportionality study). All participants gave written informed consent. The protocols were approved by the investigators' independent Medical Ethics Committees. All subjects were non-smokers, and none was on any medication during the study or in the preceding two weeks.

4.3   Fundamental pharmacokinetic properties

Absorption

The extent of absorption of eltoprazine can be assessed **a**) by comparing total excretion of labelled compounds after p.o. and i.v. admini-

stration and **b**) by comparing the absolute amount of renally eliminated radioactivity in intact animals or the sum of radioactivity in
urine and bile in bile-duct cannulated animals after oral treatment
with a certain dose.

Table IV-1

Recovery of radioactivity in the excreta after oral or intravenous administration of [U-phenyl-^{14}C] eltoprazine (label A) or [U-piperazine-^{14}C] eltoprazine (label B) to rat, mouse, dog, hamster, rabbit and human*.

Species		Sex	Dose	Route of Administr.	Label	Collection Period	Urine**	Faeces	Total Recovery
			(mg·kg^{-1})			(h)	(%)	(%)	(%)
Rat	n = 3	m	5	i.v.	B	189	72±4	17±3	89±2
Rat	n = 3	f	5	i.v.	B	189	73±5	13±2	86±3
Rat	n = 3	m	5	p.o.	B	189	69±13	24±5	92±16
Rat	n = 3	f	5	p.o.	B	189	67±4	20±5	87±7
Mouse	n = 3	m	5	i.v.	B	168	76±6	13±8	89±4
Mouse	n = 3	f	5	i.v.	B	168	38±16	43±12	80±5
Mouse	n = 3	m	5	p.o.	B	168	60±18	26±12	86±6
Mouse	n = 3	f	5	p.o.	B	168	46±23	37±22	84±2
Dog	n = 2	m	0.2	i.v	B	168	77±3	7±2	83±5
Dog	n = 2	f	0.2	i.v.	B	168	82±5	9±4	91±1
Dog	n = 2	m	0.2	p.o.	B	168	80±7	9±2	89±4
Dog	n = 2	f	0.2	p.o.	B	168	79±3	10±5	89±8
Dog	n = 2	m	0.2	p.o.	A	168	72±9	7±1	79±8
Dog	n = 2	f	0.2	p.o.	A	168	83±5	6±1	89±5
Hamster	n = 2	m	0.5	i.v.	B	192	72±1	6±1	78±2
Hamster	n = 3	f	0.5	i.v.	B	192	64±9	7±2	71±7
Hamster	n = 3	m	0.5	p.o.	B	192	64±9	13±5	77±5
Hamster	n = 3	f	0.5	p.o.	B	192	71±8	9±1	80±8
Rabbit	n = 3	m	0.2	i.v.	B	168	71±13	8±1	79±14
Rabbit	n = 3	f	0.2	i.v.	B	168	77±6	10±2	86±7
Rabbit	n = 3	m	0.2	p.o.	B	168	74±5	13±2	87±5
Rabbit	n = 3	f	0.2	p.o.	B	168	69±2	10±2	80±1
Human	n = 8	m	8***	p.o.	A	120	93±1	2±1	95±1

* values are presented as cumulated percentage of dose ± S.D.
** including cagewash.
*** fixed dose level of 8 mg per male volunteer.

In all species studied, radioactive eltoprazine was eliminated mainly in the urine (Table IV-1). In the rat, the urinary excretion of radio-activity was practically the same after oral and after intravenous administration of 5 mg·kg^{-1} (Table IV-1). Furthermore dose-corrected cumulative urinary excretion values after oral doses of 2.5, 13 and 67.5 mg·kg^{-1} were not essentially different from an oral dose of 5 mg·kg^{-1}. For these doses no effect of multiple dosing was seen in urinary excretion. Bile-duct cannulated male rats excreted more than 80% of a 5 mg·kg^{-1} dose via urine and bile. The excretion in faeces was less than 1%.

From a cascade experiment (bile-duct of one rat connected to the duodenum of a second bile-duct cannulated rat) it was concluded that between 25% and 40% of eltoprazine and/or its metabolites, excreted in the bile (about 30% of the dose), was reabsorbed, both after oral and intravenous administration. No gender-differences in biliary excretion were found. From these studies it was concluded that eltoprazine is well absorbed from the gastro-intestinal tract, in doses between 2.5 and 67.5 mg·kg^{-1} and that at a dose level of 5 mg·kg^{-1}, there may be substantial enterohepatic circulation of eltoprazine and/or its metabolites.

In the mouse, excretion of radioactivity was comparable after oral and intravenous administration suggesting complete absorption of eltoprazine (Table IV-1). At single oral doses of [phenyl-U-^{14}C]-eltoprazine at dose levels of 7.5, 22.5 and 67.5 mg·kg^{-1}, male mice excreted between 70 and 80% of the radioactive dose, female mice about 90%. After a radioactive dose preceded by eight daily doses of unlabelled eltoprazine, urinary excretion in male and female mice is about 90%, irrespective of the dose level. At the dose levels 7.5 and 22.5 mg·kg^{-1} female mice excrete significantly more via the renal route than the male mice. At the same dose levels the amount of radioactivity excreted renally by the male mice was higher after multiple dosing than after a single radioactive dose. Such differences were not found at the dose level of 67.5 mg·kg^{-1}. The percentage of the dose excreted in urine and faeces was for all three dose levels about 95%.

It was concluded that although there were apparently gender-differences in renal excretion, absorption was calculated to be complete in the mouse.

After a radioactive dose of 0.2 mg·kg^{-1} to dogs (Table IV-1), the amounts excreted via the urine were independent of the route of administration indicating complete absorption after oral administration. The same amount of urinary excretion (about 80% of the dose) was found after single oral radioactive doses of 0.5, 4 and 32 mg·kg^{-1} and also after the same doses preceded by daily dosing of non-radioactive eltoprazine. It was concluded that eltoprazine was well absorbed in doses between 0.2 and 32 mg·kg⁻¹. Dosing with (piperazine versus phenyl moiety) labelled eltoprazine results in virtually the same excretion of radioactivity in urine and faeces (mean total of 84% for phenyl label versus 88% for piperazine label recovered 168 h after oral dosing). Although for both preparations the same [¹⁴C] peak levels were found in dog plasma (see Figure IV-2), residual radioactivity is, however, much longer detectable after dosing of [U-piperazine-¹⁴C]eltoprazine.

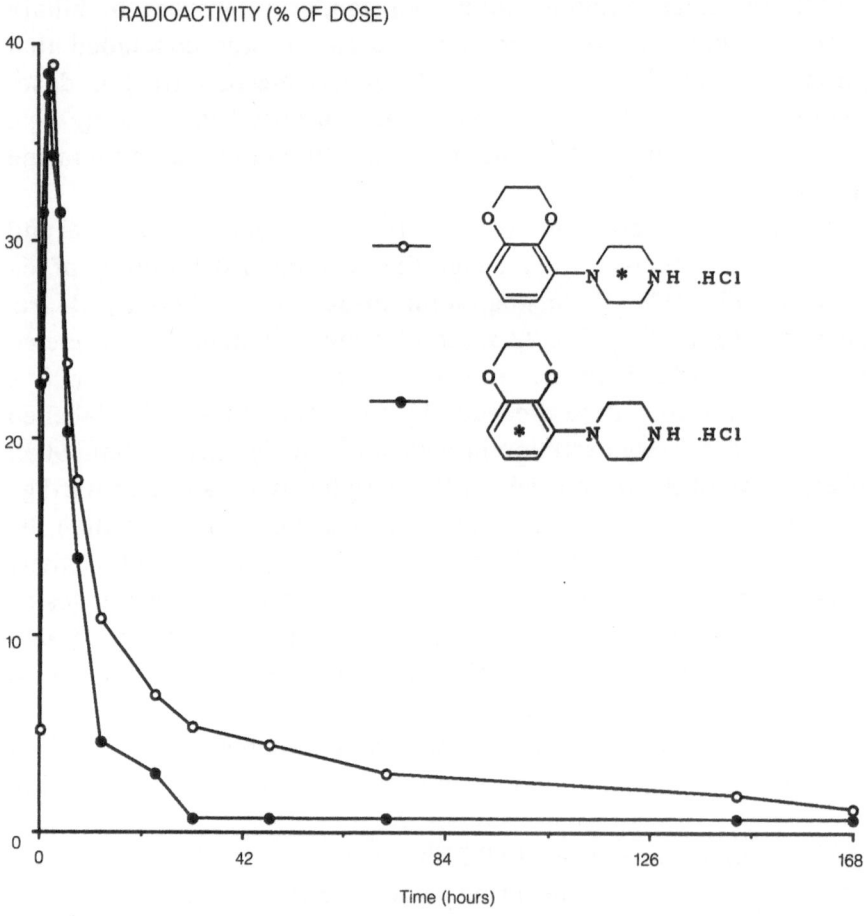

Fig. IV-2
The radioactivity-time course of [phenyl-U-¹⁴C]-eltoprazine and [piperazine-U-¹⁴C-eltoprazine] in dog plasma after single oral administration of 0.2 mg·kg⁻¹.
The radioactivity levels are expressed as % of the oral radioactive dose.

Also, in rabbits and hamsters (Table IV-1) the amounts excreted via the urine were independent of the route of administration, indicating complete absorption after oral administration.

After oral dosing with ^{14}C-eltoprazine in male human subjects, absorption is virtually complete, with 93% of the administered radioactivity excreted in the urine within 5 days (Van Harten et al., 1990). Mean plasma levels of unchanged eltoprazine, as well as mean plasma levels of total radioactivity are depicted in Figure IV-3. Plasma levels of total radioactivity were higher than levels due to unchanged eltoprazine suggesting formation of metabolites with a lower volume of distribution.

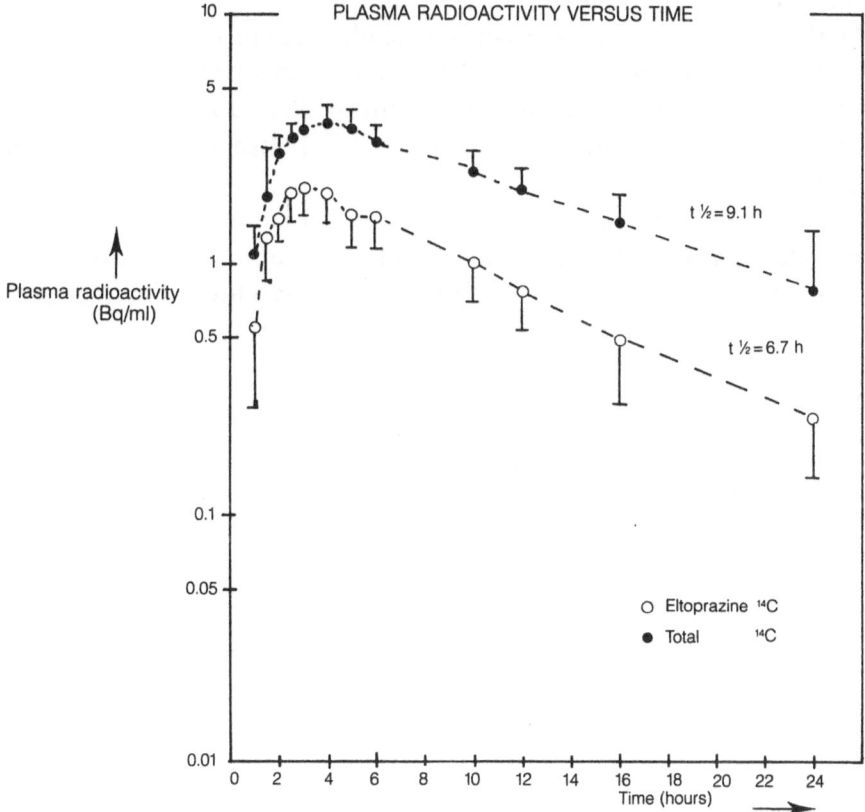

Fig. IV-3
Geometric mean (±S.D.) plasma levels of total plasma radioactivity (closed circles) and plasma radioactivity attributable to eltoprazine (open circles) versus time in eight healthy male subjects.
Taken from Van Harten et al. (1990) with permission.

The contribution of eltoprazine to total plasma radioactivity tended to decrease with time: during the first three hours dosing, between 30 and 40% of plasma radioactivity could be attributed to metabolites of eltoprazine, whereas from 5 hours after dosing and onwards, more than 50% of plasma radioactivity was due to metabolites. Maximal plasma concentrations of unchanged eltoprazine are reached within 1 and 5 hours postdose. All subjects showed irregular plasma-concentration-time curves, in some subjects a second peak was observed after oral administration (Raghoebar et al., 1990, De Vries et al., 1991). This double-peak phenomenon is dose-independent and is also described for some amines (like cimetidine), but the mechanism behind the appearance of these peaks is not clear.

At the end of the five-day study period, a mean op 95.4% [range: 94.8-96.0%] appeared in urine; 1.9% [range: 1.6–2.2%] in faeces.

Urinary excretion of radioactivity within 24, 48 and 72 hours was 78.5 ±5.4%, 91.1±2.0% and 92.9±1.0% of the total dose, respectively (Van Harten et al., 1990).

Data from pharmacokinetic studies in several animal species indicate that eltoprazine is well absorbed (Table IV-1) and that absorption is virtually complete. The drug can be classified as a low to intermediate clearance drug (extraction ratio between 0.3 and 0.7).

4.4   Distribution

Protein binding

The plasma protein binding of the base eltoprazine (pKa = 9.0) was determined in vitro by equilibrium analysis for 4 hours at 37°C with spiked samples at concentrations of 10 to 1000 ng·ml^{-1}. The plasma protein binding was 15±5%; hence, plasma protein binding is not concentration dependent in the investigated range. Due to this low protein binding, interactions of eltoprazine with other drugs for binding sites in plasma proteins as a result of competition, are not expected.

Whole-body autoradiography

The distribution of radioactivity in albino and pigmented rats has been assessed by whole-body autoradiography after single dosing. Autoradiography in male albino rats showed that one hour after oral and intravenous administration of 5 mg·kg^{-1}, high concentrations were present in the organs responsible for elimination (kidney, liver, gastro-intestinal tract), lower activity was seen in spleen, bone marrow, lymph nodes, thymus, heart and brain (fig. IV-4 and IV-5). Concentrations of radioactivity in the brain were found to be higher after two hours than after one hour. Six hours after administration a decrease of radioactivity was seen in most organs but not in lungs, spleen and adrenals. Twenty-four hours after administration practically all radioactivity was eliminated (see Figure IV-4 and IV-5). Only in liver and kidney low concentrations were seen. After oral administration to male black-hooded rats, radioactivity was observed in the pigmented parts up to 72 hours after administration. But the decrease of activity in these melanine containing parts between 6 and 72 hours after dosing is an indication that this binding is reversible (Figure IV-6).

Plasma levels of eltoprazine

Concentrations of unchanged eltoprazine in plasma were determined in the rat, mouse, dog and man. Pharmacokinetic parameters obtained from these measurements are summarized in table IV-2 and IV-3. All studies provide evidence that the oral bioavailability of eltoprazine is higher than 40% in all species tested. There were some interspecies differences. Bioavailability was lowest in the female mouse (41%). In the dog and the rat about 70% and 60% respectively, reached the systemic circulation. Man exhibited the highest bioavailability, with 110% for a dose of 8 mg, indicating that absorption from the gastrointestinal tract is complete. Peak levels in plasma were found between 0.1 and 3 hours after dosing.

The highest systemic clearance divided by body weight was observed in the mice, followed in descending order by rats, dogs and man. There was a good correlation between the logarithms of CL_s and body weight with an equation of $CL_s = 36.4 \times W^{0.695}$ (Figure IV-7).

CL_s equalled about 30 to 80% of the hepatic blood flow in the different species.

Half-lives vary from 0.5 till 3 h in animals. In man plasma levels obtained after intravenous infusion of 3 and 9 mg eltoprazine followed a bi-exponential decay with a terminal half-life of 6-9 hours. After oral administration, the terminal half-life was between 5 and 12 hours.

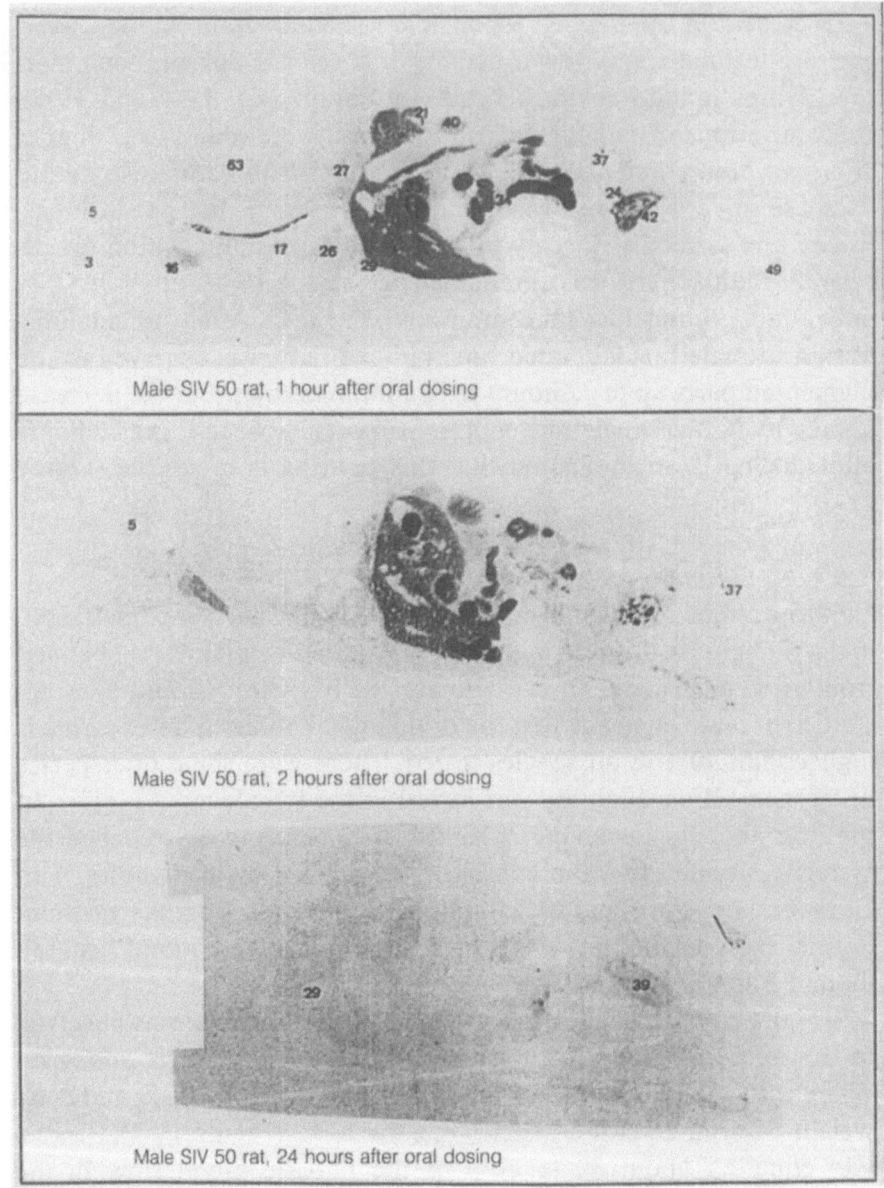

Fig. IV-4

Whole body autoradiographs obtained following oral administration of [U-piperazine-
^{14}C]eltoprazine in the male SIV 50 rat. The dose was 5 mg·kg^{-1} (4.764 MBq). The
upper, middle and lower autoradiographs represent the distribution of radioactivity at
1 h, 2 h and 24 h post dose, respectively. The black areas correspond to the presence of
radioactivity. The numbers in the figure represent: 3 = harderian gland, 5 = cerebrum,
16 = salivary glands, 17 = thymus, 21 = adrenal gland, 24 = adipose tissue, 26 = myo-
cardium, 27 = lung, 29 = liver, 33 = stomach, 34 = small intestine, 37 = colon,
39 = faeces, 40 = kidney, 42 = urinary bladder, 49 = testicle, 63 = skeletal muscle.

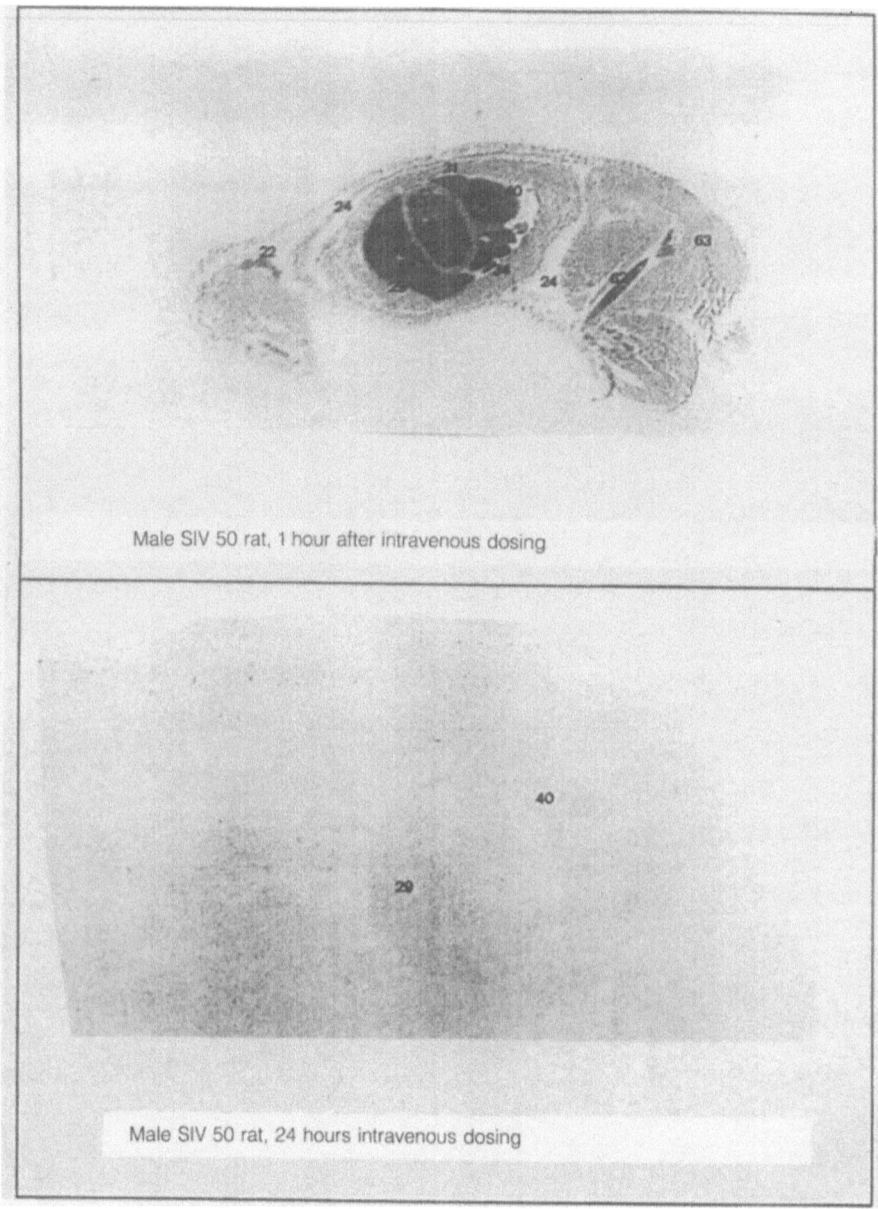

Male SIV 50 rat, 1 hour after intravenous dosing

Male SIV 50 rat, 24 hours intravenous dosing

Fig. IV-5

Whole body autoradiographs obtained following iv administration of [U-piperazine-^{14}C]eltoprazine in the male SIV 50 rat. The dose was 5 mg·kg^{-1} (4.764 MBq). The upper and lower autoradiographs represent the distribution of radioactivity at 1 h and 24 h post dose, respectively. The black areas correspond to the presence of radioactivity. The numbers in the figure represent: 22 = lymph node, 24 = adipose tissue, 29 = liver, 31 = spleen, 33 = stomach, 34 = small intestine, 40 = kidney, 62 = bone marrow, 63 = skeletal muscle.

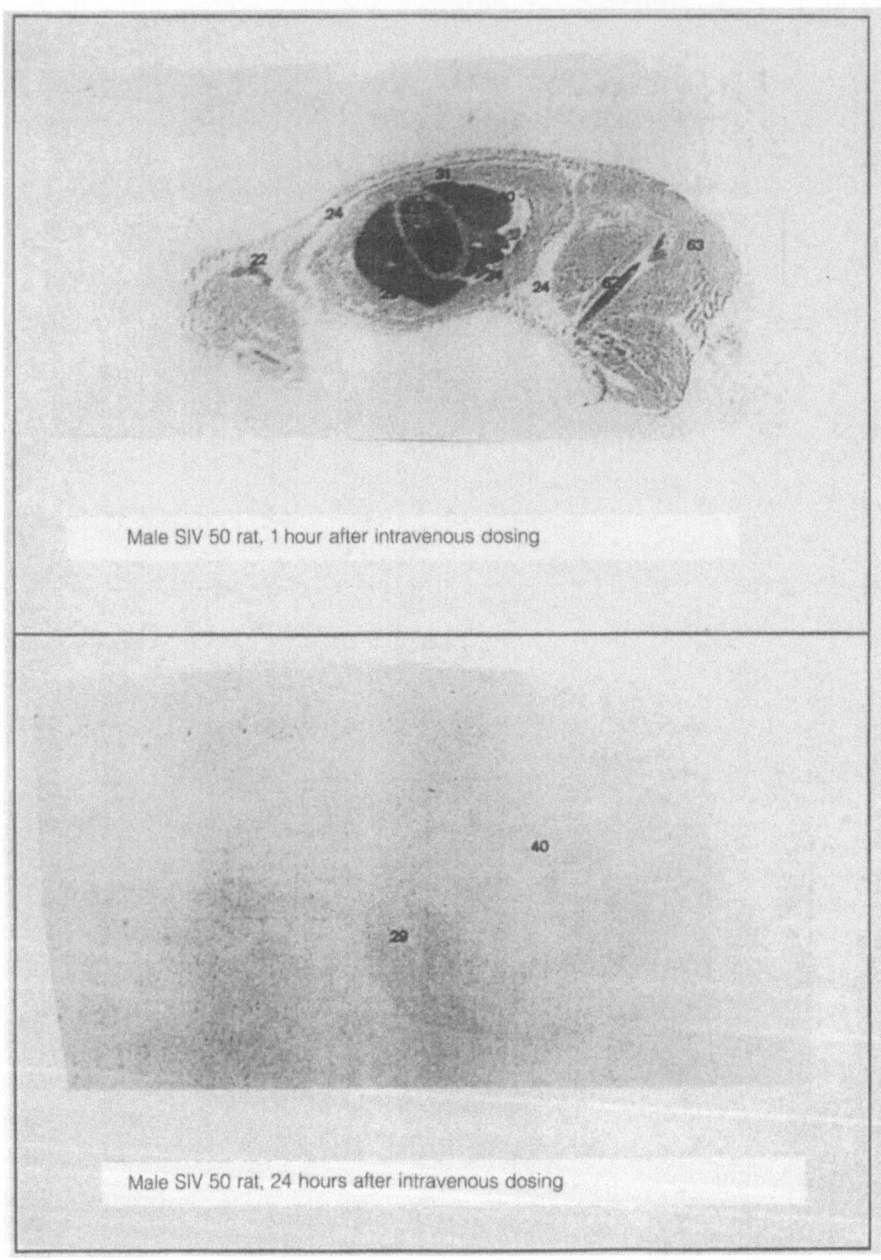

Male SIV 50 rat, 1 hour after intravenous dosing

Male SIV 50 rat, 24 hours after intravenous dosing

Fig. IV-6
Whole body autoradiograph obtained following oral administration of [U-piperazine-¹⁴C]eltoprazine in the male BDE rat. The dose was 5 mg·kg⁻¹ (4.764 MBq). The upper and lower autoradiographs represent the distribution of radioactivity at 2 h and 72 h post dose, respectively. The black areas correspond to the presence of radioactivity. The numbers in the figure represent: 1 = eye, 12 = hair follicles, 29 = liver.

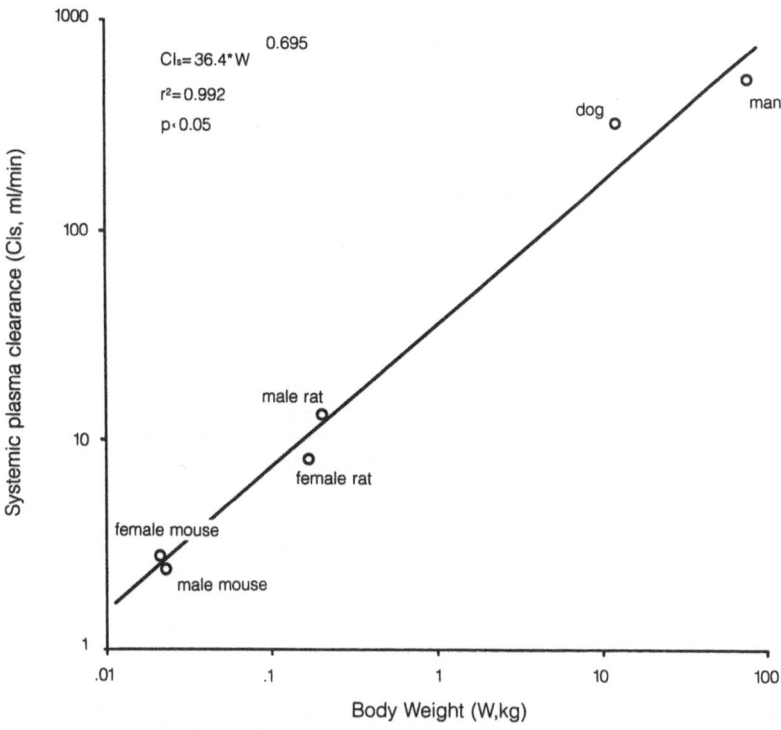

Fig. IV-7
Correlation between systemic plasma clearance (CLs) of eltoprazine and body weight
(W). The solid line was calculated by the least square method using logarithmically
transformed data.
($CL_S = 36.4 \times W^{0.695}$) ($r^2 = 0.992$, P<0.05).

In dogs and man, renal clearance is relatively high (about 8 ml·min⁻¹
in the dog and 3 ml·min⁻¹ in man) and about 40% of the dose is
excreted unchanged into the urine in dog and man, respectively. As
the renal clearance is nearly twice the glomerular filtration rate in both
species, it can be concluded that the renal excretion of eltoprazine is
characterized by net tubular secretion (Raghoebar et al., 1990, Van
Harten et al., 1990, Lammers and Van Harten, 1990).
Assuming that the difference between total and renal clearance equals
hepatic clearance, eltoprazine has to be classified as a compound with
a low to intermediate extraction ratio.
Volume of distribution was higher than 3 l·kg⁻¹, indicating extensive
distribution (table IV-2). Since plasma protein binding is low, it is
clear that eltoprazine is preferentially distributed to extravascular
sites.

Table IV-2

Pharmacokinetic parameters of eltoprazine in different species after intravenous administration.*

Species	Rat	Rat	Dog	Mouse	Mouse	Man
Dose (mg·kg⁻¹)	5	5	0.5	5	5	8***
Number of animals	12 × 2**	12 × 2**	6	26 × 2**	26 × 2**	12
Sex	m	f	3m, 3f	m	f	m
Time of observation (h)	48	48	48	48	48	72
$t_{0.5,z}$ (h)	1.7	2.1	3.0±0.9	1.7	0.6	9.3±4.4
CL_s (ml·min⁻¹·kg⁻¹)	65	48	26+7	104	132	7.9±0.9
V_{ss} (l·kg⁻¹)	8.0	6.8	6.1±1.6	8.7	5.9	3.8±0.5
AUC (ng·h·ml⁻¹)	1289	1737	336±85	801	632	247+30
CL_R (ml·min⁻¹·kg⁻¹)			7.6±4.1			3.1±0.6

* Values are arithmetic means or means ± S.D.
** n = 2/time point.
*** Dose per subject.

Table IV-3

Pharmacokinetic parameters of Eltoprazine in different species after oral administration.*

Species	Rat	Rat	Dog	Mouse	Mouse	Man
Dose (mg·kg⁻¹)	5	5	0.5	5	5	8***
Number of animals	12 × 2**	12 × 2**	6	26 × 2**	26 × 2**	12
Sex	m	f	3m, 3f	m	f	m
Time of observation (h)	48	48	48	48	48	72
$t_{0.5,z}$ (h)	1.7	2.3	2.5±0.8	1.2	0.4	9.8±3.9
C_{max} (ng·ml⁻¹)	435	371	42±13	365	545	24±6
t_{max} (h)	0.3	0.8	1.5±0.3	0.2	0.3	2.3±1.1
AUC (ng·ml⁻¹)	853	1079	231±120	483	262	282±80
F (%)	66	62	68±24	60	41	110±32
CL_R (ml·min⁻¹·kg⁻¹)			7.7±3.5			3.1±1.3

* Values are arithmetic means or means ± S.D.
** n = 2/time point.
*** Dose per subject.

In the dog and man, the kinetics are linear with dose, whereas in the mouse and in the rat, deviations from linearity at higher doses become apparent (table IV-4 and IV-5, Figure IV-8).

Multiple-dosing of 4 mg·kg⁻¹ for 8 consecutive days had no effect on the kinetics in dogs. In the rat repeated dosing for seven consecutive days at three different dose levels resulted in a non-linear increase of the AUC (see figure IV-7). At higher dose levels, the total body clearance decreased (43 ml·min⁻¹·kg⁻¹, 29 ml·min⁻¹·kg⁻¹ at 13 mg·kg⁻¹ and 15 ml·min⁻¹·kg⁻¹ at 67.5 mg·kg⁻¹, see table IV-4).

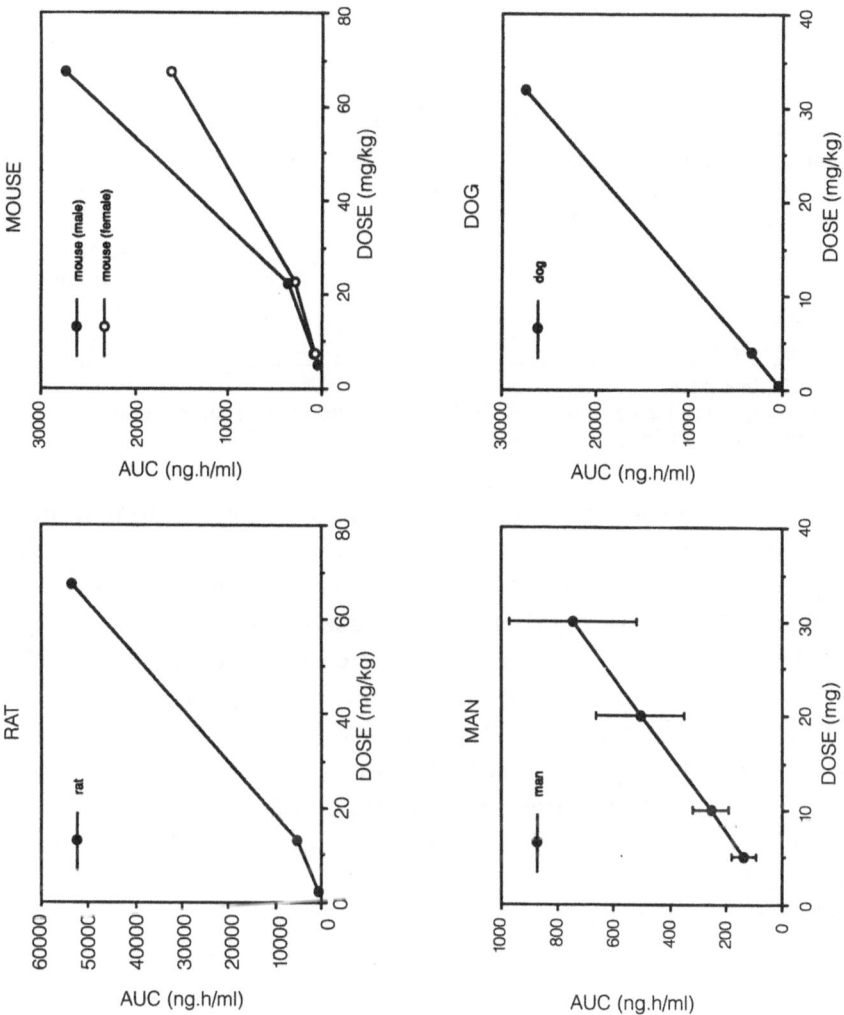

Fig. IV-8

Relationship between AUC for eltoprazine and oral dose levels. The regression equations for the fitted lines were:

Rat (male): $\text{AUC (ng·h·ml}^{-1}) = 839 \times \text{dose (mg·kg}^{-1}) - 3372$ $(r = 0.995)$
Dog (male & female): $\text{AUC (ng·h·ml}^{-1}) = 859 \times \text{dose (mg·kg}^{-1}) - 25$ $(r = 1.000)$
Mouse (male): $\text{AUC (ng·h·ml}^{-1}) = 441 \times \text{dose (mg·kg}^{-1}) - 3191$ $(r = 0.974)$
Mouse (female): $\text{AUC (ng·h·ml}^{-1}) = 258 \times \text{dose (mg·kg}^{-1}) - 1590$ $(r = 0.987)$
Man (male): $\text{AUC (ng·h·ml}^{-1}) = 24.5 \times \text{dose (mg)} + 12.2$ $(r = 1.000)$

AUC values were obtained after single oral dosing in dog, mouse and man, and followed a partly randomised, cross-over design (dog, man). The study in rats had a multiple-dose design (oral daily dosing for 7 consecutive days). On day 7 the AUC values have been estimated.

Table IV-4

Mean pharmacokinetic parameters of eltoprazine in the male albino rat after different oral doses at steady state

	Dose levels (mg·kg⁻¹)***		
	2.5	13	67.5
Number of animals	18 × 2*	18 × 2*	18 × 2*
Time of multiple-dosing (days)	7	7	7
Kinetic observations on day	7**	7**	7**
C_{max} (ng·ml⁻¹)	152	1021	5712
t_{max} (h)	0.5	0.75	1.0
AUC (ng·h·ml⁻¹)	685	5193	53620
$t_{0.5,z}$ (h)	3.4	3.5	4.8
CL_{tot} (ml·min⁻¹·kg⁻¹)	42.6	29.21	14.7

* n = 2/time point.
** Through samples collected before day 7 indicated steady state conditions.
*** once daily dosing.

This effect might be related to a certain degree of inhibition of processes involved in metabolism or elimination after repeated dosing. In the mouse disproportional kinetics at high oral doses at steady state is also observed (after chronic dosing of 7.5, 22.5 and 67.5 mg·kg⁻¹ for 8 consecutive days). The clearance decreased at higher dose levels. Multiple-dose studies in man are in progress.

Of the species studied, only rats and mice show moderate differences in handling of eltoprazine between males and females. In mice, AUC and F appeared to be larger in males than in females (table IV-2 and IV-3) while the AUC tended to be larger in females than in males in rats (table IV-2 and IV-3).

Taken together, the results of the pharmacokinetic studies indicate that eltoprazine is well absorbed and that the greater part of eltoprazine and/or its metabolites leaves the body within 24 hours. Eltoprazine is a low to intermediate clearance compound. The kidneys play an important role in the excretion of unchanged eltoprazine and its metabolites. The mechanisms of renal handling remain to be solved.

Eltoprazine tissue distribution

The degree of transient exposure of specific body targets to eltoprazine is determined by measuring the total radioactivity in major tissues and organs. A given number of mice, rats, hamsters, rabbits and dogs were administered [phenyl-U-¹⁴C]eltoprazine or [piperazine-

U-¹⁴C]eltoprazine and sacrificed at several time points for blood and tissue collection, and the mean results were used to generate the concentration-time profiles (see figure IV-9, table IV-6, IV-7).

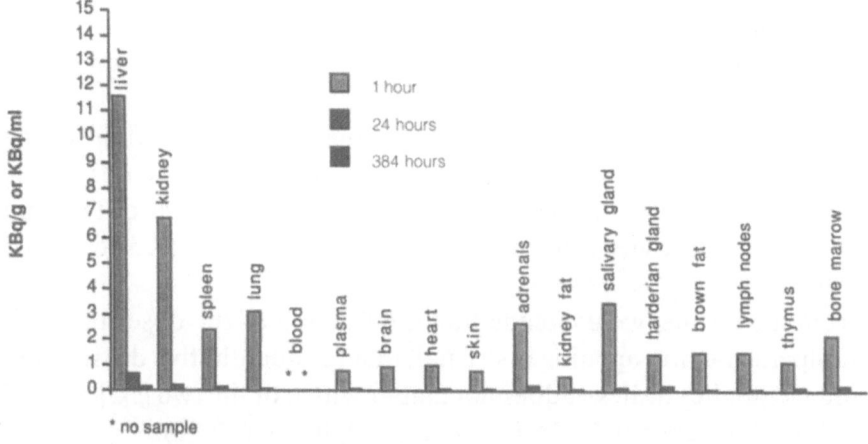

Fig. IV-9

Average distribution of total radioactivity (expressed as KBq of eltoprazine/g or ml) in tissues of rats (n = 2/time point) after a single oral dose of [piperazine-U-¹⁴C]eltoprazine (5 mg·kg⁻¹; radioactive dose 3.785 KBq/g).

The distribution of radioactivity in 17 tissues at 1, 24 and 384 hours after single oral dosing with 5 mg·kg⁻¹ [piperazine-U-¹⁴C]eltoprazine to male rats is shown in figure IV-9. At 1 hour after dosing, the excretory organs contained high concentrations of radioactivity (liver 11.6 KBq/g and kidney 6.8 KBq/g), with moderate to low concentrations being observed in all other tissues (<3.5 KBq/g). By 24 hours, the mean concentration in all tissues had declined to less than 0.2 KBq/g, except in kidney and liver which had levels of 0.21 and 0.62 KBq/g, respectively. At 384 hours after dosing, traces of radioactivity could only be demonstrated in liver, kidney, lung, heart, adrenals, brown fat and lymph nodes (at least 0.02 KBq/g).

A comparative study with eltoprazine labelled with ¹⁴C at 2 different places (in piperazine or phenyl group) resulted in similar disposition patterns in the first 24 hours after dosing (table IV-6). At later times the concentration of radioactivity originating from the [piperazine-¹⁴C]eltoprazine is higher (data not shown; see table IV-6 for data at 384 hours). These results indicate that the residual concentrations detected up to 384 hours after administration of [piperazine-U-¹⁴C]eltoprazine are not caused by retention of the entire molecule. It can be hypothesized that the piperazine ring is cleaved, resulting in small [^{14}C]labelled molecules which might be aliphatic amines. Quantitatively, the accumulation of residual radioactivity after administration of the [piperazine-U-^{14}C] labelled material is of minor importance. After 384 hours, the highest concentration was found in the liver, but this concentration was less than 1% of the peak concentration in this organ.

Comparison of the HPLC-patterns of urine radioactivity after dosing of the two preparations show only minor differences in the rat: i.e. the presence of a polar metabolite in an amount less than 1% of the total urinary radioactivity after dosing of piperazine label (Koster et al., 1990).

From the results, we conclude that the fraction of the dose subjected of piperazine ring opening is so small that for quantitative distribution and metabolic studies, it does not matter which of the two [^{14}C]labelled preparations are used (De Lange and Raghoebar, 1990).

Evidence for such a cleavage of the piperazine ring already existed for a number of phenothiazines: fluphenazine, perphenazine, perazine, prochlorperazine and trifluorperazine (Gaertner et al., 1975; Breyer et al., 1974; Breyer, 1972; Jorgensen, 1986) and was recently also described for a phenyl-piperazine (Miyamoto et al., 1988).

On the other hand, it is known from literature that a number of N-phenyl piperazines (e.g., mociprazine, urapidil, pefloxacin, trazodone, COR 3224, etoperidone, mepiprazole, antrafenine, oxypertine, milipertine, enciprazine, nefazodone, MJ-7378) are metabolised to 1-arylpiperazine metabolites with an intact piperazine ring (Caccia, 1990; Caccia et al., 1985, Vaugien et al., 1991; Fong et al., 1982; Caccia et al., 1981; Montay et al., 1984; Enreille et al., 1991; Zech et al., 1984; Franc et al., 1991). These compounds may concentrate in certain tissues including the brain at relatively high concentrations (Caccia et al., 1984), and have specific biochemical and pharmacological effects or may even antagonize the parent compound's action (Caccia, 1990; Caccia et al., 1984; Caccia et al., 1985; Caccia et al., 1987).

The quantitative distribution of radioactivity was determined in pregnant rats. The organ distribution pattern in pregnant rats corresponds to the distribution pattern in non-pregnant rats (table IV-7). Tissue levels of total radioactivity declined steadily from 3 hours to 96 hours post dose, with liver showing the highest concentrations at each time point examined. There was evidence of radioactivity crossing the blood/brain barrier and the placental barrier and at 24 hours and 96 hours post dose levels of radioactivity in the foetus were higher than those in blood. Up to 24 hours after dosing, concentrations in the foetus are lower than in maternal plasma. At later times the relatively high concentration in the foetus is probably due to cleavage of the [piperazine-^{14}C] ring of eltoprazine (see discussion above). The concentration in the amniotic fluid passed its maximum (9% of the maximum maternal plasma concentration) within 3 hours after dosing. The placental transfer appeared to be limited and highest concentrations were detected in the placenta.

Residual radioactivity in the liver, kidney, brain and bone marrow obtained from male and female rabbits (168 hours after a single dose of 0.2 mg·kg^{-1} [piperazine-U-^{14}C]eltoprazine), from male and female hamsters (192 hours after a single dose of 0.5 mg·kg^{-1} [piperazine-U-^{14}C]eltoprazine), from male and female mice (168 hours after a single dose of 5 mg·kg^{-1} [piperazine-U-^{14}C]eltoprazine, and from male and female rats (192 hours after the 11th dose (radioactive, piperazine labelled) of eltoprazine at dose levels of 2.5, 13.0 and 62.5 mg·kg^{-1}), was low but substantial. In general it can be concluded that 168 or 192 hours after dosing with piperazine labelled eltoprazine, less than 2% of administered radioactivity is still present in the animals' bodies. These results were independent of dose and gender. These findings are consistent with those in the single dosed rat (figure IV-9, table IV-6 and IV-7) and indicate the presence of breakdown products of the piperazine ring. This hypothesis is further supported by the following distribution studies which have been conducted with [phenyl-U-^{14}C]eltoprazine.

The residue of radioactivity in the above-mentioned organs in dogs is less than 0.1% (168 hours after 6th (radioactive) dose of 0.5 mg·kg^{-1}), 0.2% (168 hours after 6th (radioactive) dose of 8 mg·kg^{-1}), 1.3% (168 hours after 6th (radioactive) dose of 32 mg·kg^{-1}) per organ. In figure IV-2 it can been seen that the plasma disappearance of eltoprazine, ^{14}C-labelled in the piperazine moiety, is much slower than after dosing with the [phenyl-U-^{14}C]labelled compound.

Low concentrations of radioactivity were detected in male and female mice treated with nine daily (radioactive) doses of 7.5, 22.5 and 67.5 mg·kg^{-1} (by 96 hours after the final radioactive dose, the mean concentrations were less than 20 ng.equivalent per gram tissue or less than 0.1% of the dose).

From these data we may conclude that radioactive residues of ^{14}C-piperazine labelled eltoprazine persist somewhat longer in the body than ^{14}C-phenyl labelled eltoprazine. There was no evidence of retention or significant accumulation of radioactivity in any of the tissues in species studied.

Excretion and metabolism
a) Excretion

In order to study whether the administered eltoprazine is readily excreted from the body, mass balance studies in animals and humans have been conducted.

In all species studied, between 80 and 100% is excreted via the urine and the faeces. Excretion of eltoprazine and metabolites is mainly via the kidney (dogs and rats 70-90%, mice 40-90%, hamsters and rabbits 60-70%, man 92-94%). Excretion of radioactive eltoprazine and/or its metabolites appeared to be independent of route of administration, gender, dose level, pre-treatment with unlabelled eltoprazine and the place of ^{14}C-label in the molecule. Generally, of all radioactivity that is excreted renally, more than 90% is achieved within 24 hours. In bile-duct cannulated rats, a biliary excretion of about 30% of the dose is observed and about 30% of radioactivity excreted in bile, is reabsorbed. On average 18 and 29% of the dose was excreted unchanged after oral and intravenous dosing of 0.5 mg · kg^{-1}, respectively, to dogs (Lammers and Van Harten, 1990). In man about 40% of an oral dose is excreted unchanged in the urine (Raghoebar et al., 1990; Van Harten et al., 1990). The large renal clearances in dog and man suggest active secretion of eltoprazine in urine.

The total recovery of administered radioactivity appeared to be similar among the species tested (around 90%).

b) Metabolism

An important objective of biotransformation studies in animals is to identify species to be used in toxicological studies in which the metabolic fate of the drug is similar to that in humans.

The metabolite patterns in urine of rats, dogs, rabbits, hamsters and mice were compared with those of humans (Koster et al., 1990). Metabolite patterns of dogs and to a lesser extent also of mice resembled those of humans most closely (see figure IV-10). Urine metabolite patterns show that in rat, dog, man and mice the greater part of urinary radioactivity consists of unchanged material and two or three significant metabolites.

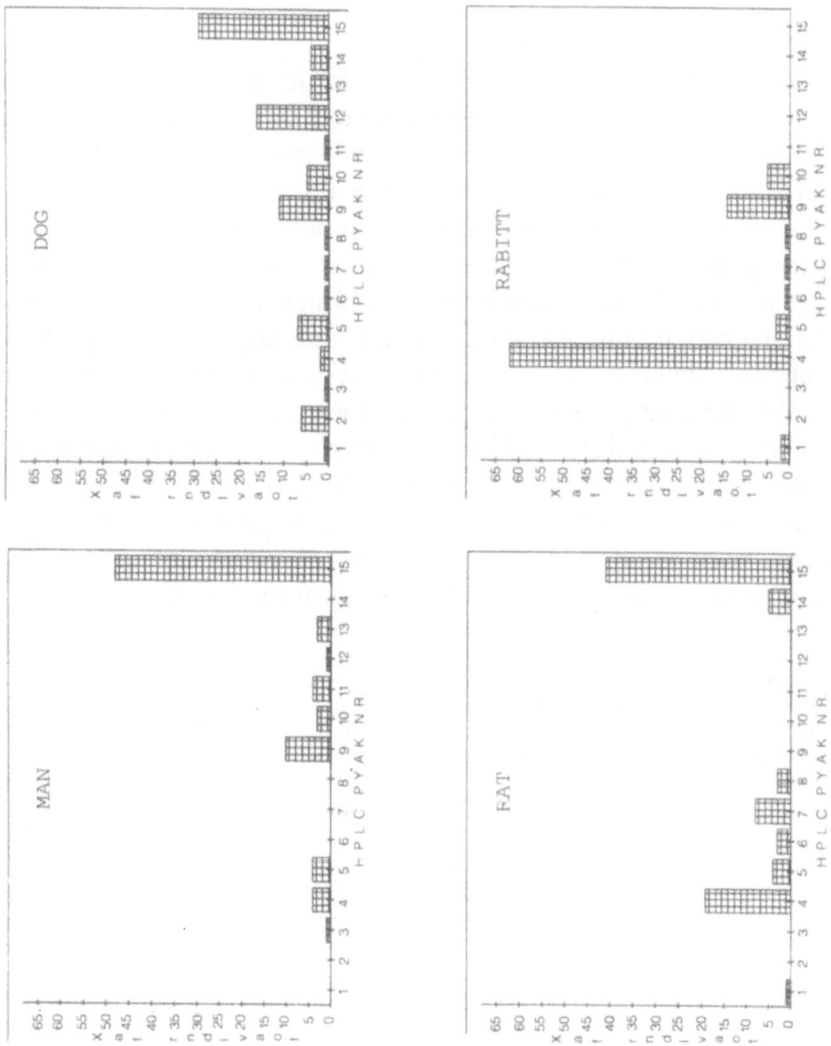

Fig. IV-10
Representative HPLC-chromatograms of human, rat, rabbit and dog urine after oral administration of [Phenyl-U-^{14}C]eltoprazine. Peak nr 18 correlates with the retention time of eltoprazine. Taken with permission from Koster et al. (1990).

The metabolite pattern of eltoprazine in man shows a large peak of unchanged eltoprazine, accompanied by a limited number of metabolites more polar than the parent compound. These metabolites are thought to be conjugated phase I metabolites. The dog appeared to be on the basis of metabolite pattern comparisons a suitable model for human exposure in long-term toxicity studies. Patterns of rabbits and hamsters are quite unlike the human patterns since they contain hardly any unchanged eltoprazine.

Therefore, these species are unsuitable for long-term toxicity studies. Patterns of rats and mice are more similar to the human patterns, but it is difficult to give clear preference. The mouse patterns show slightly more overlap than the male rat patterns, but female rats are generally better than mouse patterns. In order to better discriminate between these species, patterns of urine subjected to deconjugating enzymes were produced. This might reveal similarities in phase I metabolism between man on the one hand, and rats and mice on the other hand. From this exercise, mice patterns emerged as only slightly more suitable than rat patterns as a model for man. As an overall conclusion, there is a slightly distinct preference for using mice and not rats as the second species for long-term toxicity studies.

Metabolite structure identification is currently in progress. Pharmacokinetic studies in dog and man reveal that first-pass metabolism is not of importance for the fate of eltoprazine in the body.

Table IV-7

Average distribution of radioactivity in tissues of [piperazine-U-^{14}C]-eltoprazine to female pregnant and non-pregnant rats (5 mg·kg^{-1}; 20.46 μci·mg^{-1}). The pregnant rats were sacrificed on day 16 postconception. At each time point 2 rats were sacrificed. Of each pregnant rat 2 foetuses were collected separately.*

Tissue	Concentration (ng equiv. of eltoprazine/g or ml wet tissue)				
	Pregnant Rats			Non-Pregnant Rats	
	3 h	24 h	96 h	3 h	96 h
Plasma	969	118	19	882	33
Blood	629	88	25	608	35
Brain	679	38	22	1177	27
Liver	7474	632	221	8000	243
Kidney	2997	260	141	4311	162
Bone Marrow	774	225	84	1347	144
Lymph Node	2045	246	t**	2736	73
GI-tract	31233	1028	66	28666	98
Foetus	182	99	42		
Placenta	848	150	7		
Amniotic Fluid	84	13	4		

Data are the means of 2 rats.
** t = Trace (< 1 Bq).

Table IV-5

Mean (± S.D.) pharmacokinetic parameters derived from plasma and urine after single oral administration of 5, 10, 20 and 30 mg eltoprazine to healthy male subjects.

	Dose levels (mg)			
	5	10	20	30
n	18	18	18	12
C_{max}(ng·ml^{-1})	12.9±3.6	22.8±5.3	42.9±9.6	62.9±13.8
t_{max} (h)	2.5±1.1	2.8±1.3	3.9±1.0	3.5±1.8
AUC (ng·h·ml^{-1})	136±44.5	254±66.6	506±158	746±227
MRT (h)	11.2±1.9	10.8±1.2	10.6±1.4	10.5±1.2
$t_{0.5,z}$ (h)	6.7±1.3	6.2±1.0	5.9±0.9	5.9±0.9
CL_{tot} (ml·min^{-1}·kh^{-1})	8.7±2.4	9.0±2.0	9.2±2.6	9.3±2.2
Ae* (%)	41±9	42±10	42±9	42±6
CL_R (ml·min^{-1}·kg^{-1})	3.5±1.0	3.8±1.1	3.8±0.8	3.8±1.0

* Ae/D × 100%.

Table IV-6

Mean concentrations of ^{14}C-eltoprazine in some major tissues/organs after oral administration of 5 mg·kg^{-1} to male rats. Eltoprazine is labelled with ^{14}C either in the piperazine or in the phenyl group.
Results are the means of 2 rats and are expressed as Bq/g or Bq/ml. Mean dose was 700 KBq of piperazine label (= Pip.) and 862 KBq of phenyl label (= Phenyl).

Sampling time (h)	Liver		Kidney		Plasma		Brain	
	Phenyl	Pip.	Phenyl	Pip.	Phenyl	Pip.	Phenyl	Pip.
1	12686	11848	11528	5635	774	552	1247	647
6	2426	3470	1073	2098	115	365	100	382
24	577	762	207	261Ø 38	99	10	46	
384	4	32	5	17	t*	t*	t*	14

* t = Trace (< 1 Bq).

5   **Clinical applications of serenics and some implications of their preclinical profile for their clinical use in psychiatric disorders**

5.1   Introduction

Agonistic behaviour is the subset of social behaviours which comes into play in interactions characterized by conflict. This repertoire includes both offensive behaviours (more commonly labelled as "aggressive") and defensive behaviours. While the complexity and diversity of behavioural options vary, most species, including man, possess an agonistic behavioural repertoire.

Neither in man nor in other animals is agonistic behaviour pathological. In the framework of evolutionary theory, these behaviours are understood to encourage survival of the fittest, to disperse populations, to aid adaptation to threatening environments, and generally to improve the probability of both individual and species survival.

In human terms, we tend to understand such behaviour as "competitive" or "defensive" in ourselves and, perhaps, "aggressive" or "hostile" in others. In social terms, however, we differentiate between those agonistic behaviours which are acceptable on the one hand and those which are unacceptable on the other and we censure the latter in a variety of ways. While we find no difficulty in discriminating between the ends of this behavioural spectrum, we often find considerable difficulty in agreeing where to draw the line in the middle.

In deciding how to deal with unacceptable behaviour, we often tend to try to understand its "motivation". At least in modern Western societies, we tend to excuse the behaviour of individuals who are considered mentally incompetent by reason of great stress, mental disease, retardation, or the like.

While we know that "aggressive" behaviour is associated with a number of disease states (both somatic and psychiatric), and while such behaviour may be considered in establishing a diagnosis, there is no diagnostic category of "aggressive disease" or "offensive syndrome" per se. In the clinical literature, such behaviours may be referred to as "violent", "hostile", "agitated", "impulsive" or (indeed) "aggressive", and often become a primary focus of therapy, as they may threaten the safety of clinical staff or other patients and thus interfere with other therapeutic efforts.

For the purposes of this discussion, these problems are best referred to as "destructive behaviours" which may be defined (after Eichelman) as "behaviour which threatens or actually results in partial or complete injury to the physical, psychological or sociological integrity of a person, object or environment".

In this sense, destructive behaviours are often encountered in association with neuropsychiatric disorders, and patients will be found in a variety of settings, including psychiatric hospitals, neurologic and neurosurgical wards, rehabilitation facilities, nursing homes, community residences and institutions for the mentally retarded.

Destructive behaviours often precipitate admission to psychiatric units. For example, Tardiff and Sweillam (1980), in a survey of state hospitals in New York, found about 10% of patients had manifested assaultive behaviour in the two weeks before admission. Binder and McNiel (1986) reported 15% of patients admitted to a university-based hospital locked unit had assaulted another person within two weeks of admission. Rossi et al. (1985) reported that about 40% of patients admitted to an acute psychiatric unit in a general hospital had exhibited violent or fear-inducing behaviour immediately before hospitalization.

Destructive behaviours are also common in patients after hospitalisation. In the New York state hospital system, about 7% of patients were assaultive within a three-month period (Tardiff and Sweillam, 1982). In a one-year period, about 12,000 assaults were reported in this hospital system (New York State Senate Select Committee on Mental and Physical Handicap, 1977).

Destructive behaviour is often a problem in the management of patients with primary degenerative dementias (either Alzhelmer's SDAT, or multi-infarct, MID) and has been well documented. One way to determine the magnitude of the problem is to survey nursing home populations for the frequency of such behaviour.

Twenty-five per cent of a group of elderly patients in nursing homes in London were found to have at least weekly episodes of destructive behaviour (Mann et al., 1984). This increased to 41% of those who had mild to moderate dementia and depression.

In a random sample of residents in a large intermediate-care nursing home in the U.S., 25% exhibited active aggression, 26% showed verbal aggression and 14% were self-destructive (Rowner et al., 1986). In a survey of 1,139 nursing home patients, Zimmer et al. (1984) found that 8.3% were physically aggressive, 4.3% were self-destructive and 12.6% were verbally disruptive.

Using comprehensive rating scales to assess agitated behaviours in 66 nursing home patients, Cohen-Mansfield (1986) documented verbal aggression more than once daily for 36.8% of subjects and hitting or kicking for 21.2%. Chandler and Chandler (1988), who assessed the prevalence of neuropsychiatric disorders in 65 nursing home residents, found 72% had a dementia syndrome. Among these patients, the most common behavioural problems were agitation and aggression in almost half (48%) of the sample.

There have been studies focused on the behaviour of patients with Alzheimer's dementia. For example, Reisberg et al. (1987) studied 57 out-patients. Of the 33 (58%) with significant behavioural problems, 16 were agitated, 10 were violent and 12 had motor restlessness. Rubin et al. (1987) studied 44 patients with mild Alzheimer's dementia and found irritability in 23% and hyperactivity in 9% of these patients.

Families of patients with dementia reported a 47% incidence of physical violence (Rabins et al., 1982). This behaviour was problematic for virtually all (94%) of the families and was the most serious problem for the patient. For many families, these behavioural disturbances rather than cognitive deficits were the major source of concern leading to institutionalization.

Severely or profoundly retarded patients who require institutional care often exhibit destructive behaviour. Reid et al. (1984) reported in such a group that 33% were irritable and 20% were injurious to themselves. In a survey of patients in community residences or institutions for the mentally retarded, 30% to 40% of the residents exhibited disruptive behaviour or injury to self, others or property (Hill et al., 1985). Administration of antipsychotics was significantly associated with these behaviours. In a survey of mentally handicapped patients over age 40, Day (1985) found destructive behaviours, especially verbal abusiveness or aggression towards self, others or objects, were the most common problems and, moreover, were of long-standing duration.

Traumatic brain injury, especially frontal lobe damage, may result in a frontal lobe syndrome characterized by inability to control angry impulses (Mackinnon and Yudofsky, 1986) and the resulting behaviour interferes with rehabilitation and resocialization.

In many of these situations, it is necessary to control the destructive tendencies before therapy can be effectively applied to the underlying condition. In other cases, such as the demented or retarded, the underlying condition is essentially untreatable and moderation of the destructive behaviours is a prerequisite to reasonable and humane care in minimally restrictive settings.

5.2   Current management options

At present, there are no drugs clinically available which specifically inhibit destructive behaviours (Tupin, 1985; Sheard, 1983; Valzelli,

1979), and pharmacologic therapy aimed specifically at destructive behaviours has been reported relatively infrequently. Although lithium, propranolol or anticonvulsants have been reported to be effective for specific management of such behaviours in some cases, in general the treatment of human destructive behaviour has been only marginally successful. However, the advent of more sophisticated behavioural methodologies, the apparent, if limited, success of specific therapies, and an increasing understanding of the biological correlates have renewed optimism toward pharmacologic intervention in those individuals whose destructive behaviours represent one of the primary objectives of clinical management.

There is a clinical lore which holds that certain types of patients respond better to particular pharmacologic interventions. For example, Elliott (1978) has suggested that destructive individuals with traumatic CNS injury or ruptured aneurysm respond most favourably to beta-adrenergic antagonists. Monroe (1970, 1975 a, b) suggests that individuals with "episodic dyscontrol" (which he links to an epileptoid-like EEG) respond well to anticonvulsants or benzodiazepines. Yudofsky et al. (1987) have reviewed the pharmacologic treatment of destructive disorders. They conclude that antipsychotics have been most widely used for management of such behaviours, but with little evidence to suggest that they are specifically effective beyond their sedative effects in acutely agitated or violent patients or those whose behaviour is due to active psychosis (Valzelli, 1979; Kostowski, 1978; Delina-Stula and Vassout, 1979; Itil and Mukhopadhyay, 1978).

Yudofsky et al. (1987) consider benzodiazepines to be ineffective in chronic destructive behaviour and, indeed, that they may aggravate the behaviour or precipitate rage attacks (the "paradoxical" response observed both in animals and man) (Bond and Lader, 1979). They consider carbamazepine effective in management of behaviour related to temporal lobe epilepsy and review preliminary data suggesting its utility in other cases as well.

Lithium has proved effective in destructive behaviour related to manic excitement and, although controlled studies are contradictory, there is evidence suggesting it may also be useful in management of destructive behaviour. Finally, they review studies which suggest that beta-blockers, particularly propranolol, may have specific value in the management of destructive behaviour related to organic brain syndromes. However, it should be noted that propranolol may have a latency period, of four to six weeks and is contraindicated in a variety of conditions which are relatively common in patients with organic brain syndromes.

A few experimental drugs have been tested clinically, e.g. the benzazepine derivative Sch 12679 (Itil and Mukhopadhyay, 1978) and the indenopyridine YG19-256 (Roubicek et al., 1972; Owen, 1980). These studies suggested for the latter an anti-aggressive effect without overt sedation. Since no such specificity has been found in animal studies (Bell and Brown, 1979; Olivier and Van Dalen, 1982; Olivier et al., 1984), claims for a specific anti-aggressive profile must at present be accepted with some reservations.

Overall, it may be concluded that destructive behaviours are frequently encountered in clinical practice, that they present a significant management problem, that a variety of pharmacologic interventions have been (and are) used, and that there is much room for improvement. On this basis, it seems reasonable to search for pharmacologic agents which might specifically inhibit aggressive behaviours in animals and, therefore, might specifically inhibit destructive behaviours in man.

Such a search necessarily depends upon our crude understanding of CNS exciting and inhibiting systems; their relationship with various neurotransmitter systems; their relationship, in turn, with various in vitro and in vivo models; and finally, our own limited ability to identify from the results of such models compounds with promising effects. It is hardly surprising if this process is not especially efficient. However, because of the accumulating evidence for the association between the serotonin (5-hydroxytryptamine, 5-HT) system and behaviour, both in animals and in man, our search has focused on compounds with probable activity in the serotonin systems. In the remainder of this paper, we will trace very briefly some of the main issues considered in our search for, characterisation of and future plans for the serenics.

5.3   Serotonin and behaviour

The relationship between serotonin and behaviour (e.g., depression, anxiety, obsessive-compulsive disorders, panic) hardly needs noting and has been extensively reviewed (see, for example (Eccleston and Doogan, 1989)). Accumulating evidence suggests more or less clear

associations between some behaviours (e.g., depression) and serotonin receptor subtypes (Montgomery and Fineberg, 1989). However,
for destructive behaviours, few drugs with receptor specificity have
yet been clinically tested. Consequently, if an association does exist,
as seems likely, it has not yet been elucidated.

In considering our own work, it seems worthwhile at the outset to
discriminate between non-specific and specific suppression of aggressive behaviours (in animals) or destructive behaviours (in man). Many
drugs, among them the commonly used neuroleptics, reduce aggressive behaviour in animals, but at the expense of all other behaviours as
well, often to the point of general sedation and ataxia (Olivier and Van
Dalen, 1982; Olivier et al., 1984b; Olivier and Mos, 1986). Because
these drugs have similar effects in man, they are used in the management of destructive behaviours, but with similar suppression of other
behaviours (Sheard, 1984; Madden and Lion, 1981). This non-specific
inhibition of aggression or destructive behaviour can best be understood as "chemical restraint". In contrast, a drug with specific activity
should inhibit aggressive or destructive behaviour without significant
effects upon other behaviours or capabilities.

5.4   Animal modelling

As is customary in the search for psycho-active drugs, reliance must
be placed on the use of animal models. As long as no drugs with
demonstrable specificity in the management of human destructive
behaviour are available, the relevance of these models is difficult to
assess. However, there are several reasons for believing that such
animal models should have predictive value for human behaviour.

There are no main differences in behavioural structure between man
and animals (Baerends, 1973; Blanchard and Blanchard, 1984; Hinde,
1974) and it is suggested that man and animals possess a comparable
system (or systems) for agonistic interactions (aggression), both on a
behavioural and a neuronal level (Baerends, 1973; Moyer, 1976).

Animals and man share similar autonomic and physiological reactions during the states of high arousal which are associated with
agonistic interactions (Ursin, 1980; Brain, 1984).

In the central nervous system of mammals, including man, comparable neural substrates exist which, certainly in animals and in man,
modulate observable, aggressive behaviour (Moyer, 1976; Adams,

1979; Karli, 1981; Mark and Erwin, 1970; Valenstein, 1973). Studies of these neural substrates do not support any unitary concept of aggression. Adams (1979) and Ursin (1981) postulate that, because different brain structures are involved in defence, offence and predatory aggression, at least these three types of aggression must be recognized. However, because the brain is organized as a very complex network rather than a system of reflex chains, notions such as "neural substrates of aggression" are, in fact, over-simplified.

In our laboratory, if we are to accept a neural structure as a possible substrate for aggressive behaviour, several criteria should be fulfilled (Ursin, 1979):

- The behaviour must be elicited by electrical or chemical stimulation of the brain structure, at least when the external environment permits the expected behaviour.
- The behaviour evoked has to belong to the ordinary repertoire of the animal in its natural state.
- Units in the brain structure should change their electrical activity (EEG) during the performance of the behaviour.
- The behaviour should change as a result of lesions to the particular neural structure.
- Pharmacological manipulations should elicit, eliminate or jam the particular behaviour.
- The behavioural changes produced must be reasonably specific for the structure and should not result from interfering effects from other brain structures.

Using such criteria, there is evidence that at least the following brain structures are involved in aspects of aggression certainly in animals and probably in man as well (for most of them):

- Involvement in all three major types of aggression (i.e., offensive, defensive and predatory): Hypothalamus, Brain stem, Temporal lobe
- Involvement in offensive behaviours: Thalamus
- Involvement in defensive behaviours: Septum
- Involvement in defensive and predatory behaviours: Olfactory bulb

It has been suggested that a number of other brain structures may be involved, e.g., the hippocampus, frontal lobe and cingulate cortex, but these effects can better be attributed to the general response modulation of these structures or through changes in motivational and discriminatory functions.

In conclusion: there are a number of brain structures involved in at least offensive, defensive and predatory aggression, but it is far from clear precisely how these contribute to the behaviour. Moreover, the neurochemistry of these structures, as far as their involvement in aggressive behaviours is concerned, remains anecdotal (Cools, 1981) and detailed research is in a very early stage.

5.5   Hormones and behaviour

It is commonly accepted that hormones modulate agonistic behaviour both in animals and man. Indeed, castration has been proposed for management of some particularly serious cases. In the experimental study of agonistic behaviours it is necessary to consider the complex interplay between circulating hormones and their target areas, especially in the CNS (Svare, 1983). Hormones modulate attack and defence in a variety of ways (Brain, 1981), e.g.:
– early "programming" effects (peri- and post-natal)
– modulation of motivation
– modulation of somatic mechanisms involved in the production or detection of communicative stimuli (body size, form, colouration, vocalisation, pheromones).
While several hormones modulate to some degree effects in any model of animal aggression, androgens (testosterone) are clearly the most important (Benton, 1981; Gandelman, 1981). The effects of androgens occur both during early development and thereafter concurrently.
The early effect (early programming) occurs during pre- and post-natal development and induces permanent changes in latent (potential) behaviour. On the other hand, the concurrent effects of androgens involve activation of ongoing behaviour. The mechanism by which androgens exert their concurrent effects involves alterations in the way in which the brain processes sensory information.
A number of animal models are androgen-dependent, a number are not. In general, offensive behaviours are testosterone-dependent, while defensive and predatory behaviours are not. Thus, for example, to induce fighting in males, testosterone should be present (but, under certain conditions, is not necessary). Animals exposed to testosterone early in life require much less androgen exposure in adulthood to activate fighting, as compared with animals without such early exposure.

In conclusion, androgens are important modulators of some agonistic behaviours, especially offensive ones in males, whereas in others no effect is found. However, it is clear that hormones do not directly induce or inhibit behaviour, but do affect activational potentials. It is, therefore, unlikely that direct behavioural effects of psychotropic drugs are mediated by effects upon androgens.

Other hormones also play a role in agonistic behaviours (as well as in other behaviours), e.g., corticosteroids, prolactin, oestrogens and progestins. Their roles, however, are far from elucidated but, as with the androgens, there is no evidence of direct effects.

In the present study, various aggression models are grouped in classes representing predominantly offensive or defensive/flight aspects of agonistic behaviour. This classification does not suggest specificity for types of human aggression; rather it reflects a division now much used in animal research (Adams, 1979; Blanchard et al., 1977 a,b; Blanchard and Blanchard, 1977). Offensive behaviour is always characterized by initiative, and active attempts (attacks) to remove the attack-releasing stimulus from the environment (e.g., the territory or nesting place).

There may be some similarities in this respect between human and animal behaviours in that the offensive (animal) aggression may reflect some affective or appetitive behaviour or angry aggression (Blanchard and Blanchard, 1984). It could be assumed in many situations of human conflict that offensive or affective aggression is present in the behaviour of the attacker (Sarteschi et al., 1978). Blanchard and Blanchard (1984) postulate that the defence/flight modality in animals may be related to fear-based attack in man. Although hard evidence delineating offensive and defensive types of aggression in humans is still scarce, the face validity of the distinction is considerable and the existing evidence is not inconsistent with such an hypothesis.

Without further belabouring such issues, it seems intuitively reasonable from a biological perspective to assume that a drug, which has anti-offensive properties in animal models, may also influence some types of agonistic behaviour in man. Defensive behaviour, the other side of an animal's agonistic interactions considered in this report, probably also has its similarities in human behaviour (self-defence, flight; (Sarteschi et al., 1989). It seems possible, therefore, that drugs which are active in animal models of agonistic behaviour, whether in offensive or in defensive ones, may also prove effective in certain situations of human conflict.

Assuming, then, that animal models may have predictive value for human use, we shall discuss the properties of eltoprazine in the animal models used and compare them with those of some other putative "anti-aggressive" drugs and some other reference compounds.

5.6   Serotonin and behaviour in animals

In animals, there is general agreement that serotonin inhibits aggressive behaviours (Vergnes et al., 1986). For example, in rats, general serotonin depletions by PCPA increase offensive aggression, but leave defensive behaviours intact (Vergnes et al., 1988; Vergnes and Kempf, 1982). Localized 5-HT depletions, obtained by injections of the neurotoxin 5,7-DHT into the hypothalamus, also lead to increases in aggression. Such manipulations affect predatory aggression in a similar fashion although the biological significance of these behaviours differs. Studies in mice lead to similar conclusions about the relation between 5-HT and aggressive behaviours.

In other studies, decreased serotonergic function achieved by reducing tryptophan in the diet of rats induced predatory aggression which could be inhibited by supplying tryptophan (Gibbons et al., 1979). Increased serotonergic function achieved by injection of the immediate precursor 5-HTP reduced predatory aggression after either systemic or intraventricular application (Valzelli, 1978; Gianutsos and Lal, 1975; Nikulina and Popova, 1986).

In another approach to the study of serotonin and aggression, the correlation between serotonin turnover in various areas of the brain and aggression within and between strains was evaluated (Daruna, 1978). In particular, the hypothalamus seems to be involved since low serotonin turnover appeared to be associated with increased aggression. To a lesser extent, the hippocampus and amygdala were involved, but no correlations were found between behaviour and cortical serotonin.

In monkeys, a more complex picture emerges. Dominant and subordinate males differ in 5-HIAA and HVA levels in cerebrospinal fluid (CSF) (Yodyingyuad et al., 1985) as well as in whole blood serotonin (Raleigh et al., 1984). These status-dependent effects indicate involvement of serotonin in aggression. Although reduction of serotonin by PCPA increased aggression, various drugs which increase serotonin did not show a significant effect (Raleigh et al., 1980, 1984). However, eltoprazine, which has predominantly serotonergic activity, has proved effective in vervet monkeys.

5.7   Serotonin (5-HT) receptor subtypes

Research over the past decade has vastly expanded our understanding of the complexity of the serotonin system in animals. Several subtypes may be differentiated on the basis of radioligand binding (Peroutka, 1993). Not all the subtypes, for example, the 5-HT_{1B} receptor, are found in all species. Circumstantial evidence suggests that the 5-HT_{1B} receptor in rodents and the 5-HT_{1D} in primates and man may serve as a presynaptic autoreceptor. However, both subtypes are also found on postsynaptic neurons.

Specific agonists are available for the 5-HT_{1A} receptor, but not for the $5\text{-HT}_{1B, 1C}$ or $_{1D}$ sites; entirely satisfactory antagonists are also lacking. Nevertheless, exploration of the functional characteristics of these receptors can be undertaken with some success using the ligands which are available. Many of these serve to underline the importance of the 5-HT receptors in behaviour.

Several non-selective 5-HT receptor agonists (e.g., 5-methoxy N,N-dimethyltryptamine) as well as antagonists (e.g., methysergide) inhibit agonistic interactions in animals, but usually in a behaviourally non-specific fashion (Miczek and DeBold, 1983). 5-HT_{1A} agonists, such as 8-OH-DPAT, buspirone or ipsapirone, all reduce offensive behaviours of a resident male rat towards an intruder and maternal aggression in lactating females (Olivier et al., 1989). However, this inhibition is obtained at the cost of reductions in non-aggressive social activities, and exploratory behaviours as well as behavioural inactivity which may reflect sedative properties of these drugs.

Mixed $5\text{-HT}_{1A/B}$ agonists, such as eltoprazine, and more specific 5-HT_{1B} agonists, such as TFMPP (a metabolite of fluprazine, another serenic), inhibit offensive behaviours in several models (Olivier et al., 1990; Kruk et al., 1987) as well as in a resident animal confronting an intruder (Olivier et al., 1989 a, b; Kruk et al., 1987; Mos and Olivier, 1988; Olivier et al., 1987; Olivier and Mos, 1988, 1989). Furthermore, these compounds do not adversely affect social behaviours and may even activate exploratory behaviours.

At present, the lack of specific agonists and antagonists to the $5-HT_{1C/1D}$ receptors prevents effective exploration of their specific functions.

Behaviourally, mixed results have been obtained with $5-HT_2$ antagonists. While ketanserine reduces offensive behaviour in isolated mice (Haney and Miczek, 1989) and in the resident-intruder paradigm in rats (Olivier et al., 1989 a), albeit non-specifically in both cases, ritanserin did not significantly affect aggressive behaviours (Olivier et al., 1989 a; Olivier and Mos, 1988). Lack of selective agonists for the $5-HT_2$ site inhibits characterisation of the behavioural importance of the receptor and work with non-selective compounds gives results which are not readily interpreted.

Finally, the $5-HT_3$ receptor antagonists MDL 72222 and ondansetron (GR38032F) do not affect aggressive behaviour in male mice or in lactating female rats (Mos et al., 1989). More definitive characterisation of the behavioural importance of this site awaits development of specific agonists.

Overall, it is clear that the serotonin subtypes are important in modulation and control of agonistic behavioural interactions and that there is very considerable specificity of effect associated with selective agonists. It seems quite likely that this specificity is likely to be found also in man when suitable compounds are available for clinical use.

5.8   Serotonin and behaviour in man

In man, there is a clear, but as yet imprecisely defined, relationship between CNS serotonin function and destructive behaviours. In 1976, Åsberg et al. found in depressed patients a bimodal distribution of 5-HIAA in CSF and noted that low levels were associated with an increased risk of suicide attempts. Tråskman et al. (1981) found that suicide attempts were generally more violent in patients with depressed CSF 5-HIAA. Lidberg et al. (1985) reported similar findings in a group of suicidal subjects in whom, compared with controls, CSF 5-HIAA was significantly lower, and the lowest levels were found in those subjects who had used active, violent methods in their suicide attempts.

In a similar vein, Linnoila et al. (1983) and Lidberg et al. (1985; 1984) found CSF 5-HIAA levels significantly lower among impulsive offenders than among those whose behaviour was apparently premeditated. Virkkunen et al. (1987) found a similar association for impulsive arsonists.

In a cohort of young men with a diagnosis of personality disorder, Brown et al. (1979, 1982) found a significant negative correlation between CSF 5-HIAA and a life history of aggressive behaviour, suicide attempts and psychopathic deviate scores. Two reports by Bioulac et al. (1978, 1980) on a very small cohort (6) of particularly violent delinquents with the 47 XYY phenotype suggested that normalisation of serotonin metabolism by administration of 5-hydroxytryptophan (5-HTP) attenuated their behavioural symptomatology as effectively as the neuroleptics with which their symptoms had been controlled.

O'Neil et al. (1986) report treatment of a 22-year-old retarded man with Cornelia de Lange syndrome whose destructive behaviour was significantly moderated by treatment with trazodone and tryptophan, which markedly increased his abnormally low peripheral serotonin levels. They suggest that his aggressive behaviours may have been linked to his abnormal serotonin metabolism and that patients with similar deficits may benefit from treatment which improves serotonin function.

Finally, several drugs, including lithium and propranolol, which have been reported to moderate destructive behaviours in some patients, are known or thought to have effects which increase serotonin turnover.

Although such associations are far from elucidating the specific association between deficits in CNS serotonin function and destructive behaviour, they clearly suggest that depressed CSF 5-HIAA levels, and presumably therefore CNS 5-HT turnover, is associated with impulsiveness perhaps manifested by destructive behaviour. It also suggests that pharmacologic modulation of CNS serotonin function may specifically attenuate destructive behaviours in some patients.

It is not within the scope of this paper to contribute to the debate concerning the causes or social management of aggressive behaviours in man. Clearly, these are complex and even a consensus concerning definition of the terms used, including "aggression" itself, is often the subject of conflicting opinions arising from the enormous amount of methodological, cultural and political approaches to aggression (see, for example (Feshbach and Fraczek, 1979)).

5.9   Clinical management of destructive behaviour

In biologically oriented research into destructive behaviours in man
(by whatever name they are called), it is evident that they are
associated with and present a significant clinical problem in a number
of mental disorders and syndromes. For example, such behaviours are
not infrequently associated with schizophrenic psychosis (Yesavage,
1983), epileptic seizures, mania, depression, organic brain syndrome
and mental retardation (Sheard, 1983, 1984; Sarteschi et al., 1978).
There is in addition, violent human behaviour associated with psychiatric disorders less clearly recognised as "diseases": e.g., the personality or character disorders (Sheard, 1983; Cloninger, 1983; Eichelman, 1978) in adults and conduct disorders in children (Behar and
Rapoport, 1983; Campbell et al., 1982).
When these problems become the focus of clinical attention, treatment of the underlying disorder will always be the therapy of first
choice. However, in a number of cases, such primary therapy will be
inhibited or impossible until the gross destructive tendencies are
adequately controlled (Madden and Lion, 1981).
At present, there are no drugs clinically available which specifically
suppress aggression (Tupin, 1985; Sheard, 1983, 1984). Consequently,
reliance has generally been placed on neuroleptics and minor tranquillizers.
The taming effects of neuroleptics are closely linked with their general
inhibition of all behaviours (Valzelli, 1979; Kostowski, 1978; Delina-
Stula and Vassout, 1979; Itil and Mukhoypadhyay, 1978).
The use of minor tranquillizers, such as chlordiazepoxide, based upon
their "taming" properties, has been criticized because increased aggressiveness (paradoxical aggression) has been observed following its
use both in animals and man (Valzelli, 1979; Bond and Lader, 1979;
Essman, 1978; Mos and Olivier, 1987; Mos et al., 1987).
Eltoprazine is very active in several models of offensive aggression,
e.g., isolation-induced and inter-male aggression in male mice, territorial aggression (resident-intruder) and colony aggression in male rats
and hypothalamically-induced aggression in male rats (this volume).
The results, obtained with very extensive ethological observation and
recording techniques (Olivier, 1981), point to very specific decreases in
the offensive components of the behaviour.

Animals treated with eltoprazine (about 0.5 to 10 mg/kg by oral or parenteral route) are fully capable of normal social interactions with members of the same species, but do not display the final consummatory parts of the offensive behavioural repertoire. These changes in offensive behaviour are not secondary to any general depressant or sedative effect of eltoprazine as there is no indication at behaviourally effective doses of sedation (sitting, lying, immobility), muscle relaxation, or sensory or motor disturbances.

In fact, the inhibition of offensive behaviour was accompanied by increases in social interest and exploratory behaviour. The latter finding cannot be ascribed to psychostimulant activity such as that found with d-amphetamine. Detailed behavioural analyses (Olivier et al., 1984) showed dramatic differences in the structure of the behaviour between eltoprazine- and d-amphetamine-treated animals (Olivier and Mos, 1986), indicating that eltoprazine did not induce stereotypies. Eltoprazine has, however, some limited stimulating effects on locomotor behaviour when animals were measured in exploratory situations as, for example, in hypothalamus-stimulated locomotion, photocell activity or open-field activity. It is possible that this stimulation is also present during social interactions, but is implemented as normal behaviours without interrupting them as does d-amphetamine or scopolamine. Therefore, it can be concluded that the potent antiaggressive action of eltoprazine and other serenics is not caused by response incompatibility between locomotor stimulation and aggression.

Eltoprazine was active in play-fighting among juvenile rats. This behaviour is considered to be a form of agonistic behaviour which is a juvenile representation of later adult agonistic behaviour. Eltoprazine was active in the same dose ranges as in adult rats and showed a similar behavioural profile; i.e., the decrease in aggression was not accompanied by a decrease in activity. Eltoprazine was also active in an aggression paradigm evoked by mixing groups of piglets unknown to each other. Unlike azaperone, a neuroleptic which sedated the animals and only postponed aggression, eltoprazine inhibited fighting without sedation or other apparent side effects.

Eltoprazine was also very active in a model involving aggression of a lactating female rat confronting an intruder to her nesting area. In this model, eltoprazine, like fluprazine, exhibits a different behavioural profile than that found in most male models. In particular, the stimulation of social interest and exploration is absent (Olivier and Mos, 1986; Olivier et al., 1985, 1986). On the other hand, treated females are clearly not incapacitated as they exhibit typical maternal behaviours such as pup retrieving, burrowing of pups and pup care (suckling). The behavioural structure certainly does not point to the sedative effects characteristic of several other compounds (Olivier et al., 1986; Olivier and Mos, 1986). Eltoprazine effectively suppresses mouse-killing behaviour (muricide) in rats, a model which involves both predatory and feeding elements.

However, for a proper perspective, effects of eltoprazine in these models of agonistic behaviour in animals should be compared with other putative "anti-aggressive" drugs or other reference compounds. For this reason, a very short summary is given of the effects of representatives of the main pharmacological classes of psychotropic drugs in these models.

It is clear upon reviewing the literature (Miczek, 1987) that a considerable number of psychotropic drugs, representing various pharmacological classes, do influence aggressive behaviour in animals. Because of the different types of aggression in animals, interpretation of drug effects is often difficult, and generalisation from one type to another has to be treated with special caution.

In the past decade, several influential reviews have more or less comprehensively summarised the known effects of psychotropic drugs on aggression in animals (Valzelli, 1978; Miczek, 1987; Miczek and Barry, 1976; Miczek and Krsiak, 1979). In general, drugs may inhibit or facilitate aggressive behaviours, and the following paragraphs briefly outline the major effects.

CNS-stimulants

High doses of stimulants (e.g. amphetamine) suppress all kinds of aggressive behaviour, probably due to the stereotypy induced, leading to response incompatibility (Miczek, 1974; Miczek and Krsiak, 1981). At low or moderate doses, a confusing picture emerges, as both enhancing and inhibiting effects have been reported (Miczek, 1987). These complex effects depend upon the stimulus situation, the species, the previous behavioural experience, the dose and the type of aggression invoked.

Antidepressants

There is a wide variation in the effects of antidepressants on agonistic behaviours and it is, consequently, difficult to generalize (Miczek, 1987). After acute administration of tricyclics, aggression is generally inhibited, but this is always accompanied by non-specific side effects (Olivier and Van Dalen, 1982). On the other hand, after chronic dosing, the effects of antidepressants are often opposite to those after acute administration (Miczek, 1987; Delina-Stula and Vassout, 1981). Lithium has anti-aggressive properties (Sheard, 1978), but its use is very limited due to its toxicity.

Neuroleptics (antipsychotics)

Neuroleptics have anti-aggressive activity, but these effects are behaviourally non-specific, being secondary to the heavy sedation and severe motor debility which occur at the same dosages (Olivier and Van Dalen, 1982; Olivier et al., 1984; Miczek, 1987).

Alcohol

Low doses of alcohol may facilitate certain kinds of aggression, while higher doses inhibit agonistic behaviours (Miczek, 1987; Sheard, 1978; Winslow et al., 1987) associated with non-specific motor and sensory depression (Blanchard and Blanchard, 1987).

Barbiturates

Low doses may exacerbate aggressive behaviours, while higher doses inhibit these behaviours, due mainly to non-specific motor debility (Miczek, 1987).

Benzodiazepines

Again, low doses may increase aggression (Mos and Olivier, 1987, 1988; Mos et al., 1987; Olivier and Mos, 1986; Olivier et al., 1985, 1986), whereas high doses decrease aggression secondary to muscle relaxation. The taming effects described after benzodiazepine administration in animals and humans are mainly obtained after high doses. At lower doses, conflicting effects have been reported, including the known paradoxical increases in aggression.

Hallucinogens

Compounds such as LSD exhibit conflicting effects in animal agonistic behaviours (Miczek and Barry, 1976). There is no consistent effect and those which have been found are generally attributed to alterations in responsiveness rather than in the agonistic behaviour itself. Marijuana (Δ^9-THC) reduces all kinds of aggression in most animal species, but it also hampers the defensive capabilities of animals, which suggests that its anti-aggressive effects are non-specific (Olivier et al., 1984; Miczek and Barry, 1976).

Anticonvulsants

Leaving aside such drugs as the barbiturates and benzodiazepines, the remaining anticonvulsants (e.g., diphenylhydantoin, primidone and carbamazepine) show contradictory effects on aggressive behaviour in both animals and man. In particular, the suggestion that anticonvulsants in man decrease episodic violent behaviour due to a dyscontrol syndrome (temporal lobe epilepsy) has not been conclusively answered as most data are derived from single case reports (Monroe, 1975).

Other drugs

Recently, there have been suggestions that centrally acting β-adrenergic antagonists may have specific anti-aggressive effects in some clinical situations and in animals as well (Miczek, 1987). This area of research clearly needs much more attention, but it may be pointed out that beta-blockers may have serious side effects (Sheard, 1984).

Our preclinical results

When we compare results obtained in our laboratory using other "anti-aggressive" compounds, a very similar picture emerges. We tested some of the compounds used clinically (e.g., Sch 12679, YG19-256, chlordiazepoxide, haloperidol and chlorpromazine). It appeared that YG-19-256, Sch 12679, haloperidol and chlorpromazine all have anti-aggressive effects, but certainly coincident with and probably secondary to behaviourally non-specific effects, such as sedation (sitting, lying, immobility). Moreover, these compounds all inhibited the entire social repertoire (e.g., introductory social behaviour and avoidance in male rats) suggesting that the anti-aggressive effects were caused by highly non-specific behavioural effects (Olivier and Van Dalen, 1982; Olivier, 1981).

In our aggression paradigms, chlordiazepoxide had no anti-aggressive effect; rather it appeared even to be pro-aggressive in some models, a result which corresponds with the paradoxical increase in aggression previously observed both in animals and in man (Valzelli, 1978, 1979; Essman, 1978).

Comparison of eltoprazine with the other compounds tested shows that only eltoprazine and other serenics have a demonstrably specific anti-aggressive profile in all the offensive models. This specificity should include a dose-dependent decrease in aggression, no impairment of social behaviour, no unwanted side-effects such as sedation, motor impairment, sensory incapacity or muscle relaxation. This profile underlines the unique properties of eltoprazine which, to our knowledge, is the most specific anti-aggressive compound found so far. The anti-aggressive qualities of eltoprazine are very pronounced in offensive aggression models (isolation-induced, inter-male aggression in mice and rats, territorial aggression and brain-stimulation-induced aggression in rats), but are also present in some other models (pig, maternal and predatory aggression).

Although aggression in males is more common than in females, females can behave quite aggressively. The fact that eltoprazine reduces female aggression, strongly indicates that eltoprazine does not exert its influence via testosterone, the male hormone which has been closely coupled to the expression of certain kinds of aggression (inter-male; hypothalamic induced; territorial (Barfield et al., 1972; Bermond et al., 1982; Schuurman, 1981). In addition, fluprazine (another serenic) inhibited muricide in castrated rats, which, we believe, suggests that the behavioural effect is not mediated by any central, testosterone-dependent mechanism (Olivier et al., 1984).

Finally, it should be noted that several investigators have confirmed the specific anti-aggressive effects of the first serenic, fluprazine, in both rats and mice (Benton et al., 1984; Brain et al., 1983; Flannelly et al., 1985; Potegal and Glusman, 1983; Racine et al., 1984; Poshivalov, 1987).

In general, eltoprazine has a reasonable-to-good duration of action with results somewhat dependent upon the species and paradigm used. After subchronic administration in mice and rats, either no (mice) or some (rats) minor tolerance has been noted. This indicates that the compound remains quite active after chronic use.

Eltoprazine had no significant influence upon defensive or flight capabilities. It had no activity in a defensive behaviour model in mice or on foot-shock induced defensive behaviour. Fluprazine, on the other hand, had considerable activity in the latter model, possibly due to its analgesic properties which can interfere with the evoking stimulus, i.e., pain.

In a more ethologically valid paradigm, assessing the intruder's behavioural response to attack, eltoprazine was tested after both acute and chronic treatment to the intruders. Although acute dosing with eltoprazine shifted defensive and flight strategies from more active towards more passive forms, the absence of effects on other behaviours strongly indicates that the increase in inactive behaviours after eltoprazine has not been caused by incapacitating effects such as sedation or muscle relaxation. The unchanged aggressive behaviour of the attacker towards eltoprazine-treated intruders also suggests that the behaviour of the latter is not dramatically changed. Such an indirect drug effect on the behaviour of the attackers can be clearly observed after intruder treatment with haloperidol or d-amphetamine (Olivier and Mos, 1986). After seven days pre-treatment, and one wash-out day, intruders were not distinguishable from vehicle treated ones, suggesting that no rebound effects occur in defence/flight behaviour.

The pattern observed in defence/flight after eltoprazine is comparable to that observed after fluprazine (Olivier and Mos, 1986). The decrease in offence, concomitant with intact retention of social interest and defence behaviour, implies that serenics may be good candidates for the effective control of destructive behaviours in some clinical situations.

In summary, it can be suggested that the typical profile of the specific anti-aggressive drugs, serenics, is an inhibition of the offensive components of agonistic behaviours without interference with the social or defensive capacities of the animals. While offensive behaviours are inhibited, they engage in all kinds of social interactions, including following, sniffing, approaching, and the like. This pattern typically differs from drugs belonging to other drug classes including those most often used in attempts to manage pathological destructive behaviour in the clinic (Sheard, 1983, 1984; Madden and Lion, 1981; Sheard, 1987; Itil, 1981). The drugs used in these destructive states are largely chosen upon empirical grounds (and sedative effects) rather than by extrapolation from animal data or coherent study in patients. The non-specific effects of these drugs are clearly seen also in animal models of agonistic behaviour (Olivier et al., 1986; Miczek and Krsiak, 1981; Miczek and Winslow, 1988).

In general, by characterizing the effects of drugs in several paradigms of offensive and defensive agonistic interactions and by using ethological methodology, we believe it may prove possible to develop drugs which may specifically inhibit certain destructive behaviours, such as those which may be found associated with schizophrenia, mania, primary dementias, profound retardation and similar disorders (Sheard, 1984). The need for such drugs is further supported by some clinicians, who suggest that "the optimal pharmacologic agent has yet to be discovered" (Monroe, 1975b). Therefore, serenics, on the basis of their specific behavioural profile in animal models of agonistic behaviour, will be tested in several states associated with destructive behaviours in patients.

5.10   Our clinical results

Eltoprazine in models of aggression in volunteers

Models in volunteers have been promoted as tool for measuring the effects of serotonin agonists in provoked human aggression under laboratory conditions (Bond, 1992). Although extrapolation of the results to patients with mental pathology and aggression remains a tremendous step, such models may bridge the even larger gap between animal models and patients in the clinic. Eltoprazine has been investigated in two models presumed to test aggressive behaviours in volunteers.

The first model employed a tentative model, proposed by O'Hanlon (Van Leeuwen et al., 1988). The provocative cue consisted of a movie showing a championship boxing match to young male volunteers, interested in contact sports. As control movie a nature documentary was chosen and to verify possible anxiolytic effects a terrifying movie was shown in the last session. The 48 volunteers were randomly distributed over four treatment groups, to receive 7 or 15 mg eltoprazine, 10 mg diazepam or placebo. The neutral movie was shown during a baseline session, the aggression and anxiety provoking movies were presented at different sessions, always in this order.

The test battery was designed to measure psychomotor functions, mood and emotions (checklist and visual analogue scale) and the Spielberger State/Trait Anxiety and Aggression inventories (Dutch versions, Van der Ploeg, 1980; 1982). Neuroendocrine arousal was measured by catecholamine excretions in urine and sympathetic nervous system arousal was measured by electrodermal and electro-cardiographic recordings. Diazepam, but not eltoprazine, induced the expected sedation in the objective psychometric assessments and subjective feelings. Eltoprazine only influenced the subjective experiences in comparison with placebo. Neither drug induced changes in feelings of aggression. With the lower dose of eltoprazine an increase in the Spielberger State Anxiety Score was found in comparison with placebo after the horror movie. Since the higher dose did not increase anxiety this may be a spurious finding. (Nor)adrenaline excretions were increased during the test sessions of active drug but not less so than with placebo. In the electrophysiological variables the only interesting finding was a decrease in skin conductance at both dose levels of eltoprazine. In total the results were disappointing.

It should be realized that in this model no actions were demanded, hence only changes in feeling, neuroendocrine or electrophysiological variables could be detected. A drug which would primarily affect impulse control and block the aggressive acting out, would not show efficacy in such a model. There may be other reasons though for the lack of results. In other centres movies were found inadequate as (eliciting) cues for aggression models (personal communication, Prof. P. Netter).

The second study with eltoprazine concerns a model developed and extensively validated by Cherek and co-workers (Cherek, 1981). The data of the eltoprazine study have been submitted for publication. The model employs a simple paradigm of two optional responses: a neutral one, to collect money and an aggressive response to subtract money from a presumed competitor (in fact the computer). Psychometric tests were applied to test for selective effects. In sessions approximately one week apart subjects were tested after a dose of placebo (baseline) and 5, 10 or 20 mg eltoprazine. Results showed a dose related decrease in aggressive responses, but also in non-aggressive responses at doses of 10 and 20 mg. As the psychometric tests did not reveal sedation, the interpretation of the decrease in neutral responding remains difficult.

Patient studies with eltoprazine
a) Selection of aggressive patients

Among psychiatrists two different views are operative regarding the relation between aggression and psychiatric disorders. Behaviorally oriented psychiatrists hold the opinion aggression should be considered a disease-specific and disease-dependent phenomenon. A disease-independent hypothesis is defended by more biologically oriented psychiatrists, who partly base their arguments on the established relationship between a defective serotonergic system in the central nervous system and impulsive aggressive behaviour in many different patient populations and also in non-psychiatric subjects. In view of this controversy pilot studies have been set up both in patients with "secondary" aggressive behaviour like demented elderly, mentally retarded and psychotic patients in whom aggressive behaviour is incidental to their diagnosis. The other population consisted of personality disordered patients (borderline and anti-social) in whom the aggressive behaviour is a feature of the diagnosis. This approach also prevents premature assumptions about the generalizability of treatment effects.

b) Study design

In all patient studies a placebo-controlled baseline of three to four weeks was used to reliably establish the level of aggression in each patient and to familiarize the staff with the assessment methods. To control for the confounding influences of time and the extra therapeutic supervision, a parallel placebo-group was included during the actual study period. In the pilot studies the double-blind study period was limited to four weeks. In the follow-up studies a longer period of eight to twelve weeks was chosen and restart of (double-blind) study medication was allowed for those patients who showed a recurrence of aggressive behaviour following stop of the actual study.

c) Evaluative scales

In consequence of the hypothesised relation between primary psychiatric diagnosis and aggressive behaviour, scales used in the evaluation of treatment effects should assess both aggressive behaviour and symptoms of the underlying disease. The scales chosen for the assessment of aggressive behaviour had to be applicable in such diverse populations as demented elderly, mentally retarded and personality disordered or psychotic patients. Scales therefore had to be objective in that they examine observable behaviour. Scales used included the Staff Observation Aggression Scale (Palmstierna and Wistedt, 1987), Overt Aggression Scale (Yudofsky et al., 1986) and the

Social Dysfunction and Aggression Scale (ERAG, 1992). This latter scale combines items that address observable behaviour and items that can be assessed only in verbally competent patient groups. As in all psychotropic drug research in each study a scale allowing semi-quantification of subjective impressions was used, either the Clinical Global Impression scale or the Global Aggression Scale (Bech et al., 1986).

To assess the symptoms of the underlying disease different scales have been used, in psychotic patients the Brief Psychiatric Rating Scale, in demented elderly the Sandoz Clinical Assessment of the Geriatric Scale, in mentally retarded the Nurses' Observation Scale for In-patient Evaluation.

Pilot studies with eltoprazine in different patient populations
a) Demented elderly with aggressive behaviour

This pilot study was designed as a multi-centre parallel-group study in patients suffering from Senile Dementia of Alzheimer's Type (SDAT) or mixed SDAT/Multi-Infarct Dementia (DSM-IIIR criteria). All patients should at least have been hospitalised for two months and have shown a minimum of four episodes of hostile or disruptive behaviour per week over the four weeks preceding entry to the study. Following screening, patients were directly randomised per block of three to receive eltoprazine or placebo (2:1) in the double-blind treatment phase. Before entering the double-blind treatment phase all patients received single-blind placebo during a three-week run-in period to establish a baseline of aggressive behaviour. Other psychotropic medication should have been washed-out before the study start. Twenty-nine patients entered the study. Twenty were randomised to receive eltoprazine and nine to receive placebo. There was no influence of eltoprazine on the demented state per se that could have become evident in the scoring of the Sandoz Clinical Assessment of the Geriatric Scale. The overall level of aggression was modest and mainly of a verbal and mild physical nature. Clinically significant reductions in aggressive behaviour in eltoprazine-treated patients were especially apparent from the descriptions in the case summaries. These relevant improvements were most apparent in the more severely aggressive patients and were substantiated by the improved scorings on the Social Dysfunction and Aggression Scale in this subgroup of patients.

There were no worrying safety problems related to eltoprazine treatment. In general eltoprazine was reasonably tolerated.

b) Mentally retarded patients with aggressive behaviour

Mentally retarded patients (DSM-IIIR criteria) with a possible concurrent diagnosis of autistic disorder following screening were directly randomised per block of four to receive either eltoprazine or placebo (3:1). Before entering the double-blind phase, all patients received single-blind placebo to establish a baseline of aggressive behaviour. All other psychotropic medication was washed-out before entering the placebo run-in period. Patients who were considered for the study should have been hospitalised for at least two months and have shown a minimum of three episodes of hostile or disruptive behaviour per week over the four weeks preceding entry to the study. Recruitment of patients proved difficult due to problems in wash-out from neuroleptics. On the one hand there was a reluctance on the part of the nursing staff on the other hand some patients showed rebound aggression on stop of neuroleptic treatment. In total 22 patients entered the double-blind study period. Seventeen were randomised to receive eltoprazine and five to placebo. There was no influence of eltoprazine on the level of functioning or abilities of these patients. There was a clear hint of anti-aggressive activity of eltoprazine in those patients who on the basis of their pre-treatment Social Dysfunction and Aggression Scale scores could be considered moderately to severely aggressive. There appeared to be a poor correlation between the scale scoring number of aggressive events (Overt Aggression Scale) and the Social Dysfunction and Aggresion Scale which assesses the basal level of aggressive behaviour. Severity of aggressive behaviour is not only determined by a high frequency but also and even more by the consequences of the behaviour for the environment of the patient and the patient himself and the extent to which this behaviour is uncorrectable and unmanageable.

There were no systematic safety problems and in general eltoprazine was well tolerated.

c) Psychotic or personality disordered patients with aggressive behaviour

Patients with a history of aggressive behaviour who were either drug free or received neuroleptics in a stable regimen entered a placebo controlled single-blind baseline period of four weeks to verify the criterion of one physical aggressive event per week. All were in-patients. Following the baseline period patients were randomised per block of three to receive either eltoprazine or placebo (2:1). In total 23 patients received eltoprazine and 13 placebo.

There were no significant differences between treatment groups for the mean scores of the CGI and BPRS indicating no major influence on mental state. Analysis of the clusters for outward and inward directed aggression of the Social Dysfunction and Aggression Scale revealed a slightly greater improvement in the eltoprazine group, especially in the latter part of the study. Overall there was a considerable placebo response, underscoring the need for a placebo parallel group. The use of the Overt Aggression Scale proved cumbersome because of multiple isolation periods in many patients.

Safety and tolerance were good, except for some dreaming abnormalities and anxiety mainly during taper-off.

d) Other experiences with eltoprazine

Two small pilot studies were performed in depressed patients and chronic psychotic or personality disordered patients to asses the safety and tolerance in these populations. In the pilot study in depressed patients eltoprazine was well tolerated and appeared to equally well alleviate depressed mood as did imipramine. The small number of patients in this study (seven on eltoprazine, six on imipramine) precludes any definitive conclusion regarding the efficacy of eltoprazine in depression. The aim of the study in psychotic and personality disordered patients was to assess any possible adverse neurological effects of combined neuroleptic and eltoprazine administration. There was no evidence of eltoprazine-induced neurological abnormality. Eltoprazine added to the neuroleptic regimen induced global improvement after one week, and indications of an early effect on destructive behaviour were found in moderately or severely aggressive patients.

Further studies with eltoprazine

In the second series of studies attention was focussed on efficacy of eltoprazine in mentally retarded patients with (hetero- or auto-) aggressive behaviour and as second priority on aggressive psychotic and personality disordered patients. The choice of mental retardation was primarily based on the medical need in this patient population. Another reason was a methodological one: aggressive mentally retarded patients usually remain institutionalized, which allows follow up under more or less stable conditions.

Results in mentally retarded patients

A large study was set up to measure effects in aggressive mentally retarded patients (De Koning et al., submitted). A total of 19 centres spread over four European countries participated. The study followed a randomized parallel groups design with a 4-week baseline placebo followed by an 8-week double blind period. After extensive screening 205 patients with a diagnosis of mental retardation, some in combination with a pervasive developmental disorder, entered the baseline period. Of this cohort 160 patients who fulfilled further criteria, were randomized to receive blind medication: 119 patients were assigned to the eltoprazine group and 41 to the placebo group. The dose level of eltoprazine, after taper on, was 20 mg daily with an option to increase to 30 mg. At the end of the 8-week blind period the dose was tapered off.

Three scales were used to measure aggression, the OAS, a 20-item version of the SDAS and a 0–10 point Global Aggression Scale (Bech, 1986). In addition an overall clinical evaluation was determined at the end of the study. Six patients left the study prematurely.

When the total sample was analyzed, none of the major aggression variables showed a statistically significant difference between the groups. A decrease in scores between 20 and 35 percent was observed between baseline and week 6, the last assessment on full dose treatment in both groups. Of the separate symptoms of the SDAS, self-mutilation showed the most convincing improvement. The final clinical evaluation showed 60 percent of patients in the eltoprazine group and 49 percent of the placebo treated patients were reported to have displayed a significant improvement of behaviour. Closer analyses revealed that the difference between the groups in favour of eltoprazine was due exclusively to the response (rate) in the severely aggressive patients which was twice as high in that group as in the placebo group.

In the safety data no unexpected or drug related abnormalities were detected and tolerance was good. The data will be reported extensively elsewhere.

*Further experience in psychotic and personality
disordered patients*

The relatively large pilot study of 45 patients in psychotic and
borderline personality disordered patients had shown some early
positive effects of eltoprazine, which was most evident in patients with
a marked degree of aggressive behaviour. The entry criteria for
behaviour were very loose in that study, hence a new study was set up,
stratified for diagnosis and applying hard criteria of aggressive behaviour namely at least one episode of physical aggression during the
4-week baseline placebo period. In line with the study of mentally
retarded patients, the double-blind period lasted eight weeks, including taper on or off, with a maximum dosis 40 mg daily. The set of
aggression scales was the same as in the MR study; to check for
overall mental symptomatology the BPRS was added.

A total of 36 patients, mean age 34 years, entered the double blind
period, 18 chronic psychotic patients and 18 patients who only had an
DSM III-R axis II diagnosis of anti-social or borderline personality
disorder. Due to the unequal randomization 23 patients received
eltoprazine and 13 placebo. Three patients did not complete the study
(2 eltoprazine and 1 placebo treated patients).

Because of the small size of the study statistically significant differences were hardly expected and indeed we found no differences in the
major efficacy parameters. There were, however, positive trends in
favour of eltoprazine, specifically in the latter part of the study. This
contrasts somewhat with observations in mentally handicapped patients where improvements occurred earlier.

Placebo responses were considerable, also in this study. The scores of
the Global Aggression Scale showed a decrease of 25% in the placebo
group against 37% in the eltoprazine group.

The scores of the OAS could not be evaluated. Periods of isolation due
to behavioural problems had led to missing reports on these essential
days or weeks in the trial periods.

The BPRS total scores differed markedly between the two strata of
patients as expected. Higher scores occurred in the psychotic patients.
There was a slight trend towards improvement during eltoprazine
treatment in the psychotic patients.

There was no evidence of safety or tolerance problems. Withdrawal
effects, increased anxiety, aggression and nightmares were observed
at taper off in one patient. With reinstitution of eltoprazine treatment
these symptoms rapidly abated.

Long-term data were collected from patients in the two studies reported above, who responded well. Upon request of the investigators patients entered a 6-month extension period because of worsening after the original study. The treatment remained blind for the majority of patients in the extension treatment period. In addition an open study was set up in the same categories of patients.

Re-entry in the (extension) study produced in most patients, compared to the first 8-week treatment period, similar responses of behaviour i.e. a slight trend in favour of eltoprazine. With continued treatment, however, placebo treated patients fared at least as well as the eltoprazine group and tolerance was suspected to develop with eltoprazine. Similar experiences were reported by some, but not all investigators of the open long-term study.

Conclusion from patient studies with eltoprazine

The hints of efficacy from pilot studies in different patient populations could not be confirmed in subsequent larger studies. In these latter studies during the initial phase, eltoprazine appeared to be more efficacious in the more aggressive patients but tolerance was suspected to develop with eltoprazine. This was confirmed in the long-term extensions to these studies. Heterogeneity of behaviour for expression and basic pathology, limited range of useful scales, high placebo effects, multiple co-medications and problems in obtaining consent and Review Board approvals make the clinical aggression field a high risk arena for any clinical investigator and thus indirectly also for the sponsoring industry. Recently Eichelman has made a plea for more individual-directed research strategies in aggression and a more lenient attitude by the FDA concerning proof of efficacy in aggressive behaviours (Eichelman, 1992). If the questionable evidence from the available studies with buspirone and eltoprazine is taken at face value and the impression of some investigators based on individual patients is scrutinized, the following picture appears.

If eltoprazine acts indeed in some aggressive psychiatric patients it may be primarily through improvement in aspects related to emotions and social behaviour rather than improvement of inadequate impulse control. Remarks in this sense have been made by several investigators of buspirone and eltoprazine (Gualtieri, 1991; Realmuto et al., 1989; Tiihonen et al., 1993; Verhoeven et al., 1992).

The investigators of the larger series of patients treated with buspirone, Levy and Ratey, both report effects on aggressive behaviour and
anxiety (Levy et al., 1992; Ratey et al., 1991). In the case of Ratey's
study these effects seem to occur at a slightly different dose level and
time schedule, the effect on aggressive behaviour appearing earlier
and at a lower dose (15 mg daily). Hence anxiolytic activity of 5-HT_1
agonists may not form the basis of possible anti-aggressive effects.

In the eltoprazine studies positive effects on social attitude and
communication were noted by several investigators (Verhoeven et al.,
1992; Tiihonen et al., 1993 and unpublished data), leading to the
suggestion that this drug might be useful in autistic patients. The hints
of different and more convincing effects by eltoprazine on self-
mutilation than on hetero-aggressive behaviour, point to the need to
separate auto- and hetero aggressive behaviours in future studies with
any compound in aggressive behaviours; a feature which is clearly
supported also by the validation studies of the Social Dysfunction and
Aggression Scale (Wistedt et al., 1990; European Aggression Rating
Group, 1992).

Measurement of other effects than just pure reduction of the number
of aggressive events per time-unit, is necessary to reveal the total
spectrum of effects induced by a drug and confirm the associations
between symptoms of a psychiatric syndrome in individual patients
for whom aggressive behaviour may be only one of the intrinsic
symptoms or an incidental co-existing phenomenon.

Acknowledgements

We thank Marijke Mulder and Ruud van Oorschot for their excellent
technical assistance.

References

Adamec, R.E. and Himes, M. The interaction of hunger, feeding, and
experience in alteration of topography of the rat's predatory response to
mice. Behav. Biol. 1978; 22: 230-243.

Adams, D.B. The relation of scent-marking, olfactory investigation, and
specific postures in the isolation-induced fighting of rats. Behaviour 1976;
56: 286-297.

Adams, D.B. Brain mechanisms for offense, defense and submission.
Behav. Brain Sci. 1979; 2: 201-241.

Archer, J. The behavioural biology of aggression. Cambridge: Cambridge
University Press, 1988.

Asarch, K.B., Ransom, R.W. and Shih, J.C. 5-HT$_{1A}$ and 5-HT$_{1B}$ selectivity of two phenylpiperazine derivatives: evidence for 5-HT$_{1B}$ heterogeneity. Life Sci. 1985; 36: 1265-1275.

Åsberg, M., Tråskman, L. and Thoren, P. 5-HT in the cerebrospinal fluid: a biochemical suicide predictor? Arch. Gen. Psychiatry 1976; 33: 1193-1197.

Azcarate, C.L. Minor tranquillizers in the treatment of aggression. J. Nerv. Ment. Disease, 1975; 160: 100-107.

Baenninger, R. Some aspects of predatory behavior. Aggr. Behav. 1978; 4: 287-311.

Baerends, G.P. The ethological approach to human behaviour. In: Baerends, G.P., ed., Ethology, the biology of behaviour. Wageningen: PUDOC, 1973; 288-324.

Barfield, R.J., Busch, D.E. and Wallen, K. Gonadal influence on agonistic behavior in the male domestic rat. Horm. Behav. 1972; 3: 247-259.

Barnett, S.A. The rat. A study in behavior. Chicago and London: The University of Chicago Press, 1975.

Bech, P., Kastrup, M., and Rafaelson, O.J. Mini compendium of Rating Scales. Acta Psychiatr. Scand. 1986; 73 (suppl. 326): 7-37.

Behar, D. and Rapoport, J.L. Hyperactivity and other childhood disorders. In: Hippius, H. and Winokur, G., eds., Psychopharmacology 1, Part 2: Clinical psychopharmacology. Amsterdam, Oxford, Princeton: Excerpta Medica, 1983; 321-344.

Bell, R. and Brown, K. The effects of two "anti-aggressive" compounds, an indenopyridine and a benzothiazepin, on shock-induced defensive fighting in rats. Progr. Neuro-Psychopharmacol. 1979; 3: 399-402.

Benton, D. The extrapolation from animals to man: the example of testosterone and aggression. In: Brain, P.F. and Benton, D., eds., Multidisciplinary approaches to aggression research. Amsterdam: Elsevier/North-Holland Biomedical Press, 1981; 401-418.

Benton, D., Brain, P.F., Jones, S., Colebrook, E. and Grimm, V. Behavioural examinations of the anti-aggressive drug fluprazine. Behav. Brain Res. 1984; 10: 325-338.

Bermond, B., Mos, J., Meelis, W., Poel, v.d. A.M. and Kruk, M.R. Aggression induced by stimulation of the hypothalamus: effects of androgens. Pharmacol Biochem. Behav. 1982; 16: 41-45.

Binder, R.L. and McNiel, D.E. Victims and families of violent psychiatric patients. Bull. Am. Acad. Psychiatry Law 1986; 14: 131-139.

Bioulac, B., Benezech, M., Renaud, B., Noel, B. and Roch, D. Biogenic amines in the 47 XYY syndrome. Neuropsychobiol. 1978; 4: 366-370.

Bioulac, B., Benezech, M., Renaud, B., Noel, B. and Roch, D. Serotoninergic dysfunction in the 47 XYY syndrome. Biol. Psychiatry 1980; 15: 917-923.

Blanchard, R.J., O'Donnell, V. and Blanchard, D.C. Attack and defensive behaviors in the albino mouse. Aggr. Behav. 1979; 5: 341-352.

Blanchard, R.J. and Blanchard, D.C. Aggressive behavior in the rat. Behav. Biol. 1977; 21: 197-224.

Blanchard, R.J. and Blanchard, D.C. The organisation and modelling of animal aggression. In: Brain, P.F. and Benton, D., eds., The biology of aggression. Alphen a.d. Rijn: Sijthoff and Noordhoff, 1981; 529-561.

Blanchard, R.J. and Blanchard, D.C. Affect and aggression: an animal model applied to human behaviour. In: Blanchard, R.J. and Blanchard, D.C., eds., Advances in the study of aggression, Vol. 1: Orlando, Florida: Academic Press, 1984; 1-62.

Blanchard, R.J., Blanchard, D.C., Takahashi, T. and Kelley, M.J. Attack and defensive behaviour in the albino rat. Anim. Behav. 1977; 25: 622-634.

Blanchard, R.J. and Blanchard, D.C. Alcohol and aggression in animal models. In: Olivier, B., Mos, J. and Brain, P.F., eds., Ethopharmacology of agonistic behaviour in animals and man. Dordrecht: Martinus Nijhoff, 1987; 145-161.

Blanchard, R.J., Blanchard, D.C. and Takahashi, L.K. Reflexive fighting in the albino rat: aggressive or defensive behavior? Aggr. Behav. 1977; 3: 145-155.

Blanchard, D.C. and Blanchard, R.J. Ethoexperimental approaches to the biology of emotion. Ann. Rev. Psychol. 1988; 39: 43-68.

Blanchard, D.C., Takahashi, R., Blanchard, R.J., Flanelly, K.J. and Kemble, E.D. Fluprazine hydrochloride does not decrease defensive behaviours of wild and septal syndrome rats. Physiol. Behav. 1985; 35: 349-353.

Blanchard, R.J., Blanchard, D.C. and Takahashi, L.K. Reflexive fighting in the albino rat: aggressive or defensive behavior? Aggr. Behav. 1977a; 3: 145-155.

Blanchard, R.J., Takahashi, L.K., and Blanchard, D.C. The development of intruder attack in colonies of laboratory rats. Anim. Learn. Behav. 1977b; 5, 365-369.

Bond, A.J. Pharmacologic manipulation of aggressiveness and impulsiveness in healthy volunteers, Prog. Neuro-Psychopharmacol. Biol. Psychiat. 1992; 16, 1-7.

Bond, A. and Lader, M. Benzodiazepines and aggression. In: Sandler, M., ed., Psychopharmacology of aggression. New York: Raven Press, 1979; 173-182.

Bradford, LD., Olivier, B., van Dalen, D. and Schipper, J. Serenics: the pharmacology of fluprazine and DU 28412. In Miczek, KA., Kruk, M.R. and Olivier, B., eds., Ethopharmacological aggression research. New York: Alan R. Liss, 1984; 191-207.

Brain, P.F. Hormones and aggression in infra-human vertebrates. In: Brain, P.F. and Benton, D., eds., The biology of aggression. Alphen a/d Rijn: Sijthoff and Noordhoff, 1981; 181-213.

Brain, P.F. Biological explanations of human aggression and the resulting therapies offered by such approaches: a critical evaluation. In: Blanchard, R.J. and Blanchard, D.C., eds., Advances in the study of aggression, Vol. 1. Orlando, Florida: Academic Press, 1984; 63-102.

Brain, P.F. Alcohol and aggression. London: Croom Helm, 1986.

Brain, P.F., Jones, S.E. and Kamis, A. A preliminary ethological analysis of the effects of DU 27716 on intermale aggression in Swiss-Webster mice. Aggr. Behav. 1983; 9: 117.

Breyer, U. Accumulation and elimination of a novel metabolite during chronic administration of the phenothiazine drug perazine to rats. Biochem. Pharm. 1972; 21: 1419.

Breyer, U., Gaertner, H.J. and Prox, A. Formation of identical metabolites from piperazine and dimethylamino substituted phenothiazine drugs in man, rat and dog. Biochem. Pharm. 1974; 23: 313.

Brown, G.L., Goodwin, F.K., Ballenger, J.C., Goyer, P. and Major, L. Aggression in humans correlates with cerebrospinal fluid metabolites. Psychiatry Res. 1979; 1: 131.

Brown, G.L., Ebert, M.H., Goyer, P.F., Jimerson, D.C., Klein, W.J., Bunney, W.E. and Goodwin, F.K. Aggression, suicide, and serotonin; relationships to CSF amine metabolites. Am. J. Psychiatry 1982; 139: 741-746.

Caccia, S., Notarnicola, C., Fong, M.H. and Benfenati, E. Identification and quantitation of l-arylpiperazines, metabolites resulting from side-chain cleavance of (4-substituted aryl-1-piperazine) alkyl heterocyclic derivatives in rat plasma and brain. J Chromatogr. 1984; 283: 211-221.

Caccia, S., Conti, I. and Notarnicola, A. In vivo metabolism in the rat and mouse of antrafenine to 1-m-trifluormethylphenylpiperazine. J Pharm. Pharmacol. 1985; 37: 75-77.

Caccia, S., Conti, I., Notarnicola, A. and Urso, R. Lipophilicity and disposition of 1-aryl-piperazines in the rat. Xenobiotica 1987; 17: 605-616.

Caccia, S. In vivo metabolism of 4-substituted arylpiperazines to pharmacologically active 1-arylpiperazines. Boll. Chim. Farmaceutico 1990; 129: 183-189.

Caccia, S., Ballabio, M., Smanin, R., Zanini, M.G. and Garattini, S. (-)-m-Chlorophenyl-piperazine, a central 5-hydroxytryptamine agonist, is a metabolite of trazodone. J Pharm. Pharmacol. 1981; 33: 477-478.

Campbell, M., Cohen, I.L. and Small, A.M. Drugs in aggressive behavior. J. Am. Acad. Child. Psych. 1982; 21: 107-117.

Carlsson, A., Bédard, P., Lindqvist, M. and Magnusson, T. The influence of nerve-impulse flow on the synthesis and metabolism of 5-hydroxytryptamine in the central nervous system. Biochem. Soc. Symp. 1972; 36: 17-32.

Chandler, J.D. and Chandler, J.E. The prevalence of neuropsychiatric disorders in a nursing home population. J. Geriatr. Psychiatry Neurol 1988; 1: 71-76.

Cherek, D.R. Effects of smoking different doses of nicotine on human aggressive behaviour, Psychopharmacol. 1981; 75: 339-345.

Claassen, V., Davies, J.E., Hertting, G. and Placheta, P. Fluvoxamine, a specific 5-hydroxytryptamine uptake inhibitor. Br.J. Pharmacol. 1979; 60: 505-516.

Cloninger, C.R. Antisocial behaviour. Psychopharmacoloy 1983; 2: 353-370.

Cohen-Mansfield, J. Agitated behaviors in the elderly: II. Preliminary results in the cognitively deteriorated. J. Am. Geriatr. Soc. 1986; 34: 722-727.

Conn, J.P., Sanders-Bush, F., Hoffman, BJ. and Hartig, PR. A unique receptor in choroid plexus is linked to phosphatidylinositol turnover. Proc. Natl. Acad. Sci. 1986; 83: 4086-4088.

Conners, C.K. A teacher rating scale for use in drug studies with children, Am. J. Psychiat. 1969; 126: 152-156.

Cools, A. Psychopharmacology and aggression: an appraisal of the current situation. In: Brain, P.F. and Benton, D., eds., The biology of aggression. Alphen a/d Rijn: Sijthoff and Noordhoff, 1981; 131-145.

Da Vanzo, J.P., McConnaughy, M.M., Brooks, R., Cooke, L. Evidence that reversal of mouse aggression is not related to beta blockade. Drug Devl. Res. 1988; 13: 259-267.

Dantzer, R. and Mormède, P. Effects of lithium on aggressive behaviour in domestic pigs. J. Vet. Pharmacol. Therap. 1979; 2: 299-303.

Daruna, J.H. Patterns of brain monoamine activity and aggressive behavior. Neurosci. Biobehav. Res. 1978; 2: 101-113.

Day, K. Psychiatric disorder in the middle-aged and elderly mentally handicapped. Br. J. Psychiatry 1985; 147: 660-667.

De Vries, M.H., De Koning, P., Floot, H.L., Grahnén, A., Eckernäs, S.A., Raghoebar, M., Dahlström, B. and Ekman, L. Dose-proportionality of eltoprazine. Eur. J. Clin. Pharmacol. 1991; 41: 485-488.

De Lange, N. and Raghoebar, M. Distribution of radioactively labelled eltoprazine in rat and dog. Drug Metabol. Drug Interact. 1990; 8: 115-127.

DeBold, J.F. and Miczek, K.A. Aggression persists after ovariectomy in female rats. Horm. Behav. 1984; 18: 177-190.

Delina-Stula, A. and Vassout, A. Differential effects of psychoactive drugs on aggressive responses in mice and rats. In: Sandler, M., ed., Psychopharmacology of aggression. New York: Raven Press, 1979; 41-60.

Delina-Stula, A. and Vassout, A. The effects of antidepressants on aggressiveness induced by social deprivation in mice. Pharmacol. Biochem. Behav. 1981; 14 (suppl. 1): 33-41.

Dietrich, B., Herrmann, W.M. and Mak, M. International Congress of the

European College of Neuropsychopharmacology (ECNP), Gothenburg, Sweden, 1989; May 23-26.

Dijkstra, H., Olivier, B. and Mos, J. Dominance maintenance and intruder attack in laboratory colonies of rats: different models for the psychopharmacological control of aggression. Aggr. Behav. 1984; 10: 149.

DiMascio, A. The effects of benzodiazepines on aggression: reduced or increased? Psychopharmacologia, 1973; 30: 95-102.

Dixon, A.K. A possible olfactory component in the effects of diazepam on social behavior of mice. Psychopharmacology 1982; 77: 246-252.

Dixon, A.K and Kaesermann, H.P. Ethopharmacology of flight behaviour. In: Olivier, B., Mos, J. and Brain, P.F., eds., Ethopharmacology of agonistic behaviour in animals and man. Dordrecht: Martinus Nijhoff, 1987; 46-79.

Eccleston, D. and Doogan, D.P. Serotonin in behavioural disorders. Br. J. Psychiatry 1989; 155 (Suppl. 8): 5-69.

Eichelman, B. Animal models: their role in the study of aggressive behavior in humans. Progr. Neuro- Psychopharmacol. 1978; 2: 633-643.

Eichelman, B. Aggressive behavior: from laboratory to clinic. Quo vadit?, Arch. Gen. Psychiatry, 1992; 49: 488-492.

Elliot, F.A. Propranolol for the control of the belligerent behavior following acute brain damage. Ann. Neurol. 1978; 1: 489-491.

Enreille, A., Pognat, J.F., Galmier, M.J., Lartigue-Mattei, C., Chabard, J.L., Busch, N. and Berger, J.A. Eur. J. Drug Met. Pharmacokin. 1991; 16: 161.

Erskine, M.S., Barfield, R.J. and Goldman, B.S. Intraspecific fighting during late pregnancy and lactation in rats and effects of litter removal. Behav. Biol. 1978a; 23: 206-218.

Erskine, M.S., Denenberg, V.H. and Goldman, B.D. Aggression in the lactating rat: effects of intruder age and test arena. Behav. Biol. 1978b; 23: 52-66.

Erskine, M.S., Denenberg, V.H. and Goldman, B.D. Postpartum aggression in rats: II. Dependence on maternal sensitivity to young and effects of experience with pregnancy and parturition. J Comp. Physiol. Zool. 1980; 94: 495-505.

Essman, W.B. Benzodiazepines and aggressive behavior. Modern problems of aggressive behavior. Mod. Probl. Pharmacopsych. 1978; 13: 13-28.

European Aggression Rating Group (ERAG). Social Dysfunction and Aggression Scale (SDAS-21) in generalized aggression and in aggressive attacks. A validity and reliability study. Int. J. Methods Psychiat. Res. 1992; 2: 15-29.

Faser, D. The behaviour of growing pigs during experimental social encounters. J. Agric. Sci. Cambridge 1974; 82: 147-163.

Feshbach, S. and Fraczek, A. Changing aggression: the need and the approach. In: Feshbach, S. and Fraczek, A., eds., Aggression and behavior change – Biological and social processes. New York: Praeger, 1979; 1-5.

Flannelly, K.J., Muraoka, M.Y. and Blanchard, D.C. Specific antiaggressive effects of fluprazine hydrochloride. Psychopharmacology 1985; 87: 86-89.

Floody, O.R. and Pfaff, D.W. Aggressive behaviour among female hamsters: the hormonal basis for fluctuations in female aggressiveness correlated with estrous state. J. Comp. Physiol. Psychol. 1977; 91: 443-446.

Floody, O.R. Hormones and aggression in female animals. In: Svare, B.B., ed., Hormones and aggressive behavior. New York and London: Plenum Press, 1983; 39-89.

Fong, M.H., Garattini, S. and Caccia, S. 1-m-Chlorophenylpiperazine is an active metabolite common to the psychotropic drugs trazodone, etoperidone and mepiprazole. J Pharm. Pharmacol. 1982; 34: 674-675.

Franc, J.E., Duncan, G.F., Farmen, R.H. and Pittman, K.A. J Chrom. 1991; 570: 129.

Gaertner, H.J., Liomin, G., Villamsen, D., Birtele, R. and Breyer, U. Tissue metabolites of trifluorperazine, fluphenazine, prochlorperazine, and perphenazine. Kinetics in chronic treatment. Drug Metabolism and Disposition 1975; 3: 437.

Gandelman, R. Androgen and fighting behavior. In: Brain, P.F. and Benton, D., eds., The biology of aggression. Alphen a/d Rijn: Sijthoff and Noordhoff, 1981; 215-230.

Gianutsos, G. and Lal, H. Aggression in mice after p-chloramphetamine. Res. Comm. Chem. Pathol. Pharmacol. 1975; 10: 379-382.

Gibbons, J.L., Barr, G.A., Bridger, W.H. and Leibowitz, S.F. Manipulations of dietary tryptophan: Effects on mouse killing and brain serotonin in the rat. Brain Res. 1979; 169: 139-153.

Glennon, R.A. Site selective serotonin agonists as discriminative stimuli. Psychopharmacology, 1986; 89: (SI) 135.

Grant, E.C. and Mackintosh, J.H. A comparison of the social postures of some common laboratory rodents. Behaviour 1963; 21: 246-259.

Gualtieri, C.T. Buspirone for the behavior problems of patients with organic brain disorders (letter), J. Clin. Psychopharmacol. 1991; 11: 280-281.

Gunn, J. Drugs in the violence clinic. In: Sandler, M., ed., Psychopharmacology of aggression. New York: Raven Press, 1979; 183-195.

Guy W (Ed.). ECDEU Assessment manual for psychopharmacology. Revised. US Department of health, education and wellfare. Rockville, Maryland. Clinical Global Impression 1976; p. 218.

Haney, M., DeBold, J.F. and Miczek, K.A. Maternal aggression in mice and rats towards male and female conspecifics. Aggr. Behav. 1989; 15: 443-453.

Haney, M. and Miczek, K.A. d-Amphetamine, MDMA, and PCP effects on aggressive and conditioned behavior: 5-HT and dopamine antagonists. Soc. Neurosci. Abstr. 1989; 15 (Pt. 1): 635.

Hartog, J., Olivier, B., Krüse, C., Van Wijngaarden, I., Van der Heyden, J.A.M. and Van Dalen, D. New pharmaceutical compositions having a psychotropic activity (Duphar Intl. Res. B.V.), EP 189.612. 1986.

Hill, B.K., Balow, A.A. and Bruininks, R.H. A national study of prescribed drugs in institutions and community residential facilities for mentally retarded people. Psychopharmacol. Bull. 1985; 21: 279-284.

Hinde, R.A. Biological bases of human social behaviour. New York.: McGraw-Hill, 1974.

Horn, H.J. Simplified LD 50 (or ED_{50}) calculations. Biometrics 1956; 12: 311-322.

Huntingford, F.A. The relationship between inter- and intra-specific aggression. Anim. Behav. 1976; 24: 485-497.

Huntingford, F.A. and Turner, A.K. Animal Conflict, Chapman and Hall, London 1987.

Itil, T.M. Drug treatment in the management of aggression. In: Brain, P.F. and Benton, D., eds., Multidisciplinary approaches to aggression research. Amsterdam: Elsevier/North-Holland Biomedical Press, 1981; 489-502.

Itil, T.M. and Mukhopadhyay, S. Pharmacological management of human violence. Mod. Probl. Pharmacopsych. 1978; 13: 139-158.

Janssen, P.A.J., Jageman, A.H. and Niemegeers, J.E. Effecs of various drugs on isolation-induced fighting behaviour of male mice. J. Pharmacol. Exp. Ther. 1959; 125: 471-475.

Jorgensen, A.Metabolism and pharmacokinetics of antipsychotic drugs. In: Bridges, J.W. and Chasseaud, L.F., eds., Progress in Drug Metabolism. Taylor & Francis, London and Philadelphia 1986; 9: 111-174.

Karli, P. The Norway rat's killing response to the white mouse: an experimental analysis. Behaviour 1956; 10: 81-103.

Karli, M., Vergnes, M. and Didiergeorges, F. Rat-mouse interspecific aggressive behaviour and its manipulation by brain ablation and by brain stimulation. In: Garattini, S. and Sigg, E.B., eds., Aggressive behaviour. Amsterdam: Excerpta Medica Foundation 1969; 47-55.

Karli, P. Conceptual and methodological problems associated wilh the study of brain mechanisms underlying aggressive behaviour. In: Brain, P.F. and Benton, D., eds., The biology of aggression. Alphen a.d. Rijn: Sijthoff and Noordhoff, 1981; 323-361.

Klotz, J. A modified Cochran-Friedman test with missing observations and ordered categorical data. Biometrics 1980; 36: 665-670.

Koning De, P. and Mak, M. Problems in Human Aggression Research, J. Neuropsychiatry 1991; 3: suppl. 1., s61-65.

Koolhaas, J.M. Hypothalamically induced intraspecific aggressive behaviour in the rat. Exp. Brain Res. 1978; 32: 365-375.

Koster, H.J., De Greef, L., Klerks, F. and Raghoebar, M. The metabolite patterns of eltoprazine in man, dog, rat and rabbit. Drug Metabol. Drug Interact. 1990; 8: 129.

Kostowski, W. Effects of sedatives and major tranquilizers on aggressive behavior. Modern Probl. Pharmacopsych. 1978; 13: 1-12.

Krsiak, M. Timid singly-housed mice: their value in prediction of psychotropic activity of drugs. Br. J. Pharmacol. 1975; 55: 141-150.

Krsiak, M. Effects of drugs on behaviour of aggressive mice. Br. J. Pharmacol. 1979; 65: 525-533.

Kruk, M.R., Van der Poel, A.M. and De Vos-Frerichs, T.P. The induction of aggressive behaviour by electrical stimulation in the hypothalamus of male rats. Behaviour 1979; 70: 292-322.

Kruk, M.R. and Van der Poel, A.M. Is there evidence for a neural correlate of an aggressive behavioural system in the hypothalamus of the rat? Progr. Brain Res. 1980; 53: 385-390.

Kruk, M.R., Van der Poel, A.M., Meelis, W., Hermans, J., Mostert, P.G., Mos, J. and Lohman, A.H.M. Discriminant analysis of the localization of aggression-inducing electrode placements in the hypothalamus of male rats. Brain Res. 1983; 260: 61-79.

Kruk, M.R., Van der Laan, C.E., Mos, J., Van der Poel, A.M., Meelis, W. and Olivier, B. Comparison of aggressive behaviour induced by electrical stimulation in the hypothalamus of male and female rats. Progr. Brain Res. 1984; 61: 303-314.

Kruk, M.R., Van der Poel, A.M., Lammers, J.H.C.M., Hagg, T., De Hey, A.M.D.M. and Oostvegel, S. Ethopharmacology of hypothalamic aggression in the rat. In: Olivier, B., Mos, J. and Brain, P.F., eds., Ethopharmacology of agonistic behaviour in animals and humans. Dordrecht: Martinus Nijhoff, 1987; 33-45.

Lammers, R. and Van Harten, J. Pharmacokinetics of eltoprazine in the dog. Drug Metabol. Drug Interact. 1990; 8: 141-148.

Lehman, M.N. and Adams, D.B. A statistical and motivational analysis of the social behaviors of the male laboratory rat. Behaviour 1977; 61: 238-275.

Levy, M., Burgio, L., Davis, P., Sweet, R. and Janosky, J. Buspirone for disruptive behaviors in community dwelling patients with dementia. J. Am. Geriatr. Soc. 1992; 40: suppl. 10, SA 3.

Lidberg, L., Åsberg, M. and Sundqvist-Stensman, U.B. 5-Hydroxyindoleacetic acid levels in attempted suicides who have killed their children. Lancet 1984; 2: 928.

Lidberg, L., Tuck, J.R., Åsberg, M., Scalia-Tomba, G-P. and Bertilsson, L.

Homicide, suicide and CSF 5-HIAA. Acta Psychiatr. Scand. 1985; 71: 230-236.

Linnoila, M., Virkkunen, M., Scheinin, M., Nuutila, A., Rimon, R. and Goodwin, F.K. Low cerebrospinal fluid 5-hydroxyindoleacetic acid concentration differentiates impulsive from non-impulsive violent behavior. Life Sci. 1983; 33: 2609-2614.

Linnoila, V.M.J. and Virkkunen, M.. Aggression, suicidality, and serotonin, J. Clin. Psychiatry 1992; 53: (10, suppl.) 46-51.

Lore, R. and Flannelly, K. Rat societies. Sci. Am. 1977; 236: 106-116.

MacKinnon, R.A. and Yudofsky, S.C. Psychiatric Evaluation in Clinical Practice. New York: J.B. Lippincott Co., 1986.

Madden, D.J. and Lion, J.R. Clinical management of aggression. In: Brain, P.F. and Benton, D., eds., Multidisciplinary approaches to aggression research. Amsterdam: Elsevier/North-Holland Biomedical Press 1981; 477-488.

Mak, M., De Koning, P., Mos, J., Olivier, B. Preclinical and clinical studies on the role of 5-HT$_1$ receptors in aggression. In: Impulsive Aggression and Disorders of Impulse Control. Eds. E.Hollander and D.Stein. John Wiley & Sons, 1993 (in press).

Malick, J.B. The pharmacology of isolation-induced aggressive behaviour in mice. Cur. Dev. Psychopharmacol. 1979; 5: 1-27.

Malmberg, T. Human territoriality: Survey of behavioural territories in man with preliminary analysis of meaning. Mouton, The Hague 1980.

Mann, A.H., Graham, N. and Ashby, D. Psychiatric illness in residential homes for the elderly: A survey in one London borough. Age Ageing 1984; 13: 265-275.

Mark, V.H. and Ervin, E.P. Violence and the brain. New York: Harper and Row, 1970.

McGlone, J.J., Kelley, K.W. and Gaskins, C.T. Lithium and porcine aggression. J. Anim. Sci. 1981; 51: 447-455.

McGlone, J.J. A quantitative ethogram of aggressive and submissive behaviours in recently regrouped pigs. J. Anim. Sci 1985; 61: 559-565.

Miczek, K.A. Intraspecies aggression in rats: effects of d-amphetamine and chlordiazepoxide. Psychopharmacology 1974; 39: 275-301.

Miczek, K.A. A new test for aggression in rats without aversive stimulation: Differential effects of d-amphetamine and cocaine. Psychopharmacology 1979; 60: 253-259.

Miczek, K.A. The psychopharmacology of aggression. In: Iversen, L.L., Iversen, S.D. and Snyder, S.H., eds., Handbook of psychopharmacology, Vol. 19: New directions in behavioral pharmacology. New York: Plenum Press 1987; 183-328.

Miczek, KA. and Barry, H. III. Pharmacology of sex and aggression. In: Glick, S.D. and Goldfarb, J., eds., Behavioural Pharmacology. St Louis: Mosby, 1976; 176-257.

Miczek, K.A. and DeBold, J.F. Hormone-drug interactions and their influence on aggressive behavior. In: Svare, B.B., ed., Hormones and aggressive behavior., New York: Plenum Press, 1983; 313-347.

Miczek, K.A., DeBold, J.F. and Thompson, M.L. Pharmacological, hormonal and behavioral manipulations in the analysis of aggressive behavior. In: Miczek, K.A., Kruk, M.R., Olivier, B., eds., Ethopharmacological aggression research. New York: Alan R. Liss, 1984; 1-16.

Miczek, K.A. and Krsiak, M. Drug effects on agonistic behavior. In: Thompson, T. and Dews, P.B., eds., Advances in behavioral pharmacology, Vol. 2. New York: Academic Press, 1979; 87-162.

Miczek, K.A. and Krsiak, M. Pharmacological analysis of attack and flight. In: Brain, P.F. and Benton, D., eds., Multidisciplinary approaches to aggression research. Amsterdam: Elsevier/North-Holland Biomedical Press 1981; 341-354.

Miczek, K.A. and Winslow, J.T. Psychopharmacological research on aggressive behaviour. In: Greenshaw, A.J. and Dourisch, C.T., eds., Experimental psychopharmacology. New Jersey: Humana Press, 1988.

Middlemiss, D.N. and Fozard, J.R. 8-Hydroxy-2(di-n-propylamino)tetralin discriminates between subtypes of the 5-HT$_1$ recognition sites. Eur. J Pharmacol. 1983; 90: 151-153.

Miyamoto, G., Sasabe, H., Tominga, N., Uegaki, N., Tominaga, M. and Shimizu, T. Metabolism of a new positive inotropic agent, 3,4-dihydro-6-[4-(3,4 dimethoxybenzoyl)-1-piperazinyl]-2(1H)-quinolinone (OPC-8212) in the rat, mouse, dog, monkey and human. Xenobiotica 1988; 18: 1143-1155.

Monroe, R. Episodic Behavioral Disorders. Cambridge: Harvard University Press, 1970.

Monroe, R.R. Anticonvulsants in treatment of aggression. J Nerv. Mental Disease 1975a; 160: 119-126.

Monroe, R.R. Drugs in the management of episodic behavioral disorders. In: Fields, W.S. and Sweet, W.H., eds., Neural bases of violence and aggression. St. Louis: Warren H. Green, 1975b; 328-348.

Montay, G., Goueffon, Y. and Roquet, F. Absorption, distribution, metabolic fate, and elimination of pefloxacin mesylate in mice, rats, dogs, monkeys, and humans. Antimicrob. Agents Chemother. 1984; 25: 463-472.

Montgomery, S.H. and Fineberg, N. Is there a relationship between serotonin receptor subtypes and selectivity of response in specific psychiatric illness? In: Eccleston, D. and Doogan, D.P., eds., Serotonin in behavioural disorders. Br. J. Psychiatry 1989; 155 (Suppl. 8): 63-70.

Mos, J. and Olivier, B., Ethopharmacological analysis of the pro-aggressive action of low doses of benzodiazepines in rats. Psychopharmacology 1986; 89: 25.

Mos, J. and Olivier, B. Pro-aggressive actions of benzodiazepines. In: Olivier, B., Mos, J. and Brain, P.F., eds., Ethopharmacology of agonistic behaviour in aninials and humans. Dordrecht: Martinus Nijhoff, 1987; 187-206.

Mos, J. and Olivier, B. Differential effects of selected psychoactive drugs on dominant and subordinate male rats housed in a colony. Neurosci. Res. Commun. 1988; 2: 29-36.

Mos, J. and Olivier, B. Quantitative and comparative analyses of pro-aggressive actions of benzodiazepines in maternal aggression of rats. Psychopharmacology 1989; 97: 152-153.

Mos, J., and Olivier, B. Concepts in animal models for pathological aggressive behaviour in humans. In: Animal Models of Psychopharmacology. Eds. B.Olivier, J.Mos, JL.Slangen. Birkhäuser Verlag, Basel, 1991: pp. 297-316.

Mos, J., Olivier, B., Lammers, J.H.C.M., Zethof, T., Kruk, M.R., and Van der Poel, A.M. Pregnancy and lactation do not interact with current thresholds for brain stimulation induced aggression in female rats. Brain Res. 1987; 404: 263-266.

Mos J, Olivier B, Poth M, van Aken H The effects of intraventricular administration of eltoprazine, 1-(3-trifluoromethylphenyl) piperazine hydrochloride and 8-hydroxy-2-(di-n-propylamino) tetralin on resident intruder aggression in the rat. Eur. J. Pharmacol. 1992; 212: 295-298.

Mos J, Olivier B, Poth M, Van Oorschot R, Van Aken H. The effects of dorsal raphe administration of eltoprazine, TFMPP, and 8-OH-DPAT on resident intruder aggression in the rat. Eur. J. Pharmacol. 1993; 238: 411-415.

Mos J, B.Olivier, M.Th.M. Tulp. Ethopharmacological studies differentiate the effects of various serotonergic compounds on aggression in rats. Drug Devl. Res. 1992; 26: 343-360.

Mos, J., Olivier, B. and Van Oorschot, R. Maternal aggression towards different sized male opponents: effect of chlordiazepoxide treatment of the mothers and d-amphetamine treatment of the intruders. Pharmacol. Biochem. Behav. 1987; 26: 577-584.

Mos, J., Olivier, B. and Van Oorschot, R. Behavioural and neuropharmacological aspects of maternal aggression in rodents. Aggr. Behav. 1990; 16: 145-163.

Mos, J., Olivier, B., Van Oorschot, R. and Dijkstra, H. Different test situations for measuring offensive aggression in male rats do not result in the same wound patterns. Physiol Behav. 1984; 32: 453-456.

Mos, J., Olivier, B., Van Oorschot, R., Van Aken, H. and Zethof, T. Experimental and ethological aspects of maternal aggression in rats: five years of observations. In: Blanchard, R.J., Brain, P.F., Blanchard, D.C. and Parmigiani, S. Dordrecht, Boston, London: Kluwer Acad. Publ. 1989; 385-399.

Mos, J., Olivier, B. and Van der Poel, A.M. Modulatory actions of benzodiazepine receptor ligands on agonistic behaviour. Physiol. Behav. 1987; 41: 265-278.

Mos, J., Van der Heyden, J.A.M. and Olivier, B. Behavioural effects of 5-HT$_3$ antagonists in animal models for aggression, anxiety and psychosis. In: Bevan, P., Cools, A.R. and Archer, T., eds., Behavioural pharmacology of 5-HT. Hillsdale, NJ: Lawrence Erlbaum 1989; 389-395.

Moyer, K.E. Kinds of aggression and their physiological basis. Comm. Behav. Biol. 1968; 2: 65-87.

Moyer, K.E. The psychobiology of aggression. New York, Hagerstown, San Francisco, London: Harper and Row, 1976.

Nikulina, E.M. and Popova, N. Serotonin's influence on predatory behavior of highly aggressive CBA and weakly aggressive DD strains of mice.Aggr. Behav. 1986; 12: 277-283.

O'Boyle, M. Rats and mice together: the predatory nature of the rat's mouse-killing response. Psychol. Bull. 1974; 181: 261-269.

O'Neil, M., Page, N. and Adkins, W.N. Tryptophan-trazodone treatment of aggressive behavior. Lancet 1986; 2: 859-860.

Olivier, B. The ventromedial hypothalamus and aggressive behaviour in rats. Aggr. Behav. 1977; 3: 47-56.

Olivier, B. Selective anti-aggressive properties of DU 27725: Ethological analyses of intermale and territorial aggression in the male rat. Pharmacol Biochem. Behav. 1981; 14 (Suppl. 1): 61-77.

Olivier, B. and Mos, J. A female aggression paradigm for use in psychopharmacology: maternal agonistic behaviour in rats. In: Brain, P.F. and Martin Ramirez, J., eds., Cross-disciplinary studies on aggression. Seville: University of Seville Press 1986; 73-111.

Olivier, B. and Mos, J. Serenics and aggression. Stress Medicine 1986; 2: 197-209.

Olivier, B. and Mos, J. Serotonin, serenics and aggressive behaviour in animals. In: Swinkels, J.A. and Blijleven, W., eds., Depression, anxiety and aggression. Houten: Medidact, 1988; 133-165.

Olivier, B. and Mos, J. Serotonergic aspects of agonistic behavior. In: Lerer, B. and Gershon, S., eds., New directions in affective disorders. New York: Springer Verlag, 1989; 40-44.

Olivier, B. and Mos, J. Serotonergic and benzodiazepine modulation of agonistic behaviour: ethopharmacological analyses. Biotemas 1989; 2: 148.

Olivier, B. and Mos, J. Rodent models of aggressive behaviour and serotonergic drugs. Clin. Neuropharmacology, 1990; 13: suppl. 2, 247-248.

Olivier, B., Mos, J. and Brain, P.F. Ethopharmacology of agonistic behavior in animals and humans. Dordrecht: Martinus Nijhoff, 1987; 1-270.

Olivier, B., Mos, J., Hartog, J. and Rasmussen, D.L. Serenics: A new class of drugs for putative selective treatment of pathological destructive behaviour. Drug News Persp. 1990; 3: 261-271.

Olivier, B., Mos, J. and Rasmussen, D. Behavioural pharmacology of the serenic eltoprazine. Drug Metabol. Drug Interact. 1990; 8: 31-83.

Olivier, B., Mos, J., Schipper, J., Tulp, M.T.M., Van der Heyden, J.A.M., Berkelmans, B. and Bevan, P. Serotonergic modulation of agonistic behaviour. In: Olivier, B., Mos, J. and Brain, P.F., eds., Ethopharmacological analysis of agonistic behaviour in animals and man. Dordrecht: Martinus Nijhoff, 1987; 162-186.

Olivier, B., Mos, J., Van der Heyden, J.A.M. and Hartog, J. Serotonergic modulation of social interaction in male mice. Psychopharmacology 1989b; 97: 154-156.

Olivier, B., Mos, J., Van der Heyden, J., Tulp, M., Schipper, J. and Bevan, P. Modulatory action of serotonin in aggressive behaviour. In: Bevan, P., Cools, A.R. and Archer, T., eds., Behavioural pharmacology of 5-HT. Hillsdale, NJ: Lawrence Erlbaum, 1989a; 89-115.

Olivier, B., Mos, J., Van der Heyden, J.A.M., Tulp, M.Th.M. and Slangen, J.L. Anxiolytic properties of 5-HT$_3$ antagonists: A review. Stress Medicine 1992; 8: 117-136.

Olivier, B., Mos, J., Van der Poel, A.M., Krijzer, F.N.C. and Kruk, M.R. Effects of a new psychoactive drug (DU 27716) on different models of rat agonistic behaviour and EEG. In: Blanchard, D.C., Flannelly, KJ. and Blanchard, R.J., eds., Biological perspectives on aggression. New York: Alan R. Liss 1984; 261-279.

Olivier, B., Mos, J. and Van Oorschot, R. Maternal aggression in rats: effects of chlordiazepoxide and fluprazine. Psychopharmacology 1985; 86: 68-76.

Olivier, B., Mos, J. and Van Oorschot, R. Maternal aggression in rats: Lack of interaction between chlordiazepoxide and fluprazine. Psychopharmacology 1986; 88: 40-43.

Olivier, B., Mos, J. and Van Oorschot, R. Drugs, Neurotransmitters and offensive aggression. In: Strategies for studying CNS active compounds. T. Palomo, L. Seiden (eds.), Farrand Press (in press).

Olivier, B., Olivier-Aardema, R.L. and Wiepkema, P.R. Effect of anterior hypothalamic and mammillary area lesions on territorial aggressive behaviour in male rats. Behav. Brain Res. 1983; 9: 59-81.

Olivier, B., Van Aken, H., Jaarsma, I., Van Oorschot, R., Zethof, T. and Bradford, L.D. Behavioural effects of psychoactive drugs on agonistic behaviour of male territorial rats (resident-intruder paradigm). In: Miczek, K-A., Kruk, M.R. and Olivier, B., eds., Ethopharmacological aggression research. New York: Alan R. Liss, 1984; 137-156.

Olivier, B. and Van Dalen, D. Social behaviour in rats and mice: an ethologically based model for differentiating psychoactive drugs. Aggr. Behav. 1982; 8: 163-168.

Olivier, B., Van Dalen, D. and Hartog, J. A new class of psychoactive drugs: Serenics. Drugs Future 1986; 11: 473-499.

Orsini, J.C., Barone, F.C., Armstrong, D.L. and Wayner, M.J. Direct effects of androgens on lateral hypothalamic neuronal activity in the male rat: I. A microiontophoretic study. Brain Res. Bull. 1985; 15: 293-297.

Overall, J.E. and Gorham, D.R. The Brief Psychiatric Rating Scale. Psychol. Rep. 1962; 10: 799-812.

Owen, R.T. YG- 19-256. Drugs Future 1980; 5: 98-99.

Palmstierna, T. and Wistedt, B. Staff observation aggression scale. SOAS: presentation and evaluation. Acta Psychiatr. Scand. 1987; 76: 657-663.

Panksepp, J. The ontogeny of play in rats. Devl. Psychobiol 1981; 14: 327-332.

Panksepp, J. and Beatty, W.W. Social deprivation and play in rats. Behav. Neural. Biol. 1980; 30: 197-206.

Panksepp, J., Normansell, L., Cox, J.F., Crepeau, L.J. and Sacks, D.J. Psychopharmacology of social play. In: Olivier, B., Mos, J. and Brain, P.F., eds., Ethopharmacology of agonistic behaviour in aninials and man. Dordrecht: Martinus Nijhoff, 1987; 132-144.

Panksepp, J., Siviy, S. and Normansell, L. The psychobiology of play: Theoretical and methodological perspectives. Neurosci. Biobehav. Rev. 1984; 8: 465-492.

Payne, A.P. and Swanson, H.H. Agonistic behaviour between pairs of hamsters of same and opposite sex in a neutral observation area. Behaviour 1970; 36: 259-269.

Peroutka, S.J. 5-Hydroxytryptamine receptor subtypes: Molecular, biochemical and physiological characterization. Trends Neurosci. 1993.

Porter, D.B. and Slusser, C.A. Azaperone: a review of a new neuroleptic for swine. Vet. Med. 1985; 88-92.

Poshivalov, V.P. Pharmaco-ethological analysis of social behaviour of isolated mice. Pharmacol Biochem. Behav. 1981; 14 (suppl. 1): 53-59.

Poshivalov, V.P. Ethopharmacological and neuropharmacological analyses of agonistic behaviour. In: Olivier, B., Mos, J. and Brain, P.F., eds., Ethopharmacology of agonistic behaviour in animals and man. Dordrecht: Martinus Nijhoff, 1987; 122-131.

Poshivalov, V.P. and Khodko, S.T. Mathematical description and experimental analyslis of animal intraspecific agonistic behavior. In: Miczek, K.A., Kruk, M.R. and Olivier, B., eds., Ethopharmacological Aggression Research. New York: Alan R. Liss 1984; 59-80.

Potegal, M. The reinforcing value of several types of aggressive behavior: a review. Aggr. Behav. 1979; 5: 353-373.

Potegal, M. and Glusman, M. Effects on muricide of DU 27716 injected peripherally or into septum or dorsal raphe. Aggr. Behav. 1983; 9: 118.

Rabins, P.V., Mace, N.L. and Lucas, M.J. The impact of dementia on the family. JAMA 1982; 248: 333-335.

Racine, M.A., Flannelly, K.J. and Blanchard, D.C. Anti-aggressive effects of DU 27716 on attack and defensive behaviours in male mice. In: Flannelly, K.J., Blanchard, R.J. and Blanchard, D.C., eds., Biological perspectives on aggression. New York: Alan R. Liss, 1984; 281-293.

Raghoebar, M., Mak, M., Cournot, A., Pistorius, M.C.M., Van Harten, J. and Roseboom, H. Pharmacokinetics of eltoprazine in healthy male subjects after single dose oral and intravenous administration. Br. J. Clin. Pharmacol. 1990; 30: 879-883.

Raleigh, M.J., Banner, G.L., Yuwiler, A., Flannery, J.W., McGuire, M.T. and Geller, E. Serotonergic influences on the social behavior of vervet monkeys (Cercopithecus aethiops sabaeus). Exp. Neurol. 1980; 68: 322-339.

Raleigh, M.J., McGuire, M.T., Banner, G.L. and Yuwiler, A. Social and environmental influences on blood serotonin concentrations in monkeys. Arch. Gen. Psychiatry 1984; 41: 405-410.

Ratey, J.J., Sovner, R., Parks, A. and Rogentine, K. Buspirone treatment of aggression and anxiety in mentally retarded patients: a multiple baseline, placebo lead-in study. J. Clin. Psychiatry 1991; 52: 159-162.

Realmuto, G.M., August, G.I. and Garfinkel, B.D. Clinical effect of buspirone in autistic children. J. Clin. Psychopharmacol. 1989; 9: 122-125.

Reid, A.H., Ballinger, B.R. and Heather, B.B. The natural history of behavioural symptoms among severely and profoundly mentally retarded patients. Br. J. Psychiatry 1984; 145: 289-293.

Reisberg, B., Borenstein, J. and Slalob, S.P. Behavioral symptoms in Alzheimer's disease: phenomenology and treatment. J. Clin. Psychiatry 1987; 48 (Suppl. 5): 9-15.

Rodgers, R.J. Neurochemical correlates of aggressive behaviour: Some relations to emotion and pain sensitivity. In: Brown, K. and Cooper, S.J., eds., Chemical influences on behaviour. New York: Academic Press 1979; 374-419.

Rodgers, R.J. Drugs, aggression and behavioral methods. In: Brain, P.F. and Benion, D., eds., Multidisciplinary approaches to aggression research. Amsterdam, New York-Oxford: Elsevier/North-Holland Biomedical Press, 1981; 325-340.

Rossi, A.C. The "mouse-killing" rat: ethological discussion on an experimental model of aggression. Pharmacol. Res. Commun. 1975; 7: 199-216.

Rossi, A.M., Jacobs, S. and Monteleone, M. Violent or fear-inducing behavior associated with hospital admission. Hosp. Comm. Psychiatry 1985; 36: 643-647.

Roubicek, J., Klos, A. and Tschudin, A. YG-19-256: EEG and clinical study in aggressive oligophrenics. Psychopharmacologia 1972; 26 (suppl.): 71.

Rowner, B.S., Kafonek, S. and Filipp, L. Prevalence of mental illness in a community nursing home. Am. J. Psychiatry 1986; 143: 1446-1449.

Rubin, E.H., Morris, J.C., Siorandt, M. and Berg, L. Behavioral changes in patients with mild senile dementia of the Alzheimer's type. Psychiatry Res. 1987; 21: 55-62.

Sànchez, C., Arnt, J., Hyttel, J. and Moltzen, E.K. The role of serotonergic mechanisms in inhibition of isolation-induced aggression in male mice, Psychopharmacology 1993; 110: 53-59.

Sarteschi, P., Longo, E. and Baglivo, S. Pathological aggressiveness in man: some theoretical and practical considerations. Modern Probl. Pharmacopsychiatry 1978; 13: 159-174.

Sbordone, R.J., Gorelick, D.A. and Elliot, M.L. An ethological analysis of drug-induced pathological aggression. In: Brain, P.F. and Benton, D., eds., Multidisciplinary approaches to aggression research. Amsterdam, New York-Oxford: Elsevier/North-Holland Biomedical Press, 1981; 369-385.

Schipper, J., Tulp, M.Th.M., Sijbesma, H. Neurochemical profile of eltoprazine. Drug Metabol. Drug Interact. 1990; 8: 85-115.

Schouten, W.G.P. Rearing conditions and behaviour in pigs. PhD Thesis, Wageningen 1986; 1-151.

Schuurman, T. Endocrine processes underlying victory and defeat in the male rat. Groningen: PhD Thesis, 1981; 1-109.

Scott, J.P. Agonistic behaviour in mice and rats: a review. Am. Zool. 1966; 683-701.

Scott, J.P. and Fredericson, E. The causes of fighting in mice and rats. Physiol Zool 1951; 24: 273-309.

Sheard, M.H. Shock-induced fighting (SIF): Psychopharmacology studies. Aggr.Behav. 1981; 7: 41-49.

Sheard, M.H. The effect of lithium and other ions on aggressive behavior. In: Valzelli, L., ed., Modern problems of pharmacology: psychopharmacology of aggression. Basel: Karger, 1978; 13: 82-102.

Sheard, M.H. Psychopharmacology of aggression. In: Hippius, H. and Winokur, G., eds., Psychopharmacology 1. Part 2: Clinical Psychopharmacology. Amsterdam, Oxford, Princeton: Excerpta Medica, 1983; 188-202.

Sheard, M.H. Clinical pharmacology of aggressive behavior. Clin. Neuropharmacol. 1984; 7: 173-183.

Sheard, M.H. Psychopharmacology of aggression in humans. In: Olivier, B., Mos, J. and Brain, P.F., eds., Ethopharmacology of agonistic behaviour in animals and humans. Dordrecht: Martinus Nijhoff, 1987; 257-266.

Siegel, S. Non-parametric statistics for the behavioral sciences. New York: McGraw-Hill, 1956.

Sijbesma H, Schipper J, Cornelissen J.C.H.M., de Kloet ER. Species differences in the distribution of central 5-HT$_1$ binding sites: a comparative autoradiographic study between rat and guinea pig. Brain Research, 1991; 555: 295-304.

Sijbesma H., Schipper J., de Kloet ER. Eltoprazine, a drug which reduces aggressive behaviour, binds selectively to 5-HT$_1$ receptor sites in the rat brain: an autoradiographic study. Eur. J. Pharmacol. 1990; 177: 55-61.

Sijbesma H., Schipper J., de Kloet ER, Mos J, van Aken H, Olivier B. Postsynaptic 5-HT$_1$ receptors and offensive aggression in rats: a combined behavioural and autoradiographic study with eltoprazine. Pharmacol. Biochem. Behav. 1991; 38: 447-458.

Svare, B. Maternal aggression in mice: influence of the young. Biobehav. Rev. 1977; 1: 151-164.

Svare, B. Models of aggression employing female rodents. In: Brain, P.F. and Benton, D., eds., The biology of aggression. Alphen a.d. Rijn: Sijthoff and Noordhoff, 1981; 503-508.

Svare, B. Hormones and aggressive behaviour. New York and London: Plenum Press, 1983.

Svare, B. and Gandelman, R. Postpartum aggression in mice: experimental and environmental factors. Horm. Behav. 1973; 4: 323-334.

Svare, B. and Mann, M. Hormonal influence on maternal aggression. In: Svare, B., ed., Hormones and aggressive behavior. New York: Plenum Press, 1983; 91-104.

Svare, B., Mann, M. and Samuels, 0. Mice: Suckling stimulation but not lactation important for maternal aggression. Behav. Neural. Biol. 1980; 29: 453-462.

Symoens, J. and Van den Brande, M. Prevention and cure of aggressiveness in pigs using the sedative azaperone. Vet. Rec. 1969; 85: 64-77.

Takahashi, L.K. and Lore, R.K. Intermale and maternal aggression in adult rats tested at different ages. Physiol. Behav. 1982; 29: 1013-1018.

Tardiff, K and Sweillam, A. Assault, suicide, and mental illness. Arch. Gen. Psychiatry 1980; 73: 164-169.

Tardiff, K. and Sweillam, A. Assaultive behavior among chronic inpatients. Am. J. Psychiatry 1982; 139: 212-215.

Tedeschi, R.E., Tedeschi, D.H., Mucha, A., Cook, L., Mattis, P.A. and Fellows, E.J. Effect of various centrally acting drugs on fighting behaviour of mice. J. Pharmacol. Exp. Ther. 1959; 125: 28-34.

Tiihonen, J., Hakola, P., Paanila, J. and Turtiainen, M. Eltoprazine for aggression in schizophrenia and mental retardation (letter). The Lancet 1993; 341: 307.

Timmermans, P.J.A. Social behaviour in the rat. PhD Thesis. University of Nijmegen 1978; 1-298.

Traskman, L., Åsberg, M., Bertilsson, L. and Sjöstrand, L. Monoamine metabolites in CSF and suicidal behavior. Arch. Gen. Psychiatry 1981; 38: 631-636.

Tuinier, S. Clinical aspects of aggression. In: Swinkels, J.A. and Blijleven, W., eds. Depression, anxiety and aggression. Factors that influence the course. Houten: Medidact, 1988: 181-193.

Tupin, J.P. Psychopharmacology and aggression. In: Roth, L.H., ed., Clinical treatment of the violent person. Rockville, MI): US Department of Health and Human Services, 1985; 83-99.

Ulrich, R.E. and Azrin, N.H. Reflexive fighting in response to aversive stimulation. J. Exp. Anal. Behav. 1962; 5: 511-520.

Ursin, H. Aggression and the brain: reflex chains or network? Behav. Brain Sci. 1979; 2: 227.

Ursin, H. Affective and instrumental aspects of fear and aggression. In: Koukkou, M. and Lehmann, D., Eds., Functional states of the brain: their determinants. Amsterdam: Elsevier/North Holland, 1980.

Ursin, H. Neuroanatomical basis of aggression. In: Brain, P.F. and Benton, D., eds., Multidisciplinary approaches to aggression research. Amsterdam: Elsevier/North-Holland Biomedical Press, 1981; 269-293.

Valenstein, E.S. Brain control: a critical examination of brain stimulation and psychosurgery. New York: John Wiley and Sons, 1973.

Valzelli, L. The "isolation syndrome" in mice. Psychopharmacologia 1973; 31: 305-320.

Valzelli, L. Psychopharmacology of aggression. Basel: S. Karger 1978.

Valzelli, L. Effects of sedatives and anxiolytics on aggressivity. In: Boissier, J.R., ed., Modern problems of pharmacology of anxiolytics and sedatives. Basel: S. Karger, 1979; 143-156.

Valzelli, L. Psychopharmacology of aggression: an overview. Intl. Pharmacopsychiatry 1981; 16: 39-48.

Valzelli, L. and Bernasconi, S. Psychoactive drug effect on socioenvironmental deprivation in rats. Pharmacol. Res. Commun. 1980; 12: 279-282.

Van der Ploeg, H.M., Defares, P.B. and Spielberger, C.D. Handleiding bij de Zelf-Beoordelings Vragenlijst, Swets and Zeitlinger BV, Lisse, The Netherlands 1980.

Van der Poel, A.M., Mos, J., Kruk, M.R. and Olivier, B. A motivational analysis of ambivalent actions in the agonistic behaviour of rats in tests used to study effects of drugs on aggression. In: Miczek, K.A., Kruk, M.R. and Olivier, B., eds., Ethopharmacological Aggression Research. New York: Alan R. Liss, 1984; 115-135.

Van der Poel, A.M., Olivier, B., Mos, J., Kruk, M.R. and Meelis, W. and Van Aken, J.H.M. Anti-aggressive effect of a new phenylpiperazine compound (DU 27716) on hypothalamically induced behavioural activities. Pharmacol. Biochem. Behav. 1982; 17: 147-153.

Van Harten, J., Mathlener, I.S. and Raghoebar, M. Pharmacokinetics of eltoprazine in healthy subjects. Drug Metabol. Drug Interact. 1990; 8: 149-158.

Van Leeuwen, C.J., Riedel, W.J. and O'Hanlon, J.F. Assessment of the antiaggressive effects of a putative anxiolytic, CGP 361A, versus those of diazepam and placebo in humans using a novel experimental approach, Psychopharmacology 1988; 96: (suppl. 232) S358.

Van Praag, H.M. Serotonergic dysfunction and aggression control (Editorial), Psychol. Med. 1991; 21: 15-19.

Vaugien, B., Descas, P., Gomond, P., Lambrey, B., D'Arnoux, C., Jarry, C., Mosser, J., Panconi, E., Saudubray, F. and Roux, J. COR 3224. Drugs of the Future 1991; 16: 893-894.

Vergnes, M. and Kempf, E. Effect of hypothalamic injections of 5,7dihydroxytryptamine on elicitation of mouse-killing in rats. Behav. Brain Res. 1982; 5: 387-397.

Vergnes, M., Depaulis, A. and Boehrer, A. Parachloro-phenylalanine induced serotonin depletion increases offensive but not defensive aggression in male rats. Physiol Behav. 1986; 36: 653-658.

Vergnes, M., Depaulis, A., Boehrer, A. and Kempf, E. Selective increase of offensive behavior in the rat following intrahypothalamic 5,7-DHT-induced serotonin depletion. Behav. Brain Res. 1988; 29: 85-91.

Verhoeven, W.M.A., Tuinier, S., Sijben, N.A.S., Dosen, A. and Van den Berg, J.W.H.M., Pepplinkhuizen, L., and Van Nieuwenhuizen, O. Eltoprazine in mentally retarded selfinjuring patients (letter), The Lancet 1992; 340: 1037-1038.

Virkkunen, M., Nuutila, A., Goodwin, F. and Linnoila, M. CSF monoamine metabolites in male arsonists. Arch. Gen. Psychiatry 1987; 44: 241-247.

Winslow, J.T., DeBold, J.F. and Miczek, K.A. Alcohol effects on the aggressive behaviour of squirrel monkeys and mice are modulated by testosterone. In: Olivier, B., Mos, J. and Brain, P.F., eds., Ethopharmacology of agonistic behaviour in animals and man. Dordrecht: Martinus Nijhoff, 1987; 223-244.

Wise, D.A. Aggression in the female golden hamster: effects of reproductive state and social isolation. Horm. Behav. 1974; 5: 235-250.

Wistedt, B., Rassmussen, A., Pedersen, L., Malm, U., Traskman-Bendz, L., Wakelin, J. and Bech, P. The development of an observer scale for measuring social dysfunction and aggression. Pharmacopsychiatry 1990; 23: 249-252.

Ybema, C.E., Slangen, J.L., Olivier, B. and Mos, J. Discriminative stimulus properties of the serotonergic compound eltoprazine. J. Pharmacol. Exp. Therap. 1992; 260: 1045-1051.

Yen, C.Y., Stanger, R.L. and Millnam, N. Ataractic suppression of isolation-induced aggressive behavior. Arch. Int. Pharmacodyn. Ther. 1959; 123: 179-185.

Yesavage, J.A. Inpatient violence and the schizophrenic patient. A study of Brief Psychiatric Rating Scale scores and inpatient behavior. Acta Psychiatr. Scand. 1983; 67: 353-357.

Yodyingyuad, U., de la Riva, C., Abbott, D.H., Herbert, J. and Keverne, E.B. Relationship between dominance hierarchy, cerebrospinal fluid levels of amine transmitter metabolites (5-hydroxyindole acetic acid and homovanillic acid) and plasma cortisol in monkeys. Neurosci. 1985; 16: 851-858.

Yoshimura, H. Ethopharmacology of agonistic behaviour in male and female mice. In: Olivier, B., Mos, J. and Brain, P.F., eds., Ethopharmacology of agonistic behaviour in animals and man. Dordrecht: Martinus Nijhoff, 1987; 94-109.

Yudofsky, S.C., Silver, J.M. and Hales, R.E. Pharmacologic management of aggression in the elderly. J. Clin. Psychiatry 1990; 51: supl. 22-28.

Yudofsky, S.C., Silver, J.M., Jackson, W., Endicott, J. and Williams, D. The Overt Aggression Scale for Objective Rating of Verbal and Physical Aggression. Am. J. Psych. 1986; 143: 35-39.

Yudofsky, S.C., Silver, J.M. and Schneider, S.E. Pharmacologic treatment of aggression. Special Issue: Treatment of aggressive disorders. Psychiatric Annals 1987; 17: 397-407.

Zech, K., Eltze, M., Kilian, U., Sanders, K.H. and Kolassa, N. Arch. Int. Pharmacodyn. Ther. 1984; 272: 180.

Zimmer, J.G., Watson, N. and Treat, A. Behavioral problems among patients in skilled nursing facilities. Am. J. Public Health 1984; 74: 1118-1121.

Progress in Drug Research, Vol. 42
Edited by Ernst Jucker
© 1994 Birkhäuser Verlag Basel (Switzerland)

Transfer factor 1993: New frontiers

By H. Hugh Fudenberg[1] and Giancarlo Pizza[2]

NeuroImmuno Therapeutics Research Foundation[1], Spartanburg, SC, USA, and S. Orsola-Malpighi Hospital[2], Bologna, Italy

1   An overview
1.1   Historical perspective

Adoptive transfer of antigen-specific cell-mediated immunity in humans, first demonstrated by Lawrence [1] in 1949, opened a new avenue of research that has led both to increased understanding of basic immune mechanisms and to the development of many forms of immunomodulant therapy, alone or in combination with other immunotherapeutic or chemotherapeutic agents. Lawrence originally showed that transfer of intact viable lymphocytes from a normal tuberculin skin test-positive donor for a given antigen to a normal recipient, skin test-negative for that antigen, resulted in a conversion ("transfer") of the recipient to skin-test positivity; however, this observation created little interest in the immunologic community for several reasons. In 1955, the lymphocyte was mentioned for the first time as an immunologic organ. (Before this, the lymphocyte had been studied in hematologic rather than in immunologic terms.) In 1955, in the third edition of his classic textbook on the anatomy of the lymphoid system [2], Professor A. Joffy of the University of Bristol proposed three questions to lymphocytes: "Where do you come from, where do you go; and what do you do, if anything?" In 1962 [3], J. Miller showed that the immune system in chickens could be divided into two components, namely, the B-lymphocyte, derived from the bursal system (B cell, producing antibodies that protect against infection from classic micro-organisms *(pneumococcus, meningococcus, streptococcus, gonococcus,* etc.) and thymic-dependent (T cell) systems that protect against fungi, parasites, viruses, mycobacteria, and cancer metastases. Previously, Lawrence [4] demonstrated that delayed cutaneous hypersensitivity (DH) responsiveness could also be *transferred* by soluble extracts of leukocytes from 20 ml of blood and termed the factor responsible for this phenomenon "transfer factor" (TF) (fig. 1a). TF could transfer DH of a given specificity from a skin test positive individual to a normal skin test negative individual, hereafter termed primary recipient. Within six months, white cells obtained from this primary recipient could be similarly fed and the leukocyte extract given to a secondary recipient negative by skin test. This secondary recipient, too, would become positive in accordance with the specificities of the first donor (fig. 1b). At that time, the significance of DH was unknown so TF received little attention. All

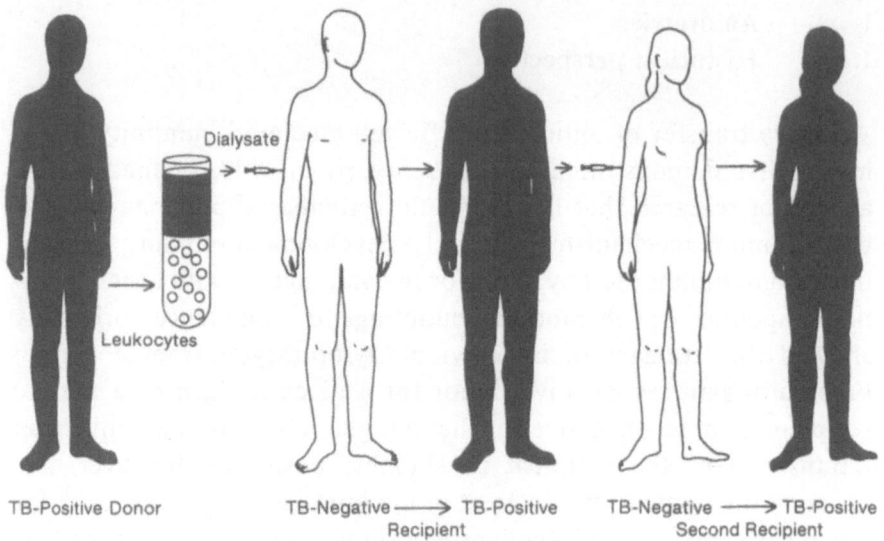

Dialysate

Leukocytes

TB-Positive Donor   TB-Negative ⟶ TB-Positive   TB-Negative ⟶ TB-Positive
                                Recipient   Second Recipient

Figure 1a
Transfer of skin test reactivity from a normal individual, positive by skin test to tuberculin-purified protein derivative (PPD), to a normal recipient previously negative by delayed hypersensitivity skin test to PPD, using a cell-free extract derived from donor leukocytes.

Figure 1b
Note that the cell-free extract derived from the primary recipient after transfer converted a second normal subject previously skin-test negative to PPD to skin-test positive. PPD positive status in black, PPD negative status in white.

immunological phenomena were thought to be an effect of antibodies; such antibodies had molecular weights (MW) of 150000 to 1000000 daltons or greater. DH was postulated to be due to antigen-binding at the skin injection site by antibodies of very high affinity [5]. Therefore, no attention was paid to Lawrence's finding of transfer of DH by a soluble factor of a MW < 20000 daltons, as demonstrated by passage through dialysis membrane which retained molecules > 20000 daltons. Secondly, skin tests were used by allergists for whom immunologists had no respect at that time. Hence, Lawrence's observations did not excite the immunologic scientific community. Thirdly, the pH Lawrence used to obtain the blood to process human white cells was one pH (due to the anti-coagulant) that did not permit cells of other species (e. g., rats, mice, guinea pigs and rabbits) to produce TF (for example, certain $\alpha 1$ proteases have optimum pH at 3, 5, and 7 for activitiy of this enzyme); furthermore, skin tests were used by allergists for whom immunologists at that time had little respect. Thus the immunologic community paid little attention to Lawrence's observation. Substitution of the anti-coagulant EDTA-sodium to obtain blood from other species has now made it possible to obtain dialyzable leukocyte extract from a host of non-human species *(vide infra)*. In any event, because of these negative factors, for many years Lawrence's observations were ignored; that is, until our first paper in 1970. No one had thought of putting into clinical use and monitoring its effects by tests of CMI. By that time it had been shown that DH was equivalent to in vitro measures of systemic cell-mediated immunity in man by 1968 and laboratory tests for human MIF had been derived in 1968; therefore, when we saw a child with an insoluble immunologic

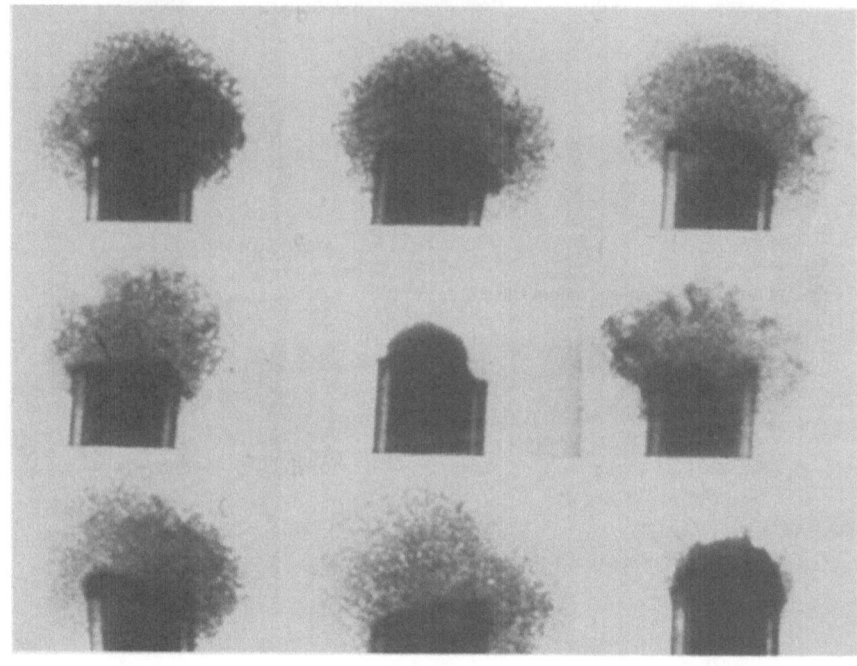

Figure 2
Macrophage migration inhibition produced when PBL, from individuals either non-immune (normal cells, a and b) or sensitive to tuberculin (tuberculin-sensitive cells c and d) were incubated with medium alone (no antigen) or with PPD added. The extent of migration inhibition can be calculated after measuring the areas of migration either as:

$$\% \text{ migration} = \frac{\text{average migration of cells in the presence of antigen}}{\text{average migration of cells without antigen}}$$

or as: % inhibition = 100 – % migration.
Generally, inhibition > 20% is significant in MMI systems.

problem; namely, Wiskott-Aldrich Syndrome, a rare X-linked disease, with recurrent infections, especially with viruses, molds, and fungi, and death during puberty, we decided to use "transfer factor" *in vivo* accompanied by *in vitro* tests to see if this "agent", really a mixture of many substances, could be used to transfer systemic CMI to immuno-compromised individuals.

Lawrence thought the dialyzate contained only one moiety. We now know that the extract obtained by the Lawrence method contains at least 200 different moieties with MW from 1 to 20 kilodaltons (K. D.) and that only one of them is antigen-specific TF (hereafter referred to as $TF_{a.s.}$) with a MW of approximately 3.5 to 6. K. D. *(vide infra)* [6].

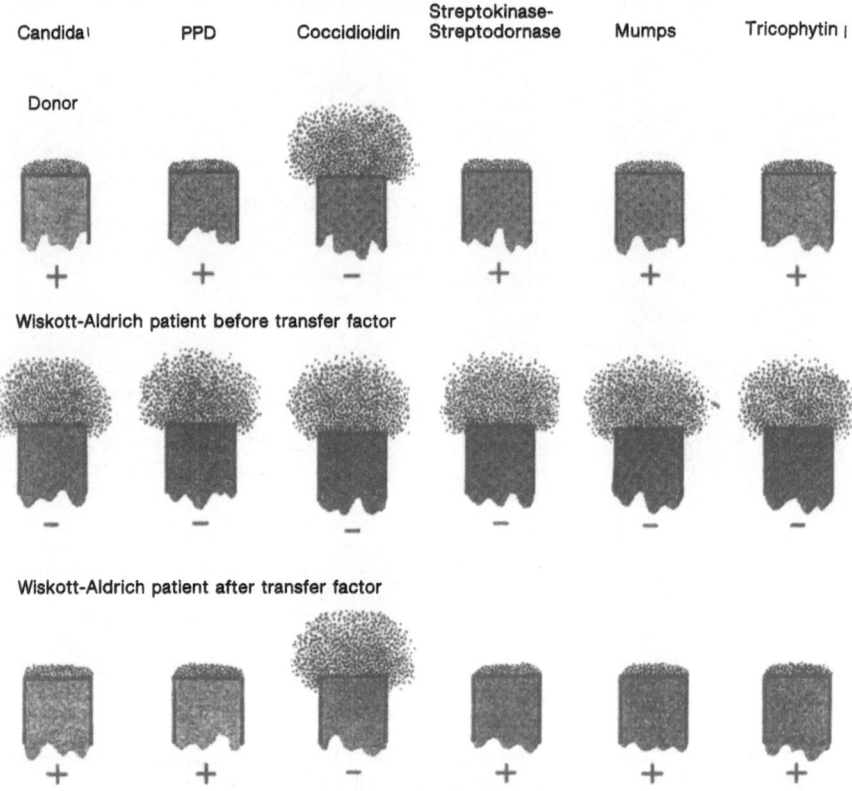

Figure 3

The specificity of TF using the macrophage migration inhibition factor (MIF) using a donor positive by MIF assay for five of six antigens. TF was administered to a Wiskott-Aldrich patient anergic for all six antigens listed above. Top: The donor was positive for all but coccidioidin. Middle: Before therapy, the patient was negative for all six antigens. Bottom: After TF therapy, the patient remained negative for cocci antigens, but positive for all of the other five.

Hence, we call preparations made by the Lawrence method dialyzable leukocyte extract (DLE). In 1970, we showed [7a] that DLE could not only transfer skin-test positivity but also produce or initiate other cell-mediated immunity (CMI) reactions, such as inhibition of macrophage migration (fig. 2) in an antigen-specific fashion in various immunodeficiency states (e.g., in Wiskott-Aldrich syndrome patients [7b], the antigen-specific transfer of CMI (fig. 3) provides protection for a period of approximately six months, paralleled by antigen-specific production of lymphokines, such as macrophage migration inhibitory factor (MIF) [8] and leukocyte migration inhibition factor (LIF) for granulocytes. The generalized term "leukocyte migration inhibition" was adopted because the target cell was then unknown; when the target cell was later found to be the granulocyte, the old term, LIF, was unfortunately retained.) DLE can also transfer the ability to produce MIF and LIF in an antigen-specific fashion from one normal individual who has this ability to another individual, normal or diseased, (e.g., a normal who has never been exposed to the specific antigen, or an abnormal who cannot produce it upon exposure respectively); these functions generally exactly parallel the skin test reactivity. However, both the nature and mechanisms of action of TF and its potential as an immunotherapeutic agent were until 1987 highly controversial, partly because of semantic confusion [9] of the terms defined below.

1.2   Definition of terms

Disruption of buffy coat cells or lymphoid cells into aqueous solution, followed by dialysis to obtain a low MW fraction, yields of crude preparation Dialyzable Leukocyte Extract (DLE). As stated above, this extract contains more than 200 distinct moieties, of which a number have been identified, for example thymosin [10], prostaglandin [11a], hypoxanthine [11b], and nicotinamide [11c]. Certain components of DLE possess adjuvant properties [12] (nonantigen-specific immunostimulation effects) whereas others have been shown to suppress immune responsiveness. (An immunosuppressant factor has been obtained from DLE by V. E. M. Rosso di San Secondo et al. [13] and also by others and it eventually will certainly be of great clinical use. It inhibits IL-2R expression in cultured lymphocytes, inhibits DNA and RNA synthesis of isolated nuclei and in a cell-free system.

These data suggest that TFs may act directly at the level of DNA polymerization processes with a mechanism of action similar to those of cyclosporine A and FK-506. Whether the mechanism is "switch-off" of cell proliferation is conjectural.) We now reserve the term TF for the components of DLE that transfers T-lymphocyte responses in an antigen-specific fashion; that is $TF_{a.s.}$[6]. This fraction, in turn, contains a multitude of TFs corresponding to the sum of immune experiences of the individual subject. We now use the terms DLE-TF to describe a dialyzable leukocyte extract and DLyE to describe a dialyzable lymphocyte extract (DLyE enriched in TF is made by adding an additional procedure namely, micropore vacuum filtration, that eliminates molecules >6,000 daltons MW). Furthermore, we use the term $DLE-TF_{a.s.}$ for DLE-TF which is known to be specific for a desired antigen, e.g. $DLE-TF_{ova}$ (for ovalbumim). As stated above, some immunologists, especially the British, used the term TF to describe the entire DLE. This resulted in much semantic confusion [9] since DLE contain non-specific immunologic adjuvant moieties (and unfortunately to abandonment of research on TF in Great Britain; the absence of presentations by British investigators at the International Symposia on Transfer Factor during the last 10 years has been noticeable). More recently, we have used mononuclear cells obtained by lymphopheresis using a cell separator to exclude granulocytes; we termed this resultant material DLyE-TF [6].

1.3   General characteristics of transfer factor

Human, mouse, and bovine TFs, all well studied, are small molecules approximately 3500 to 6000 daltons. TF is heat labile but cold stable; indeed, the biologic activity of the factors remains unimpaired after several years of storage at $-20\,°C$ to $-70\,°C$. Most studies of the effect of enzymes on the antigen-specific biologic activity of TF indicate that the factors contain RNA bases attached to small peptides [e.g., 14]. Although Kirkpatrick, using the mouse footpad assay recently reported TF to be "proteinaceous" in nature, that is, devoid of RNA [15a, b, c], other investigators, e.g. those at the University of Leipzig, Germany [16a], as well as Chinese [16c], Japanese [16d], and Russian investigators [16b], using in vitro assay methods confirmed the oligoribonucleotide-peptide structure. (Editorial comment: Perhaps the reason for the differences in results between Kirkpatrick and all others is in the method of obtaining the dialyzates; namely ultra pressure filtrate versus chromatographically precleaning dialyzates. The Elution profile of an ultra pressure filtrate differs from the chromatographically pre-clean dialyzates in the considerably higher nucleotide content of the former.) At present, it appears that the RNA and peptide are complexed *in vivo* and that breaking of the RNA peptide bond destroys their biologic activity [16 e]. Groups at the University of Leipzig, China, and Russia have recently confirmed our previous findings that the low MW ultrafiltrate from human leukocytes is mainly hybrid molecules, namely, oligoribonucleotides – linked to peptides, in keeping with our own observations [14]. Further, data on TF structure is given in Section IV.B *(vide infra).*

If indeed a unique TF exists of each antigen specificity, then it is likely that individual TFs differ structurally in a manner similar to the subtle variations in antigen-binding sites at the hypervariable region of immunoglobulins, or in T-cell receptors for antigens. In view of the MW and composition, it is likely that each TF contains at least eight amino acids [17]. Therefore, if one considers the possible combinations of the 20 known amino acids, there are at least several billion variations in the primary structure, e.g., 8^{20}, and thus at least several million TFs specific for different antigens exist in every normal immune inventory [17]. (Actually, 18 of the 20 known amino acids have been found in various semi-purified TFs, so the value is 8^{18}).

2   Current status
2.1   Immunotherapy with DLE containing TF
2.1.1   *Indications for therapy*

The criteria for selection of suitable candidates for therapy depend to some extent on the nature of the disease under consideration. Thus, treatment with DLE containing TF would be indicated in "broad spectrum" defects in CMI, e.g. Wiskott-Aldrich syndrome, ataxia telangiectasia, partial DiGeorge syndrome, etc. [6]. It would also be useful in patients with an "antigen selective defect" in cell-mediated immunity (e.g., familial chronic mucocutaneous condidiasis) or in certain neoplastic diseases refractory to other therapy, e.g. DLE-TF specific for osteosarcoma. However, encountering such patients who have not already had prior therapy with other medications is relatively rare. Hence, we have used DLE or DLyE only in patients with diseases unresponsive to any conventional prescription medications or patients who fail to respond to, or developed severe toxicity to, standard prescription medications. Such a clear-cut indication is, however, relatively rare. More frequently, an antigen-specific defect may be suspected but not proven, as in certain patients with chronic or recurrent severe viral infections. A more uncertain area includes diseases of unknown etiology but presumed by many to be initiated by viral infection (e.g., Behçet's syndrome), in which evidence of cell-mediated immune abnormalities have been obtained and in which the only currently used therapy is prolonged high-dose steroids with or without immunosuppressive agents (e.g. immuran); we have treated such patients only after severe adverse effects. Results of reported therapeutic trials with DLE must therefore be interpreted with caution, as the activity of adjuvant or inhibitory factors present in crude preparations of DLE may in certain instances be responsible for any therapeutic effect unless "control DLE", devoid of TF of desired specificity, has previously been administered to the recipient without clinical benefit (i.e., unless each patient served as his or her own control, as described below). We believe this a far better control than placebo double-blind studies in these dread diseases for which there is no current prescription therapy.

2.1.2   Side effects of dialyzable leukocyte extract therapy

DLE is usually administered by subcutaneous or intramuscular injection, although oral administration appears equally effective, [e.g., 18 a, b], can be given by suppository [18 c] and incorporated into liposomes [18 d] so that the biologic activity persists for a longer duration. For rapid action, it can also be administered intravenously (vide infra). DLE is remarkably free from adverse side effects. When given intramuscularly or subcutaneously, it may cause pain at the injection site for 10 to 20 minutes. Transient low grade pyrexia may occur, but there have been no reports of hypersensitivity reactions or of long-term adverse effects. Patients with osteosarcoma or breast cancer with bone metastases treated with (and responding to) DLE containing TF of appropriate specificity have experienced severe pain at the site of primary or metastatic lesions, caused by necrosis of tumor cells; whereas, DLE devoid of TF of corresponding specificity did not cause pain [17]. This is analogous to the flare reaction (increased pain) on successful treatment of bone metastases by chemotherapy and endocrine therapy [19].

2.1.3   Choice of donor

The selection of suitable donors of DLE is a major factor in the efficacy of therapy. Clearly, all potential donors must be screened to confirm general immunocompetence, but of equal importance is the investigation of donors for antigen-specific immune responses where appropriate, for example, when the patient is known to have an antigen-selective defect for a given microbial agent or tumor antigen. In our early studies, lack of MIF production was used as the criteria for an antigen-selective defect in the patient (see fig. 3a and 3b), but in the last 10 years, we have used lack of LIF production.
LIF production is measured by the direct assay for inhibition of random leukocyte migration in agarose (LMI) [20] (see fig. 4). Peripheral blood leukocytes, or PBL (2.0×10^8 cells/mL), are incubated with medium 199 only (control) or with medium plus test antigen at 37°C

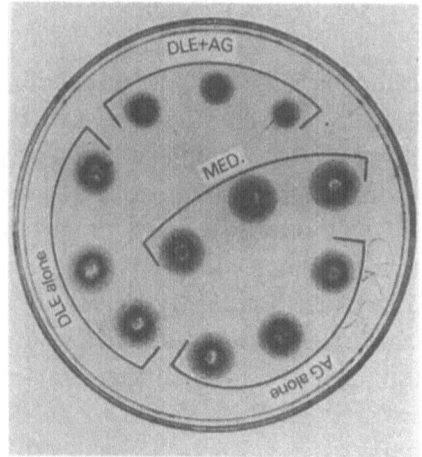

Figure 4
Standard plate pattern for testing effects of DLE *in vitro* by leukocyte migration inhibition in agarose (LMI). MED = PNL incubated with medium only. AG = PBL incubated with antigen. DLE = PBL incubated with DLE containing $TF_{a.s.}$. DLE + AG = PBL incubated with DLE plus specific antigen. The migration areas shown were obtained after 18 hours. PBL were initially nonresponsive to the antigen, as shown the MED and AG diameters of migration. At the concentration of DLE used. DLE alone had no effect ($MI_A = 1.00$). Note, however, the decreased migration when PBL were incubated with DLE + AG.

[20]. During this incubation period, the granulocytes (polymorphonu-clear neutrophils, or PMN) randomly migrate out of the application wells under the agarose to form a circular zone of cells. Respon-siveness to antigen or mitogen is expressed as a migration index (MI). Note that migration can also be expressed as percentage inhibition by the equation:

$$\% \text{ inhibition} = (1 - MI) \times 100$$

For the highest concentrations of each test substance used, an MI < 0.80 (i.e., $>20\%$ inhibition) indicates responsiveness (induction of LIF production [20]. When the patient is known to have an antigen-selective defect, the potential donor is identified by laboratory tests as having CMI for the relevant antigen by the same assay: direct leukocyte migration inhibition in agarose. When the relevant antigen is unknown, potential donors of DLE should be selected from close household contacts of a least 6 months duration (not necessarily relatives of the patient) on the premise that such contacts have shared exposure to the agent and mounted a normal cell-mediated immune response to it, and therefore have not developed the disease [6].

2.1.4   Preparation of dialyzable leukocyte extract

We usually obtain 10^{10} mononuclear cells (0.1% of total body immuno-cytes [0%–8% granulocytes]) by lymphophoresis, using an IBM/Kobe cell separator, with the collection bag placed on a tray contain-ing ICB. The cells are then disrupted by freeze-thawing and sonica-tion. The leukocyte lysate is subsequently dialyzed through tubing with pore size that prevents substances with MW > 13 K.D. to pass through the pores and further fractionated (lysozyme, 12 K.D. and horse myoglobin 17.7 K.D. are used in one tube as a control for the dialyzate and retentate, respectively); then further fractionated by micropore dialysis with pore sizes of 6000 K.D. to 8000 K.D.; then lyophilized. An aliquot of the DLE is then subjected to two-week culture to ensure sterility and also tests for absence of endotoxin. As mentioned above, this material, now enriched in TF, we term DLE-TF; it is then lyophilized $\times 3$ in distilled water devoid of protein or growth medium. To permit some comparison between batches, one international unit (I.U.) of DLE has been (somewhat arbitrarily) defined as that amount of extract derived from 5×10^8 leukocytes [21] and is usually placed in a 1-ml vial. Thus, since the ratio of polymorphonuclear cells to mononuclear cells in normal buffy coat is approximately 2:1; our preparations (95% mononuclear cells) are made from 10⁹ immunocytes; each batch therefore contains approximately 30 I.U. The batch is divided so that two South Carolina units are placed in each of 15 vials. It should be emphasized that unit standardization provides no information on potency of either the TF moiety or of antigen-nonspecific fractions of the extract. Two batches of extract containing TFs of the same specificity and prepared from the number of lymphocytes may differ twenty-fold in potency. We determine potency units using production of LIF [22] (fig. 5). That dilution of the DLE preparation which produces 10% inhibition of LIF production [23] in an antigen-specific manner determines the potency index [20, 22] (fig. 5). Although for scientific purposes purification and structure for the TFs of differing specificities is mandatory, for clinical purposes a mixture of at least several moieties is probably preferable since nature has designed, at least in the immune system, molecules that work synergistically when combined. An example is provided by experience with interferon. The first product

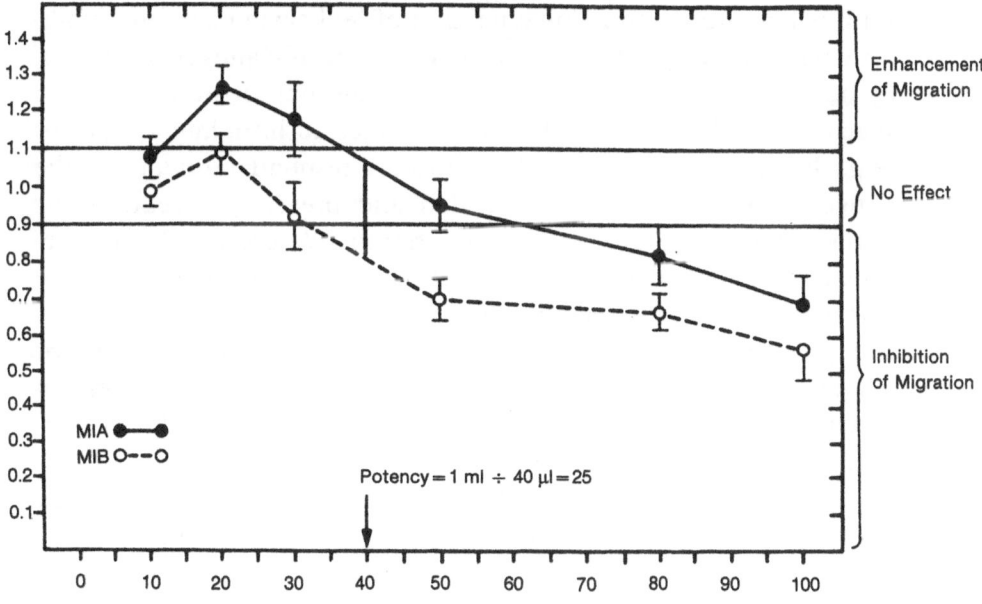

Figure 5
Potency assay. Direct leukocyte migration in agarose. In each panel, the top line represents random migration; the bottom line represents inhibition of migration by one or another activity of the Sephadex G 25 fractions.

termed gamma-interferon was provided by the Helsinki Blood Bank, which shipped leukocyte extracts to Sweden for clinical trials [24]. In clinical trials, this material was reported to benefit 50% of patients with a wide variety of cancers. Great emphasis (and much research funding) was placed on purifying gammainterferon free of contaminants. However, when this was finally achieved, and recombinant γ interferon became available, it produced clinical benefit in only 1% of cancer patients. Presumably, the "contaminants" were responsible, at least in part, for the favorable results of the original mixtures (we found TF and LIF among them) [25].

2.1.5   *In vitro determination of potency*

As noted above, many years ago, we demonstrated that batches of dialyzable leukocyte extract, prepared from different donors and standardized in identical manner by LMI assay, varied markedly in their ability to induce lymphokine production by immunologically normal cells exposed to specific antigen [26]. This fact necessitated the standardization of TF by potency units. The LMI assay for potency of DLE is based on a direct investigation of leukocyte migration inhibitory factor (LIF) produced in response to specific antigen used [27a, b]. It is useful, not only for studies in humans, but for studies in other species as well. This assay has been applied to infra-human species (e.g., burro) as well. If the lymphocytes respond normally to the antigenic challenge, LIF is liberated and prevents or reduces the normal PMN leukocyte random migration. We use this LMI assay extensively in the diagnosis of antigen-specific cell-mediated immune defects and in donor selection. The addition of DLE to this system has two potential effects: first, an antigen-independent inhibition of migration at low concentrations of extract, and second, antigen-specific induction or enhancement of LIF production at lower concentrations of extract [27a, b].

The method for determining DLE-TF potency is briefly summarized as follows: (α) Aliquots of target cells (PBL) from three normal donors previously shown to be nonresponsive to the test antigen (in this case PPD) by LMI (MI ≥ 0.90) are incubated in either (1) medium alone, (2) medium plus antigen (100 g/ml), (3) DLE (in at least ten different concentrations) in medium, and (4) DLE (in the same ten concentrations) plus antigen plus medium for 30 min at 37 °C in a humidified incubator gassed with 5% CO_2 in air, before neutrophil migration. (b) After neutrophil migration (18 hr), the effects of antigen alone, DLE alone, and DLE plus antigen are quantitated by determining three migration indices termed, respectively, the MI, MI_A, and MI_B. The MI_A value quantitates antigen-independent (LIF-independent) LMI produced by non-TF components. MI_A values ≤ 0.80 indicate significant antigen-independent effects. The MI_B value quantitates antigen-dependent LMI induced by LIF released from T lymphocytes newly sensitized by TF in the presence of specific antigen [27 a]. An MI_B value < 0.90 indicates meaningful antigen-dependent LMI. All concentrations of DLE are tested in six replicate cultures. The MI, MI_A, and MI_B values given are the mean $\pm$ SEM for all determinations. DLE preparations are initially tested over a concentration range of 1 to $50 \mu l$ (we store DLE frozen in 1-ml vials); for example, if 40 μl provide MI_B of 0.90, 1 ml of this DLE preparation contains 25 south Carolina potency units; that is $1000 \div 40$ (fig. 5). A similar system in which the mitogen phytohemagglutinin (PHA) is substituted for antigen can be used to standardize preparations of extract intended for therapy of patients with immune defects of unknown specificities. This LMI assay also identifies batches of DLE that for unknown reasons contain significant amounts of immunoinhibitory factors (about 10% to 15% of DLE preparations). In many of these, the RNA peptide bond has been cleaved, presumably by enzymes from disrupted contaminating granulocytes [16 e]. These preparations inhibited IL-2 receptor expression in cultured lymphocytes and inhibited lymphocyte DNA and RNA synthesis in response to PHA. The effect was reversible in that the cells when incubated with suppressive factor were washed prior to addition of PHA; furthermore, no suppression could be seen when the factor was added to culture 24 hours after PHA addition [16 e].

2.1.6   *Laboratory monitoring of clinical response*

Striking differences in clinical response to DLE therapy occur between individual recipients [28]. Responses vary according to (a) the disease process, (b) the severity of disease, (c) the potency of the extract preparation (as discussed above), and (d) the amount of antigen burden [28]. Thus, two patients with the same disease may well display quite disparate responses to the same batch of extract. It is therefore imperative that appropriate *in vitro* laboratory evaluation of patients is performed in any trial of DLE so that the scheduled amount and frequency of therapy may be titrated against both the clinical and immunologic responses. Many *in vitro* immunologic assays are currently available for monitoring recipients; and, in general, their use has superseded that of skin testing for monitoring immunologic response, since skin testing (a) is time-consuming and difficult to evaluate in a quantitative manner and (b) introduces antigen (possibly for the first time) in the recipient [29 a], which by itself may influence CMI to that antigen [29 a, b].

2.1.6.1   Antigen-specific responses

The previously mentioned direct LMI test is, in our opinion, the best way available at present to investigate antigen-specific immune response. Certain patients showed clinical improvement in response to the adjuvant moieties of DLE in the absence of an antigen-specific response [30]; the LMI test clearly identifies such patients. Although antigen-specific TF confers on the previously unresponsive individual the ability to produce lymphokines in response to specific stimulation, it does not produce *de novo* the ability to respond to antigen by lymphocyte DNA synthesis [31 a, b]. However, DLE-TF will enhance antigen-dependent DNA synthesis in already committed lymphocytes [31 b]. The activity referred to in [31 b] is found in the adjuvant moiety of DLE that is quite distinct from the moiety responsible for the *de novo* induction of mediator production. Thus, antigen-dependent lymphocyte DNA synthesis is not an appropriate test either for *in vitro* screening of preparation of extract or for monitoring of recipient response [31 b]. Indeed, no improvement in deficient DNA synthesis was found in a few patients who responded well to extract therapy in terms of skin-test conversion, lymphokine production, and clinical improvement [31 b, 32]. In addition, DLE contains immunologically active peptides IMREGs *(vide infra)* that boost the recipient's own CMI in an antigen-specific manner [33 a, b, c]. These moieties, MW approximantely 1500 to 2000 daltons, have greatly increased CMI to antigens previously encountered by the recipient (e. g., upper respiratory viral infections) [34 a, b]. In this respect, the observations of Peng et al., are especially important. 100 patients with a variety of malignant tumors (e. g., lung, breast, esophageal, gastric, nasopharyngeal, etc.)

were simultaneously given combination chemotherapy and placental dialyzable placental lymphocyte extract (DPE). "The frequency of catch cold was markedly decreased in many patients by ... DPE and the symptoms were much abated even if they caught cold. [In addition] their appetite and physical strength increased in spirit, higher ...; immunological indexes of 39 cases increased after [immunotherapy] treatments even if under violent chemotherapy." Furthermore, "... all patients successfully passed the chemotherapy without severe side effects." (Editor's comment: The decreased frequency and severity of the viral upper respiratory infections in these 100 cancer patients was undoubtedly due to IMREGs in the placental extract; whereas, resistance to chemotherapy was probably due to either TF and/or the adjuvant moiety in the extract). Several other authors [e. g., 63 b] have commented that patients receiving TF have an unusual decrease in the incidence and severity of viral upper respiratory infections *(vide infra)*, as have we [34 c].

Another valuable immunologic test is antigen-specific T-cell cytotoxicity – a test frequently employed in the investigation of patients with a variety of neoplastic diseases [35]. Purified T-lymphocytes are cultured with viable tumor cells at ratios of 40:1 (labeled with ^{51}Cr) derived either from the patient's own tumor or from a cell line of the same tumor type. Tumor cells of other types plus matching fibroblasts are used as controls. The specific cytotoxic activity of the lymphocytes results in lysis of the tumor cells and release of the radioisotope into the medium in amounts far greater than release of radioisotope from cells of other tumor types. Addition of DLE derived from a donor proven by this test to be responsive to the relevant tumor antigens enhances the specific cytotoxicity of the patient's lymphocytes in a dose-dependent manner [35].

2.1.6.2 Rosette formation by active T-cells with sheep red blood cells (SRBC)

This test enumerates a subset of T-lymphocytes that form immediate rosettes with sheep erythrocytes; this active percentage (a measure of function) of T-cells usually correlates more closely with cell-mediated immune status than does the percentage of "total" T-cells as measured by rosette formation with SRBC at 18 hr. The two tests are performed at different temperatures and different T-cell/SRBC ratios [36]. We

[37], and others [e. g., 38] have demonstrated that in immunodeficient patients suffering from recurrent viral, fungal, or mycobacterial infections, or from certain malignancies, response to DLE-TF therapy is associated with a normalization of the active T-cell population. *In vitro* investigations have shown that the fraction of DLE-TF that mediates this effect is also responsible for the transfer of antigen-specific reactivity [39 a, b]. Tests for active T-cells in the guinea pigs and pigs have been reported [39 c, d]; this test has the same utility in animal models as does the test for "active" T-cells in humans.

2.1.6.3   Interactive T-cells

We have increasing evidence that the enumeration of so-called "interactive" T-cells (IAT) is of particular value in monitoring response to DLE therapy in certain diseases [40]. This subpopulation of T-cells is identified by its ability to form rosettes with human transformed B lymphocytes (such as cells from the RAJI cell line) (fig. 6). This reaction appears to involve a membrane receptor on the lymphoblastoid cell that is distinct from, for example, Fc receptors. Function of Interactive T-cells (numbers since currently a numerical test is used only functional T-cells bind to the B-cell line) are frequently reduced in patients with recurrent viral and/or fungal infections and in subsets of retinitis pigmentosa (RP), Alzheimer's disease (AD), and the

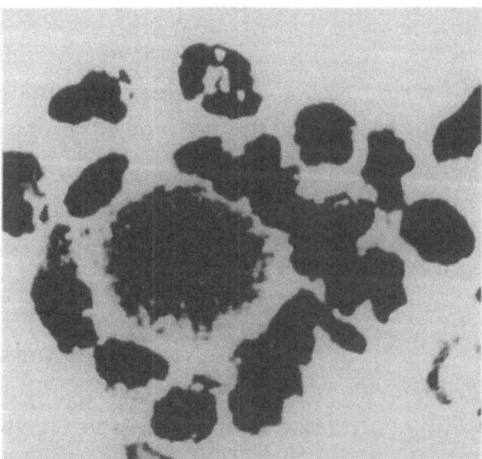

Figure 6
Picture of interactive T-cells binding to a central B-cell (obtained from the RAJI cell line to form an interactive rosette.

so-called Florence Nightingale Disease (FND). The membrane markers of interactive T-cells do not correspond to any known T-cell subpopulation (e. g., CD4+, CD8+, etc.), but these cells appear to be those that "accept" antigens (epitopes) presented to them by B-cells [34a]. A reduction in circulating IAT correlates in several diseases with deficient mitogen-dependent lymphokine production [e.g., 41] and low percentages in this subset are frequently observed in many cell-mediated immunodeficiency states, as described below. When decreased, normalization of the IAT population is one of the first

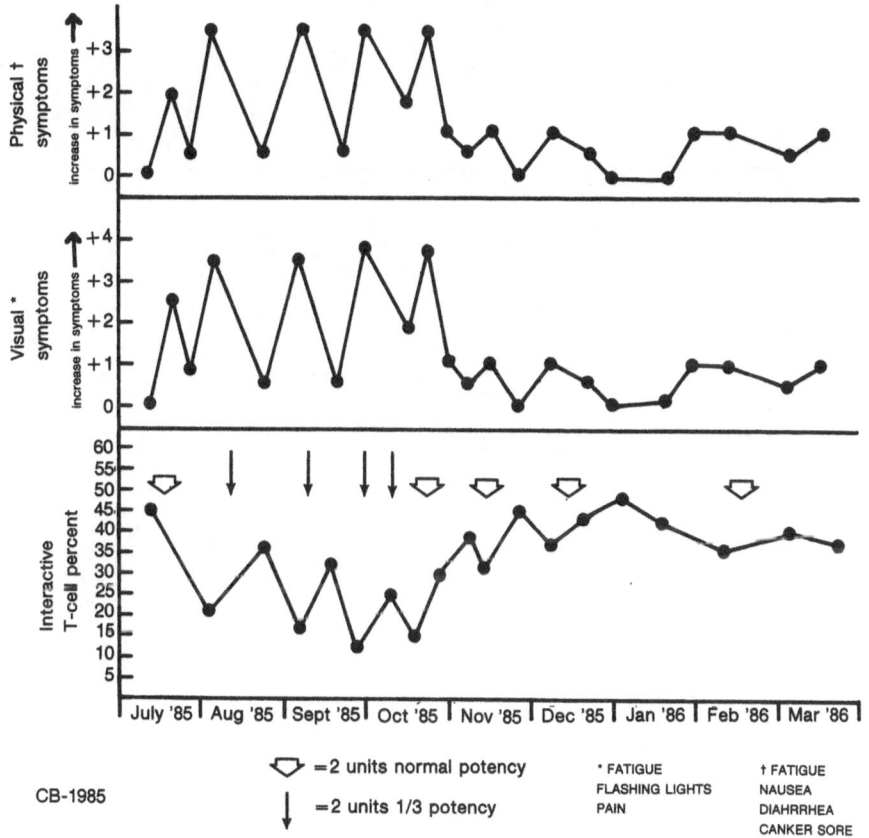

CB-1985

⬇ = 2 units normal potency   * FATIGUE   † FATIGUE
                              FLASHING LIGHTS   NAUSEA
↓ = 2 units 1/3 potency   PAIN   DIAHRRHEA
                                                   CANKER SORE

Figure 7

DLE, interactive T-cells, and clinical symptoms in a 40-year old white female patient, first seen in 1981, with retinitis pigmentosa and recurrent viral infections, many of which triggered visual symptoms.

7a.   Interactive T-cells and visual and physical symptoms in response to DLE from cells of husband and DLE from cells of random donors. Note that following administration of DLE from husband, visual and physical symptoms were completely eradicated and there was a marked increase in IAT to supranormal levels.

events to occur following administration of DLE containing TF of the relevant specificity. An example of the value of such tests is illustrated by the course of one representative patient with RP followed for 7 years [42]. The DLE derived from the lymphoid cells in her spouse was far more effective than that derived from cells of a normal random donor. Clinical improvement by DLyE-TF was repeatedly administered and always was reflected in a rise in IAT after DLyE. Furthermore, of at least a dozen batches of DLE obtained from immune cells of her husband, one (obtained shortly before an onset of a mild viral

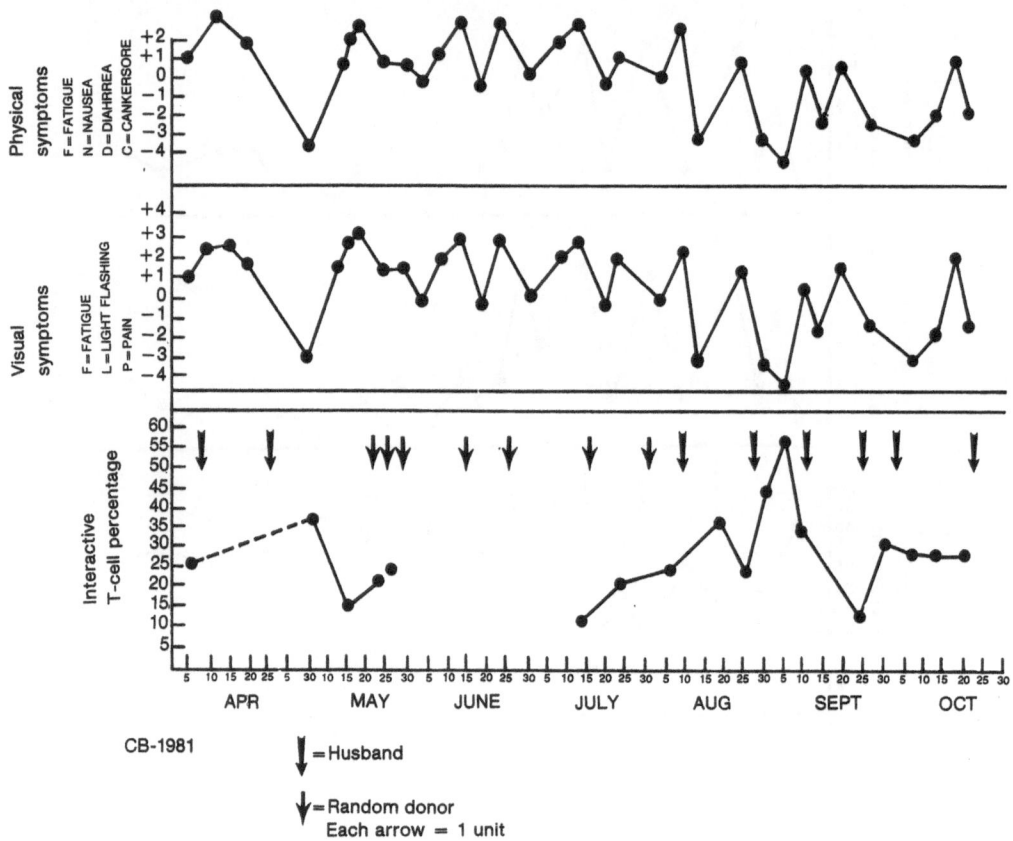

7b. Interactive T-cells and visual and physical symptoms in response to DLE from husband, normally, and DLE from husband, obtained five days prior to viral infection. Note that one batch of DLE from husband during the five years had approximately ⅓ the usual potency, and administration of this material raised IAT and reduced visual and physical symptoms far less than did DLE obtained from husband on other occasions. For example, note the difference between September 1, 1985, mid-October 1985, and December 1985 to March 1986. Symptoms are lower and IAT are higher.

infection) was only one-third as potent as the usual DLE; fig. 7a depicts clinical and laboratory response to the usual DLE and to that obtained shortly before onset of viral infection in husband and compares the clinical response obtained to DLE prepared from cells of a normal control (fig. 7b) compared to that of DLE prepared from cells of her husband. During the time she received the DLE-TF$_{random}$, she suffered recurrent viral infections and loss of visual fields.

2.1.6.4   Other *in vitro* effects of DLE

Although little is known of the mechanisms of action of TF, much has been learned of the results of activity of both TF and DLE both *in vivo* and *in vitro*. *In vitro*, DLE increases macrophage activation and IL-1 production [43] both highly important in CMI. In the opinion of this author, these are the two most important properties of TF; a third important is the switch-on of T-suppressor cells, probably via an IL-1 mediated mechanism. Nekem et al. have shown that TF also augments resynthesis of the receptors (the CD11 site) for trypsinized sheep RBC (Trypsin destroys these receptors [39b, 44]. This has been confirmed by others. The CD11-antigen site of T-cells is one site involved in T-cell activation). DLE inhibits spontaneous loss of such receptors; it also enhances antibody-dependent cell-mediated cytotoxicity (ADCC) activity of normal peripheral blood lymphocytes [45]; it augments DNA synthesis by normal lymphocytes [46]; it stimulates mixed lymphocyte culture reactivity [47] and enhances defective leukocyte chemotaxis [48] and deficient natural killer (NK) cell function [49] the latter perhaps also via IL-1 production. *In vivo*, the extract enhances graft rejection [50] and augments lectin-dependent ADCC activity [51]. This wide variety of effects of crude DLE reflects the activities of its many different moieties of crude DLE, including non-specific adjuvant or inhibitory functions. Antigen-specific properties due to the TF moiety within the dialyzable extract include the ability to confer on non-responsive lymphocytes the potential to react with the relevant antigen *in vivo*, to produce lymphokines *in vitro* [51] (and presumably *in vivo* as well) and to enhance antigen-specific T-cell cytotoxicity against tumor antigens by previously non-responsive cytotoxic cells [52]. These effects must be considered in both *in vitro* testing of preparations of DLE and monitoring of patient response to therapy with DLE and/or DLyE, as discussed below.

2.2   Results of therapy with DLE containing TF (Table 1)

Since DLE contains many moieties in addition to TF and since these other moieties may account for 10%–15% of immunologic activity in DLE, we used each of the first 100 patients as his or her own control. This was accomplished by making TF from the cells of a donor lacking immunity to the given antigen; e. g., herpes 1, *Mycobacterium fortuitum,* cytomegalo-virus. DLE lacking CMI for the relevant antigen was administered over 6 weeks. No improvement was noted either clinically or in immunologic parameters during this period or over a subsequent 6 weeks without DLE. Each patient was subsequently given DLE from a donor with high CMI to the relevant antigen DLE$_{a.s.}$ over a 6-week period; 80% of patients improved dramatically; improvement was always preceded by improvement in formerly deficient laboratory parameters. The above experiments where the patient served as his or her own control provide compelling evidence that TF is directly responsible for the clinical and laboratory improvements [53, 54a, b, c, d]. Several double-blind placebo control studies have shown definite benefit of DLE-TF$_{a.s.}$ over DLE-TF$_{random}$ versus saline; e. g., McMeeking [72b].

We have published several detailed reviews of DLE therapy in a wide variety of diseases [e. g., 6, 42, 54a, b, c, d]. Thymus-derived lymphocytes ("T-cells") acting by production of soluble mediators of cell-mediated immunity, in some undefined manner protect us against protozoal (e. g., *pneumocystis cariini, cryptosporidia),* infection, fungal infections (e. g., candida albicans), mycobacterial infections (e. g., human, avian, and bovine tuberculosis, M. Fortuitum pneumonia, leprosy, etc.), parasitic infection (e. g., leishmaniasis), viral infections (e. g., cytomegalovirus), and protect us, at least partially, against cancer metastases *(vide infra).* The next section describes the results of DLE-TF therapy in selected disorders.

2.2.1   *Fungal diseases*
2.2.1.1   Chronic mucocutaneous candidiasis (CMC)

CMC, a fungal disease, has been frequently cited as a classic example of an antigen-specific cell-mediated immunodeficiency that may respond to DLE-TF$_{a.s.}$ therapy [e. g., 8, 54–56]. We first described the therapeutic use of DLE in CMC in 1972 [8]. Since then, many reports

Table 1
DLE-Transfer factor – Beneficial results

Reported by us, confirmed by others

1. Familial T-lymphocyte dysfunction with severe recurrent infection
2. Herpes infection
3. Cytomegalovirus infection
4. Candidiasis
5. Parasitic infection (e.g., pneumocystis carinae, cryptosporidiosis, etc.)
6. Mycobacterium tuberculosis infection refractory to antibiotics
7. Behçet's syndrome
8. Lupus erythematosus
9. Pemphigus vegetans (skin disease)
10. Wiskott-Aldrich Syndrome
11. Florence Nightingale Disease (a.k.a. Chronic Fatigue Immune Dysfunction Syndrome)
12. Bone metastases after surgical removal of breast cancer
13. Bone metastases after surgical removal of kidney cancer
14. Guillian Barre
15. Amyotrophic lateral sclerosis (one subset)
16. Retinitis Pigmentosa (one subset, 50%; DLE-TF does not reverse the disease but prevents additional visual loss)

Reported by us

1. Mycobacterium fortuitum infection
2. Mycobacterium avian infection
3. Alopecia totalis
4. Alzheimer's disease (one subset)
5. Autism (one subset, 70%)
6. Osteosarcoma (DLE-TF prevents metastases to lungs)
7. Epidermal dysplasia (multiple cutaneous malignancies)
8. Certain food and chemical hypersensitivities
9. Coccidiosis
10. Burkitt's lymphoma, etc.

Reported by others

1. Lepromatous leprosy
2. Leishmaniasis
3. Rat diabetes (Type I-immunologic) (trials in humans not yet reported)
4. Myasthenia gravis
5. Subacute sclerosing panencephalitis
6. Atopic dermatitis
7. Bronchial asthma
8. Recurrent otitis media
9. Varicella
10. Hepatitis B – acute and chronic
11. Myasthenia gravis
12. Brucella
13. Asthma
14. Nasopharyngeal carcinoma
15. Stomach carcinoma
16. Colon carcinoma
17. Non-small cell lung carcinoma
18. Spontaneous abortions

from other centers have indicated that DLE prepared from candida-sensitive donors frequently improves the immunologic response of the CMC patient, but has a variable effect on the patient's ability to eliminate the pathogen [e.g., 55, 56]. In our first report of 11 cases of CMC treated with DLE, about half of the patients responded clinically [57]. Good results were obtained with suppositories [18 c] in five patients with systemic candidiasis. It seemed to be as effective as did patients with the same degree of disease treated with DLE derived from human blood. Immunologic parameters were also normalized to approximately the same extent by the suppository therapy as with subcutaneous therapy. Fig. 8a and 8b show the hands of a representative patient with severe CMC who responded dramatically to DLE-TF, administered after amphotericin had produced nephrotoxicity (18 months). We administered DLE-TF obtained from the cells of a candida-negative donor for six weeks without clinical benefit, then placebo for six weeks without change in renal function and slight increase in lesion size; then DLE-TF derived from the cells of a donor with strong CMI for candida albicans. This figure shows the patient's hands before (fig. 8a) and after therapy (fig. 8b); the patient's face and feet were affected to the same degree. Fig. 8c shows a partial response half way through the two month course of DLE-TF$_{a.s.}$ to candida. It is now recognized that CMC is not a single disease entity but rather a syndrome consisting of several entities, each with a distinct immunologic profile [58]. A retrospective analysis of our own data indicates that only patients with one of these entities (about 60%) respond to DLE therapy – furthermore, large doses of DLE containing TF after the antifungal therapy were required. More recently, the influence of other immunologic factors in CMC has been recognized, such as the presence of circulating inhibitory factors (in some cases antigen [candida]-antibody complexes). One patient who apparently fulfilled the criteria for potential DLE-TF$_{a.s.}$ therapy for candida had a circulating suppressor factor; therefore, a trial of therapeutic plasma exchange was performed. After the second exchange, the patient's immune response became normal, and after three weeks of continued antifungal therapy, the patient was disease free and remained so for at least a year [59]. These examples illustrate both the disease-specificity and recipient-specificity of potential response to antigen-specific DLE therapy (hereinafter termed TF$_{a.s.}$), and probably explains in part the variable results of such therapy, at least in CMC. Antigen-specific TF

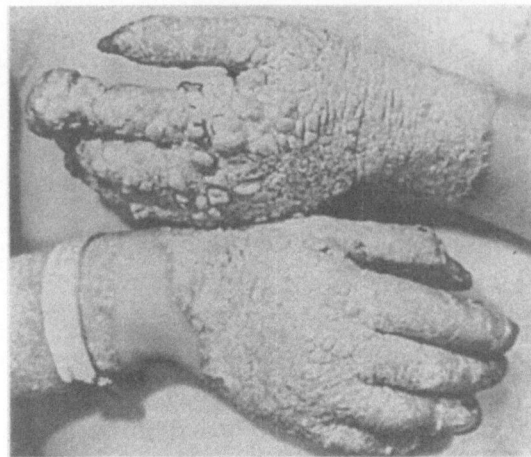
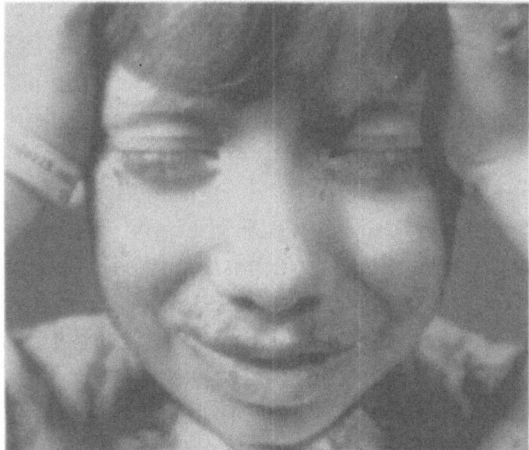
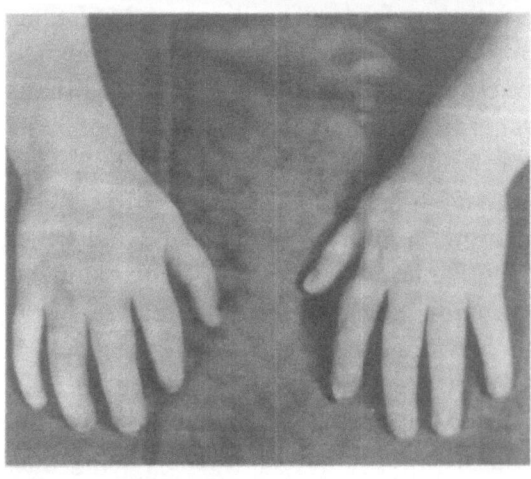

Figure 8
Efficacy of DLE containing TF$_{a.s.}$ for candida prepared from lymphocytes of a donor with high CMI to candida on the first patient with chronic mucocutaneous candidiasis so treated. Photographs show the hands of child before (Figure 8a) and 3 months after (Figure 8b) TF. Feet show similar change in appearance. Candidiasis also involved lower half of face (Figure 8c) and this, too, cleared with therapy (photograph taken two months after initiation of therapy).

has also proved useful in other fungal diseases (e.g., disseminated coccidiomycosis [e.g., 60]).

2.2.2   *Mycobacterial diseases*
2.2.2.1   Lepromatous leprosy

This manifestation of the disease caused by *Mycobacterium leprae* is characterized by absent cell-mediated immune responses to the lepromin-antigen derived from the mycobacterium or to the organism itself [61]. Other cell-mediated immune defects complicating this disease include reduction in peripheral and lymph node T-cells, impaired response to mitogens, and the anergy to common recall antigens. These latter defects are reversed by successful antimycobacterial therapy, although apparently cured patients often remain anergic to lepromin. An early report of the effect of lepromin-specific DLE in this disease described induction of lepromin-responsiveness in six of nine patients following one injection [62]. In a later report, four patients treated with a 12-week course of antigen-specific DLE in conjunction with antimycobacterial therapy had enhanced elimination of mycobacteria from lesions during DLE therapy and also became leprominpositive as determined by skin testing [63 a]. Thirty-one lepers were selected for the study; 17 cases of lepromatous leprosy, 10 cases of tuberculoid leprosy, and 4 cases of borderline leprosy – 22 were treated with TF one ampule once weekly for three months, then one ampule twice weekly for eight additional months (Editorial comment: These are really quite low doses for a disease in which the body is teaming with hundreds of millions of M. Lepra; nonetheless, there were significant increases in E. Rosette formation in the treated group and none in the control group). DNA synthesis increased significantly after therapy in the treated group but not in the control group. Before therapy IgG and IgA were elevated; with treatment, a 10% drop occurred (22.65 ± 147 to 232.7 ±137). In general, the sum of the patients felt more comfortable, vigorous, had better appetites, and better moods. Of interest is the following statement: "The incidence of coryza (common cold) reduced markedly over the corresponding period of the previous year" [63 b].
Subsequently, Leser et al. [64] performed a double-blind trial of DLE therapy in 15 patients with lepromatous-leprosy, using non-antigen-specific therapy in 15 patients with lepromatous-leprosy, using non-

antigen-specific DLE prepared from spleen and cadaveric kidney donors. Five patients received sulfone therapy in conjunction with saline placebo injections, five received sulfones and DLE, and five received placebo tablets and DLE. Clinical and bacteriologic improvement occurred in patients in all three groups. Immunologic studies revealed no changes in T- or B-lymphocyte numbers following therapy in any group. Therapy with DLE containing TF corrected previously defective mitogen-dependent lymphocyte DNA synthesis; however, there was no conversion of negative lepromin skin tests in any of the patients. This is not surprising, since antigen-specific DLE was not used. However, these results and those reported previously suggest that extract may be therapeutically beneficial in lepromatous leprosy, and that larger trials of therapy with DLE prepared with lepromin-sensitive donors are indicated.

We have also successfully treated one patient with lepromatous leprosy, acquired by a Texan who shot and killed, but did not thoroughly cook, an armadillo (one of the few infra-human species which carries leprosy), with $DLE_{a.s.}$ for leprosy [34a].

Other mycobacterial diseases that have responded dramatically to DLE containing $TF_{a.s.}$ include *tuberculosis vulgaris* (fig. 9a and 9b) and pulmonary tuberculosis refractory to all antibiotics [65a], confirmed by Pekárek et al. [65b] and *Mycobacterium fortuitum* (MF)

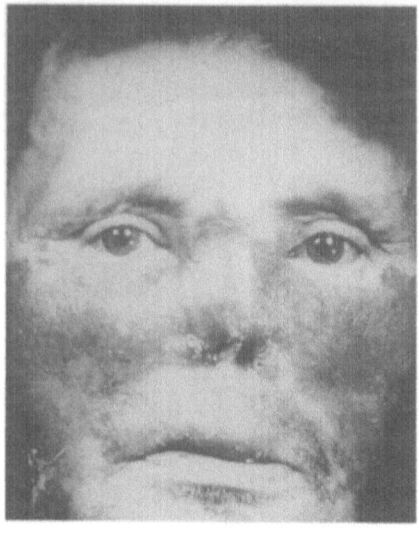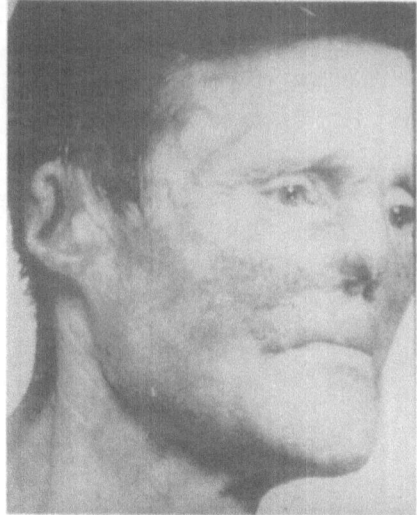

Figure 9
Face of patient with lupus vulgaris before (9a) and after (9b) DLE-$TF_{a.s.}$ therapy.

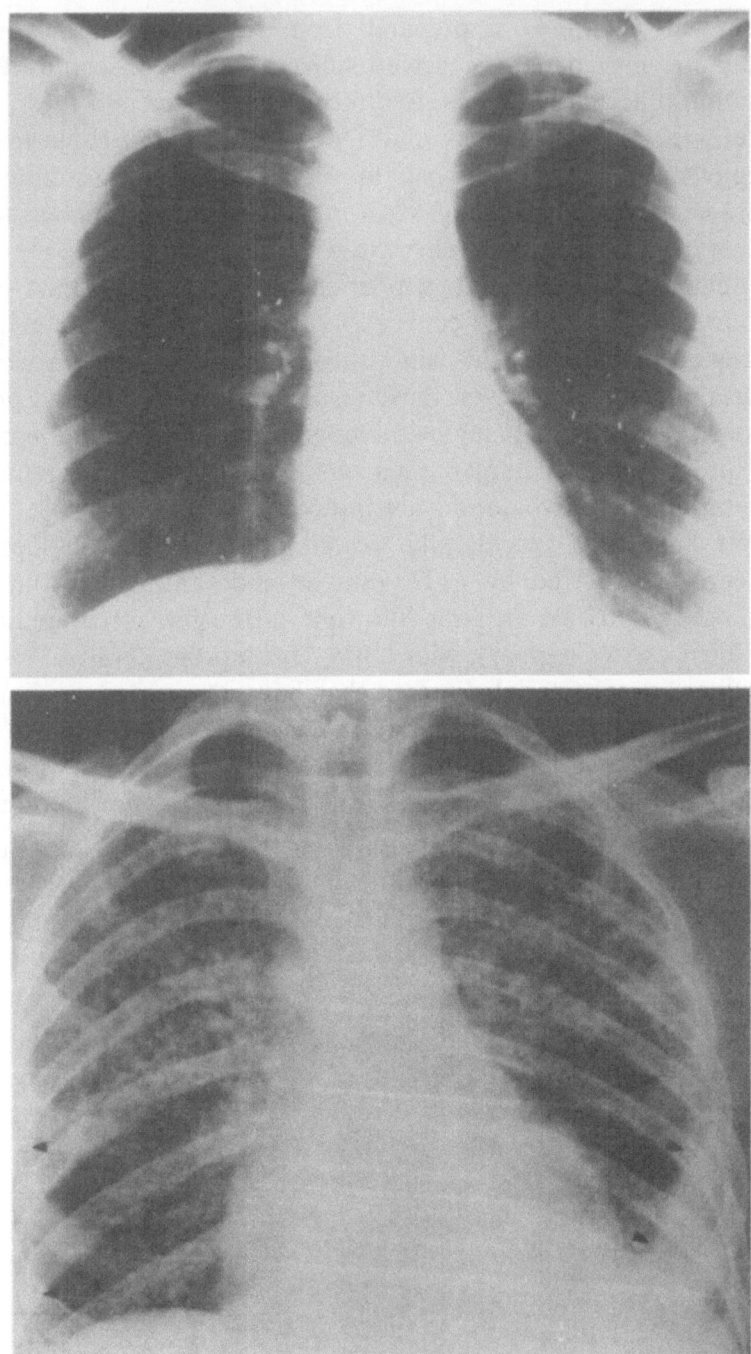

Figure 10
X-rays of chest of patient with miliary T. B. before (10 a) and after (10 b) DLE-TF$_{a.s.}$.

pneumonia refractory to antibiotic therapy [66, 67] (see fig. 10a and 10b). (M. Fortuitum is present in 50% of South Carolina soils.) It is noteworthy that DLE-TF obtained from cells of a donor with high CMI for *Mycobacterium tuberculosis* (PPD Standard), but no detectable CMI for (PPD-MF) antigen, produced no improvement in the patient with M. Fortuitum pulmonary disease, but DLE-TF positive for PPD-MF and negative for PPD-S produced dramatic improvement in both immunologic tests and clinical symptoms.

2.2.3   *Parasitic infections*
2.2.3.1   Cutaneous leishmaniasis

Cutaneous leishmaniasis, a parasitic infection which is usually self-limiting in humans, may in certain patients persist for years. It is generally presumed that an antigen-specific defect underlies the persistent disease. Sharma [68] reported the effects of $DLE_{a.s.}$ in cutaneous leishmaniasis; intensive therapy with DLE-TF for several months produced dramatic healing of lesions in three patients whose disease had existed for 8–30 years. At our suggestion, Sharma then conducted a therapeutic trial of extract in 23 patients [69]. Her exemplary study is one of the few well-controlled trials of DLE therapy reported. Patients received either placebo (saline injections), or non-antigen-specific DLE or $DLE_{a.s.}$ prepared from patients who had recovered from leishmaniasis. Eight patients with acute infection showed no response to non-specific DLE, although healing was observed in three patients with acute disease. The non-responders in this group were all negative to the pathogen by skin testing, whereas all three responders were skin-test positive, suggesting a nonantigen-specific adjuvant effect of DLE in these patients. Finally, twelve patients were treated with $DLE_{a.s.}$, i.e., DLE containing TF specific for the referenced antigen. In this group, all eight patients with acute disease rapidly responded to therapy as did two of four with persistent infection. Similar results were obtained in a subsequent study by Delgado et al. [70]; they administered DLE prepared from leishmania-responsive healthy donors to seven patients without antigen-specific CMI response. Four of the seven with acute leishmaniasis had complete resolution of their disease; this was accompanied by conversion to antigen responsiveness. None of the other three patients, all of whom had the disease for at least 10 years, responded.

2.2.3.2   Schistosomiasis

$DLE_{a.s.}$ completely eradicated schistosomiasis in a rhesus monkey model [71a, b, c].

2.2.3.3   Cryptosporidiosis

Bovine DLE specific for cryptosporidiosis administered orally, eliminated the diarrhea and parasites and ova in the stool in patients with diarrhea associated with this organism and with no other obvious disease. An exciting finding occurred in a trial, double-blind placebo cross-over of cryptosporidiosis with four patients assigned to each of two groups. The first group initially received $DLE-TF_{a.s.}$ for cryptosporidiosis whereas the other group initially received $DLE-TF_{a.s.}$ for coccidioides. In four of eight patients with AIDS and severe diarrhea caused by this parasite, the diarrhea disappeared as did the presence of ova in the stool. The clinical benefits lasted for the four weeks that $B-DLE_{a.s.}$ for cryptosporidiosis was given and for four weeks thereafter. Only small doses (1 International Unit/week) for four weeks were given [72a, b]. Half the responders were in the first group which received $DLE-TF_{a.s.}$. After the eight weeks, the animals on $TF_{a.s.}$ for coccidioides were then given $DLE-TF_{a.s.}$ for cryptosporidiosis; two of four in this second group responded clinically. Incidentally, as noted earlier, oral TF appears to be equally effective as DLE administered IM or subcutaneously. DLE has been used successfully in many other parasitic diseases in man and also in animal models of human parasitic diseases (e. g., schistosomiasis in monkeys) and in disases of sheep and cattle [e. g., 71 c.].

2.2.4   Viral infections
2.2.4.1   Varicella

The dramatic prophylactic use of $DLE_{a.s.}$ in *Varicella zoster,* a significant cause of mortality and morbidity in children with acute lymphocytic leukemia who are immunosuppressed by the leukemia chemotherapy, is a dramatic example of DLyE potential for prevention of disease and complications thereof. Many children with leukemia in remission die of cerebral varicella. In a well-designed prophylactic trial, Steele et al. [73] administered either placebo or antigen-specific

DLE in a double-blind to 61 children with leukemia and devoid of immunity to chickenpox as assessed by both skin testing and serum antibody levels. DLE, prepared from adults convalescing from chickenpox and with skin-test positivity. Of the 15 children in the placebo group, 13 became infected; of these, 3 had disseminated varicella. Only 1 of the 16 exposed patients in the group receiving DLE contracted disease, which was clinically not severe. It is noteworthy that 7 of 11 patients treated with DLE containing TF specific for varicella zoster but not exposed to chickenpox became skin-test positive to varicella zoster antigen. Furthermore, of the 15 patients receiving DLE and exposed to chickenpox but who did not become clinically infected, 7 acquired skin-test positivity. These dramatic results indicate that DLE containing antigen-specific TF induced antigen-specific CMI to varicella zoster that prevented overt clinical infection in these children.

2.2.4.2   Herpes

We have had excellent results with DLE-TF$_{a.s.}$ for herpes in treatment and prevention of other recurrent herpes infections; such therapy promptly eradicated lesions and subsequent prophylactic DLE-TF$_{a.s.}$ markedly decreased the frequency of recurrence. The most dramatic example of DLE-TF$_{a.s.}$ in herpes was the eradication of ophthalmologic herpes within six hours of administration [74a]. BN-DLE also has been used with similar success in the treatment of herpes infections [74b]. Viza has also used TF for prevention and/or treatment of herpes simplex infection in both mice and men [75a, b]. Excellent results have also been obtained in herpes zoster by Czechoslovakian [75c] and in herpes simplex keratitis by Chinese investigators [75d]. In 15 patients with herpes zoster who were given DLE$_{a.s.}$ lesions disappeared rapidly in all of the treated groups, but were still present by five days in the untreated group. None of the untreated group developed post herpes radiculopathy although seven of the fifteen in the control group developed this syndrome [75c].

In terms of genital herpes, 35 patients were treated with 1 unit of TF IM three times weekly for six weeks then 1 unit weekly for six weeks (total dosage 24 units); lesions disappeared on an average of three days, much shorter when given DLE$_{a.s.}$ for herpes. Controls (untreated) were given non-specific DLE; they had a much longer duration of lesions and much more persistent pain; whereas, the pain disappeared rapidly in the treated group. In terms of recurrences, during the first year of observation, ten patients had no recurrence and in the others, the periods between the appearance of one outcrop and the next was lengthy [75 e].

2.2.4.3   Liver disease and TF

Special emphasis will be paid to this section in view of the groundless fears of the public (inspired by the FDA) that properly prepared DLE or DLyE can transmit hepatitis and/or other viruses; e. g., AIDS. Not only has treatment of hepatitis with DLE, dialyzable placental leukocyte extract (DPLE), and bovine spleen dialyzable extract (BS-DLE) been successful, but no cases of viral disease resulted, nor did flare-ups of previous disease. Furthermore, in DLE obtained from Hepatitis B virus (HBv) positive spleen or placenta, or DLE from bovine spleen of cows inoculated with HBv appeared more effective in reducing or alleviating clinical symptoms, lowering elevated serum hepatic enzymes, decreasing the size of enlarged liver, and converting positive tests for HBe and HBs antigens than did DLE from household contacts in that less was required. This model will surely have applicability to AIDS [76 a].

HBv-TF obtained from spleens of pigs immunized with HBv was used in 97 cases of chronic HBsAg carriers, chronic active hepatitis (72 cases), and chronic persistent hepatitis (25 cases); all subjects improved or became asymptomatic; all normalized hepatic function, improved immunologic status, and seroconversion to negative for HBeAg and in HBsAg occurred in 53% and 56%, respectively, of the subject cases; no relapses were seen during 2½ years of follow-up and no toxic reactions were observed. DLE obtained from leukocytes of eight random individuals was ineffective *in vivo* and *in vitro;* whereas, PBL obtained from nineteen blood donors with HBsAg+ hepatitis enhanced PHA-induced lymphocyte proliferation in the presence of HBvirusAg and produced some beneficial clinical effect.

In 260 cases of Hepatitis B treated with placenta (P-DLE) [control 145 cases (used laser irradiation)] with P-DLE–TF$_{a.s.}$ from Hepatitis B Ag ± placenta; 2 mg I.M. daily for an average of 44 days.

Raised CD-1 and CD-4 cells, lowered CD-8 cells, and increased rosette forming cells. 100% clinical recovery; no side effects HBsAg and

HBeAg seroconversion rates to negative were 75.6% and 45.6% respectively. Liver biopsies showed obvious improvement; no relapse during 4½ month follow-up. Since such placenta is easy to obtain in China, the author proposes to use this exclusively in the future for acute hepatitis.

Fifty-two cases of chronic hepatitis were treated with 4 mg bovine spleen (B.S.) TF (obtained after HBv injection) every day for two to three months. All had chronic persistent hepatitis, chronic active hepatitis, and cirrhosis after hepatitis with HBsAg in serum. Symptoms improved or disappeared in all, especially fatigue and common cold (author's emphasis). High SGPT 16/28 decreased or returned to normal. HBsAg became negative or dropped at least 3 two-fold dilutions; HBeAg 19/35 dropped or disappeared. The authors also cited clinical cure rate of 35/52 reported by Hubei Medical College treated with poly-IC/therapy. These 35 had decreased titer or negative HB antigen [76b].

Random placebo control study of fifteen patients, seven received DLE, eight albumin as control. After end of study, the placebo group switched to DLE using 12 units over six months. (Chronic active and chronic persistent HBsAg + hepatitis B). There was an additional six months of follow-up. Random non-specific DLE was then used with no significant change in liver enzymes, HQ-Ag positivity, or histologic status (Author's comment: What a waste of time. Of course pooled DLE from Germany's fewer HBv+ individuals (in contrast to Japan's 3% and China's 33%) won't work [76c]).

Two groups of 29 patients each with chronic hepatitis 0.5 to 8 years:

Group A: BS TF$_{a.s.}$
Group B: Poly-I.C.
Group A: BSTF 2 mg subcutaneous twice weekly for two to three months
Group B: Poly-I.C. 4 mg twice weekly for two to three months

Comparison:

Group A: Cured or improved 97.5%
Group B: Cured or improved 74.1%

HBe negative or diminished at least four fold:

Group A: 91.6%
Group B: 66.7%

HB DNA P:

Group A: 50%

Group B: 0/9 tested

Patients studied were all chronic virus carriers with long medical history and impaired immunity with high HBsAg level and active reproduction of virus. The short duration of treatment with BS-DLE$_{a.s.}$ for HBv was as effective as human HBv + spleen for a longer period; it caused the interferon level to increase by six hours after injection, Poly-I.C. is an interferon inducer, mechanism unknown, perhaps direct, perhaps by stimulating production of TF. It is a good adjuvant; however, TF rich in inosine may explain why ampligen (one strand inosine DLE, one strand poly-inosine), a double-stranded mismatched RNA (one strand is poly-inosine), is beneficial in mild cases of CFIDS [76 d].

Many other articles in many countries attest to the efficacy of TF$_{a.s.}$ for HBv, whether derived from bovine or human spleen, placenta, pig spleen, or bovine lymph nodes [76 e–q].

In China, more than 6 000 000 people are receiving DLE from one of the sources above in an attempt to prevent, not only hepatitis, but the chronic active hepatitis which can follow and which can result in carcinoma of the liver [76 o]. These studies are being followed with great interest as they may prove a means of preventing other forms of cancer which follow viral infection.

2.2.4.4   Miscellaneous viral infections

Other viral infections (e. g., cytomegalovirus) have also been shown to respond to DLE containing TF of appropriate specificity [e. g., 77 a–d], prepared from human donor leukocyte or lymphocytes or to calf TF derived from a calf with bovine rhino tracheitis and CMI to CMV, administered orally [77 d]. DLE obtained from a lymphoid cell line prepared from cells from donors with CMI to EB virus has been used to treat chronic infectious mononucleosis [78 b]. Potent ox TF derived from cells of both peripheral blood and spleen, highly potent for the EB-virus has also been developed [78 c].

In terms of use of TF for viral diseases, the most exciting results have been obtained in AIDS using TF$_{a.s.}$ in three patients [79 a] and in the simian model of AIDS; in the latter the TF was derived from a lymphoblastoid cell line [79 b]. Indeed, it has been shown that TF$_{a.s.}$ for

HIV reverse transcriptase inhibits reverse transcriptase *in vitro* [e.g., 79c]. Indeed Viza et al. have made the $DLE_{a.s.}$ for the HIV virus and presumably preliminary results in three patients are dramatic; T-4 counts rose from 60 to 80 to 500 to 650, although the doses administered were quite small by our standards [79a]. Borvák et al. have also shown that HPLC fractions of $DLE\text{-}TF_{a.s.}$ inhibit HIV-1 reverse transcriptase activity *in vitro* [79c]. Surely extensive trials of DLE in this disease are highly warranted due to the results described in these few patients reported elsewhere herein.

2.2.5   *Putative viral diseases*
2.2.5.1   Behçet's syndrome (BS)

This syndrome, which we and others [e.g., 80–84] believe to be of viral origin, is characterized by severe urogenital ulceration and inflammation of the large joints (e.g., knee joints); because of blood vessel involvement, many organs may be involved, but the ophthalmologic and neurologic consequences are the most serious. Although the syndrome is rare in the United States, it is relatively common in the Mideast (e.g. Turkey and Lebanon) and Japan; several of our patients first developed BS after a prolonged (3–6 months) febrile illness while traveling in Japan or the Mideast [34a]. In two BS patients, one in California, one in New Orleans, DLE-TF cells of random normal donors were ineffective, whereas DLE-TF prepared from lymphocytes of a household contact of a BS patient in New Hampshire induced clinical and immunologic normalization in a BS patient in California, implying that a similar, if not identical, environmental agent (presumably viral) is involved in the etiology or pathogenesis of most or all cases of BS [34a]. We, and others [84], have found that patients with Behçet's syndrome and also all with recurrent aphthous stomatitis (RAS) had autoreactivity to mucosal antigens. Our most consistent finding was diminution in function of interactive T-cells in peripheral blood [85]. The CMI defect may be a predisposing factor; alternatively, the diminution of function of interactive T-cells or a defect resulting from the disease permits its persistence. Another explanation is that Behçet's patients form an aberrant immune response to the putative virus.

We first began therapeutic trials of DLE in patients with Behçet's initially employing DLE prepared from random donors, but have

subsequently used household-contact donors, since the putative etiologic agent is unknown but presumed environmental. These trials
were uncontrolled, and the therapeutic regimen was tailored for each
patient according to clinical and immunologic responses. Despite
these deviations from the ideal trial protocol, the clinical results were
most encouraging [86a]. Subsequent trials using household contact
donors in patients requiring prednisone decreased from 60–80 mg/
day to 0.5 mg/day in nine patients with severe Behçet's syndrome
[86b]. Many others have reported similar success [e.g., 56b]. We have
since treated 14 patients with Behçet's with DLE-TF, in ten patients
made from cells derived from household contacts, in others from
random donors. Disease presentation and severity varied widely in
these patients, although all required high doses of cortico steroids.
Seven of these ten had both normalization of immunologic parameters
and dramatic clinical improvement. In two of the ten, remission was
short-lived, one becoming unresponsive to therapy after six months
and one 2 months after discontinuing therapy, when exacerbation of
disease occurred. In the remaining eight patients with Behçet's,
long-term remission was obtained with continued DLE-TF therapy;
high-dose prednisone therapy (80 mg/day) was gradually discontinued in six and much reduced in two without exacerbations for at least
six months of follow-up. Similar results have been observed in this
disease by subsequent investigators. In two patients with acute neurologic Behçet's with symptoms resembling stroke, but presumably due
to involvement of cerebral blood vessels, and not improved by 100 mg
prednisone intravenous administration of DLE-TF$_{a.s.}$ for Behçet's
induced rapid remission, within 20–30 minutes [34a].

Six patients with severe Recurrent Aphthous Stomatitis of several
years duration who were treated with household-contact DLE-TF
showed rapid and dramatic clinical responses within two weeks of
onset of therapy and enhanced cell-mediated immunity and were able
to gradually reduce prednisone from 80 mg/day to 0 mg/day over a
four-week period. One patient remaining in remission with monthly
injections of extract for six months, when therapy was discontinued
because the patient became pregnant and exacerbation of severe
disease occurred. The other patient has remained in partial remission
for over one year, with occasional episodes of oral ulceration only
[85]. As mentioned above, enumeration of interactive T-cells has
proved to be the most reliable index of immunologic response in these

patients; their function became normal shortly before patients noted clinical improvement. Others have reported variable effect of DLE in double-blind trials; the variability probably was due to poor selection of donors. Different pools of cells of normal individuals were used, rather than one household contact per batch of DLE.

2.2.5.2   Alopecia totalis

This disease, presumably caused by a virus, is characterized by hair loss that involves the entire body. The frequent personal or family history of autoimmune phenomena suggests that the pathogenesis of alopecia totalis is itself autoimmune, although the evidence is far from conclusive [87] and autoreactivity to hair follicles has not been convincingly demonstrated; mononuclear cell infiltration has been found at the scalp biopsy site. We believe that in certain patients, especially college-age women with a genetic predisposition, the disease process is triggered by an environmental agent (probably viral), as in Behçet's syndrome. This subpopulation with alopecia totalis has concomitant thyroid autoreactivity in the absence of thyroid dysfunction; consistent CMI defects were found in this population, including diminished function of interactive T-cell populations and deficient mitogen-dependent lymphokine production [85]. We have recently performed an open-labeled trial of DLE therapy in nine patients with severe alopecia (totalis or universalis) and documented CMI defects, using DLE prepared from household contacts [88]. The therapeutic regimen was determined according to the individual patient responsiveness; in general, an initial course of 9–12 international units administered over a five-day period was followed by booster injections of one unit every three to four weeks. All patients responded immunologically to therapy, with normalization of interactive T-cell percentages and conversion to positivity of mitogen-dependent LIF production, with one exception to the latter. No significant clinical response was observed in three patients. However, in the others, regrowth of hair between 1 and 3 months following onset of therapy, and growth persisted. The first patient included in the trial received therapy for 18 months 9 years ago, and has had no noticeable hair loss since. In three patients, therapy was discontinued during regrowth (at 3–6 months following the onset of therapy). In each patient, acute hair loss was noted within 1 month of withholding DLE, and growth returned with continued therapy. Good results were also noted in some patients given isoprinosine, an alkylated inosine compound [86 a] (TF is rich in inosine; DLE plus isoprinosine appear to be synergistic in this disorder and in immunologic tests *in vitro* [89 a–c].

2.2.5.3   Other putative viral diseases

Other putative viral diseases in which DLE has produced dramatic clinical improvement include *pemphigus vegetans* [90]; chronic discoid *lupus erythematosus* [91]; chronic systemic epidermodysplasia [92], a widespread dermatologic malignancy (caused by one form of papovavirus). DLE has also produced marked clinical benefit in an animal model of immunologic (Type I) diabetes [95]; namely, the obese rat. In this model, there are no antibodies to pancreatic islet cells, but histology of the pancreas indicates that these cells are replaced by a characteristic feature of CMI; namely infiltration by monocytes and lymphocytes.

2.2.6   *Malignant diseases*
(These are reviewed in the accompanying paper by Pizza et al., but are summarized herein.)
2.2.6.1   Melanoma

The immunologic aspect of malignant melanoma has been widely studied, and information available to date suggests that patients with melanoma respond immunologically to the tumor and that immune mechanisms may influence the disease course [96]; Melanoma would thus appear to be a disease suitable for therapy with specific DLE. Several therapeutic trials with DLE have been performed; however, the results obtained were highly variable, with overall poor clinical response to therapy [97–99]; in the treated group, 17 of 20 had extended life span. Average duration of survival of those given $TF_{a.s.}$ was 49 months, those given non-specific TF, 37 months, and those given placebo 18 months. (These investigators believe that negative results were due to use of DLE derived from random normal donors.) These early trials, including our own, were performed before the development of many of the assays used for the selection of donors and monitoring of response, and the significance of the results obtained is questionable. Perhaps because of this, the investigation of antigen-specific DLE therapy in melanoma has not been pursued.

2.2.6.2   Osteosarcoma (OS)

We previously reported clinical and immunologic parameters in osteosarcoma patients who received OS-specific DLE [12, 35] as well as parameters in household contacts of these patients and of patients with breast cancer [100]. Among seven patients bearing primary tumors (surgically removed prior to the beginning of OS-specific DLE therapy), 80% were dead by 24 months with single agent chemotherapy, radiation therapy, or no therapy. These had no improvement in survival time as compared with historical controls [35]. However, five of six patients apparently free of overt metastases after tumor resection treated with OS-specific DLE for 24 months, were alive and disease-free at the end of that period and also at last follow-up, 100–120 months after therapy [101]. Compared with 5-year survival computed from historical controls, this data is statistically significant (>0.008). This increase in survival time is due to prevention of pulmonary metastases in patients treated with $DLE_{a.s.}$ for O.S. In seven patients without surgical removal of the primary, there was no clinical benefit prior to DLE administration; use of DLE devoid of TF-specific for OS antigen (e.g., $TF_{a.s.}$ for fibrosarcoma and $TF_{a.s.}$ for breast cancer) failed in all cases to prevent death from lung metastases within 24 months [35].

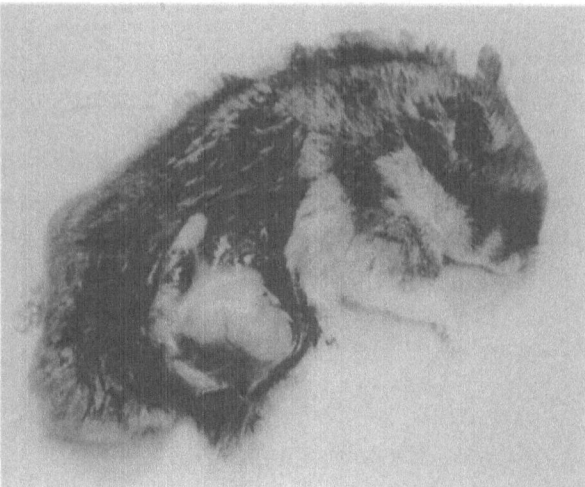

Figure 11
Chromosome marker of human osteosarcoma cell line found in metastases in lung of dead hamsters.

These results have been reproduced in an animal model of human osteosarcoma [12, 102]. Fetal hamsters at day 14 of fetal life were tolerized to OS antigen in utero with purified human osteosarcoma antigen; they were inoculated with 2 million live human osteosarcoma cells at day 3 after birth. By day 14, palpable tumors were present. Untreated hamsters or hamsters without surgical removal of the primary were all dead of pulmonary metastases by day 60. In all instances, as is true in humans with osteosarcoma, death was due to metastases to the lungs; the metastatic cells were of human origin as shown by cytogenetic studies. Osteoid formation was also present (fig. 11) in microscopic examination. DLE-OS extended life span to normal (12 months) in 60% of the animals by preventing lung micro-metastases; whereas, DLE specific for fibrosarcoma, breast cancer melanoma, etc., had no effect on extension of life span [103]. (50% survival 60 to 75 days) (fig. 12). As in humans, the DLE-OS was effective only if the primary was removed prior to therapy [12, 103]. DLE$_{osteo}$ but not DLE specific for other tumors also normalized DTH, lymphocyte DNA synthesis in response to semi-purified osteo-antigen

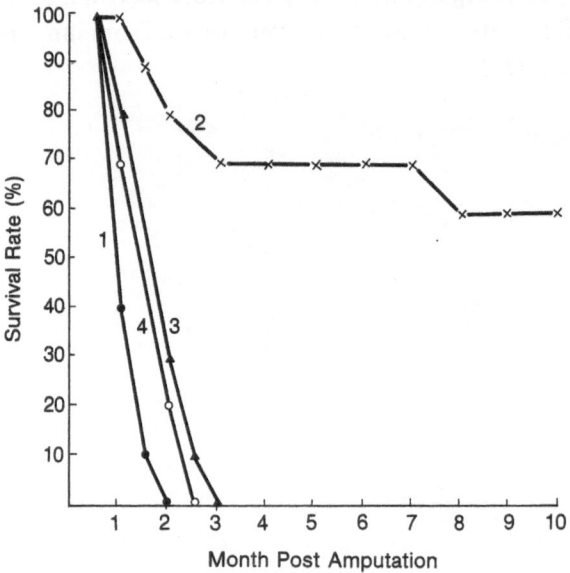

Figure 12
Survival rate *in utero* tolerized hamsters treated with DLE-TF OS compared with that

but not other cancer antigens, and leukocyte adherence inhibition in the presence of osteo antigen but not other cancer antigens [103]. DLE-TF$_{a.s.}$ has proved remarkably successful in bladder [104] and renal malignancies [105] and in preventing relapse in Burkitt's lymphoma after induction of remission by chemotherapy [106]. DLE in neoplasia and AIDS is covered in detail in the accompanying chapter (Pizza et al.). Bovine spleen TF$_{a.s.}$ has proved highly useful for preventing immunosuppression and/or recurrence in patients with cancer of the colon [107a, b] and in nonsmall cell lung carcinomas [108a–c]. Of particular interest is the study described in 108a, since lung cancer is rapidly increasing in Japan. A total of 1139 patients with these types of lung cancer were studied and divided into stages I, II, and III and pathologically into T–1, T–2, T–3, and T–4. A randomized control trial post-operatively evaluated in no therapy versus chemotherapy versus DLE versus a.s. and chemotherapy plus immunotherapy and chemotherapy plus IL–2 plus LAK (killer cells activated *in vitro* by IL–2 show that in stage 1 patients the survical rate with immunotherapy was considerably greater than with chemotherapy or no therapy or chemotherapy plus (IL–2 plus LAK). Prolongation of life was considerably extended in this group in terms of 5-year survival. However, in the dosage used, there was no increase in survival of patients in Stage 2 oder 3. It has also prevented immunosuppression due to chemotherapy in patients with a wide variety of malignant tumors [109a, b, c].

2.2.6.3   Distant metastases following amputation of primary tumor

We have treated two patients with breast carcinoma who developed two or three femoral metastases three to four years after removal of primary tumor. Breast cancer-specific DLE-TF caused eradication of metastases within seven days. The two patients arrived via air ambulance and stretcher, but walked out unaided two weeks later [34a]. We have also treated two patients with hypernephroma (HN) who developed cerebral metastases, as shown by pineal shift, on pneumoencephalogram three to four years after resection of the primary. In both cases, DLE-TF (HN) caused disappearance of cerebral symptoms, and disappearance of pineal shift to normal within 24 hours [54a]. One other patient who developed HN and bone metastases after surgical removal of the primary (HN) is still alive ten years later, receiving DLE-TF (HN) every two weeks. (When this was stopped for six weeks, additional metastases occurred and DLE-TF (HN) was reinstituted; examination six months later showed no new metastases nor increase in size of old metastases, and stable clinical status [110 a].) Pizza has had good effects with the use of antigen-specific TF in bone metastasis from prostate cancer [110 b].

Bukowski et al. have noted objective regression of tumor in one of 25 patients with metastatic hypernephroma using DLE-TF, 16 with and 9 without other immunostimulants [98]. We have kept one patient with surgically resected hypernephroma but with bone, lung, and liver metastases, alive for four years without deterioration in status; he died five months after his physician moved to a distant city, and his new physician refused to administer DLyE for fear it was unsafe [110 a].

It is conceivable that the beneficial action of $TF_{a.s.}$ in malignancy is that it antagonizes the immunosuppressant effects of human alpha-feto-protein on RNA and protein synthesis of lymphocytes; that is, prevents its immunosuppressive effect.

2.2.7   *Neurologic diseases*

DLE-TF has also been effective in subsets of certain neurologic disorders which are probably syndromes rather than distinct entities, with immunologically aberrant subsets, perhaps autoimmune. Among these disorders are Alzheimer's disease [111 a–c, 112], autism [113, 114], amyotrophic lateral sclerosis (Lou Gehrig's Disease) [115], and retinitis pigmentosa [116 a]. Approximately 20% of patients with Alzheimer's disease, 70% of patients with autism, and 50% of patients with retinitis pigmentosa [111 a–116 b] have antibodies to neuron axon filament proteins (NAFP), presumably the hallmark of unconventional virus infection of the central nervous system [117]. These antibodies are not etiologic or pathogenic in these disorders, but rather a result of therapies, since about 50% of household contacts have such antibodies and without disease [34 a]. Whether or not the donor is a blood relative is immaterial. If the blood relative lives far away and has not been continually exposed to the recipient for six months, his or her DLE-TF is ineffective. Six of nine AD patients with such antibodies were given DLE derived from household contacts and showed considerable improvement; e.g., regain of speech, regain of capacity to recognize spouse, improvement in cognitive function, and in one instance regain of ability to walk unaided (previously in a wheel chair). Twenty-five "South Carolina units" (roughly equivalent to 800 international units) were given over a 5-day period. Beneficial effects lasted about one month; after a subsequent month without therapy, the patients regressed to baseline levels. Three patients without antibodies had no clinical improvement. This series of events was repeated three times with exactly the same results. Use of DLE from non-household contacts had no beneficial effect. Again, patients with antibodies in NAFP (predominantly 70 K.D.) improved while those lacking such antibodies did not.

Fifteen of nineteen patients with sudden infantile onset of severe autism (with cessation of verbalization and sudden loss of attention span, marked hyperkinesis, sleep disorder, repetitive movements, self-mutilation behavior, etc.), onset usually at age 15 months, treated with DLE-TF from cells of parental or sibling donor, showed considerable improvement, including normalization of sleep (8–10 hours of sleep per night rather than 2), marked decrease in hyperkinesis, regain of verbalization capacity, some marked increase in attention span, etc. [113]. Some became completely normal and able to earn their own living (e. g., house painters), moved out of their parents house, and did their own cooking, cleaning, laundry, etc. It is noteworthy that patients with autism have recently been shown to have antibodies, presumably auto-antibodies, to a neuronal protein (myelin basic protein) [118].

In *retinitis pigmentosa,* nine of ten patients treated with DLyE from a household contact have had no further visual loss during the five-year period [34a]. The patients usually do not notice visual difficulties until 65%–70% of visual fields are lost and usually lose 15% of their remaining visual fields thereafter [119]. (The retina is the end of the second cranial nerve so that, though located in the eye, it is really part of the central nervous system and probably its most rapidly metabolizing portion.)

We have had numerous instances where TF from household contacts was effective but TF from "friends" was not. For example, we have had dramatic success with DLyE-TF administration with 20 "South Carolina units" over 3 days, every 6 to 8 weeks in one of three patients with severe (severe bulbar symptoms, inability to walk) amyotrophic lateral sclerosis, one of three such patients with antibodies to NAFP in serum and spinal fluid [34a]. One other patient with such antibodies remained stable for several years, but did not receive as much DLE as the patient referred to above. (The latter patient had only one household contact donor; the first patient referred to above had three household contact donors.) Seven patients with severe ALS without such antibodies derived no benefit from household contact DLyE. The first patient referred to above is of particular interest since he improved dramatically clinically (e.g., eventually became able to ambulate without aid after previously being first confined to bed, then to use of a wheel chair, then to cane poles, then to crutches, then to a cane. He arrived via air ambulance on a stretcher). After the first coarse of therapy "total T-cells" a functional test measured by rosette formation with SRBC rose from 30% to 50% (normal 64%–77%). After five years of DLE-TF obtained from three close contacts, he was able to work a 40-hour week. The only failure to improve (and indeed a decline) occurred when the patient, without his knowledge, received the usual amount of DLE-TF, but on this occasion derived from the cells of the spouse of a patient with multiple sclerosis. Administration of this DLE-TF resulted in a decline in both immunologic function tests and clinical status for six weeks. Thereafter, the usual DLE from one of these three household contacts was reinitiated and steady improvement followed [115]. At one point, DLyE derived from cells of a son who lived 2,000 miles away and who visited home for only 7–10 days during the Christmas season in each of the three preceding years was used; it was completely ineffective [34a, 115]. Pekárek et al. have reported considerable slow-down of clinical progression in 12 of 12 patients treated with the isolated suppressor portion of TF, isolated by absorption and elution. These patients all had a diminution in CD-8 positive cells. In contrast to the untreated control patients who lived only one to two years, these 12 have been alive for 3 to 5 years (immunologic status being sustained by administration of the suppressor TF every month).

We have treated one patient with a familial neuro-degenerative disease, namely, Creutzfeld-Jacob's disease (both mother and sister died of CJD, at age 42 and age 36, respectively) and with antibodies to NAFP with good results [34a]; after three days, the patient's symptoms disappeared for four to six weeks. She has received injections approximately every six weeks for 8½ years, is now 37 years old, and her clinical status has improved markedly compared to when first seen here (e.g., can drive both car and boat, play the piano, knit, etc.). On placebo therapy for 12 months (her husband – donor – had a coronary, followed by severe gastric hemorrhage), she gradually deteriorated and is now in a wheel chair. DLE immunotherapy has just been re-instated. One other patient, an eighteen-year-old French boy, twelve years after receiving pooled pituitary growth hormone for dwarfism (donor: father), improved dramatically with one batch of our TF (40 S.C. units), which caused marked improvement from a semi-comatose condition for three months; symptoms had begun seven months earlier. However, without further therapy, (blocked by governmental bureaucracy), he died 12 months later [34a].

We have used DLE-TF from household contacts in the so-called post-viral chronic hyperfatigability-cognitive dysfunction syndrome (formerly and erroneously termed chronic Epstein-Barr virus disease in the U.S.) [120] and myalgic enkephalitis in the British Common-wealth countries [121a] and spasmophilia in France [121b] and more recently termed Florence Nightingale Disease (FND) by us [6, 122a], and also by Hyde [122b]. Thirty-nine patients, almost all previously unable to work (all patients with this disorder have severe chronic hyperfatigability and marked cognitive impairment; e.g. temporary amnesia, inability to think clearly, etc.) received household-contact DLE-TF for one year or more. These patients had experienced severe symptoms for time spans of 1–5 years. Thirty-five of thirty-nine improved considerably on DLE-TF and seven of the eight have returned to work 40 hours per week after 18 months. Of eleven without household contacts, four were secondary recipients, receiving DLyE from a primary recipient, analogous to the primary recipient in Lawrence's experiments (see fig. 1b); of the other seven, none improved on DLyE from random donors but two improved when given DLyE from donors carefully selected so that immunologic parameters were closely matched, e.g., antibody to antigen(s) of hepatitis were present in both donor and recipient [34a]. We have followed 20 additional patients for less than one year, and although some have already shown considerable clinical improvement, we hesitate to draw conclusions before one year of therapy. Of the 39 patients treated with DLyE derived from household contacts, 35 were immunologically normal by 15 months and working 40 hours weekly; prophylaxis was continued for another six months. All five patients who had been off therapy for five years or more remained in excellent condition and without relapse, except for one patient who had a very gradual but severe exacerbation following 62 injections of a very potent cortisone analogue by a dermatologist for an unrelated condition (This, of course, caused marked immunosuppression.) [122 c]. Another 11 patients with severe FND who lacked household contacts because of death or divorce of marital partner were also studied. Two, both with previous histories of hepatitis, and high titers of antibody to hepatitis C antigen and to cytomegalovirus responded dramatically to DLE obtained from cells of normal donors who had high CMI to cytomegalovirus and antibodies to hepatitis C-antigen but not to normal donors who lacked these laboratory findings. Of the remaining 11, seven were treated using DLE derived from a normal primary recipient ("immunologically stimulated donor") who had received DLE prepared from the cells of a former donor barred from further donation because of age. This "educated" DLE from the primary recipient was administered to seven patients (secondary recipients). Five of the seven improved significantly during the next year. Thus, of the total of 50 patients, only 8 did not have dramatic clinical and laboratory response. The primary recipient (secondary donors) noted marked diminution in frequency and severity of viral upper respiratory infections as compared to previous years, presumably because of the effect of Imregs. These effects cannot be due to placebo because (1) a placebo effects, that is clinical "improvement" starts immediately. In these patients, all responders to any given batch of DLE had an exacerbation of symptoms for five to seven days following each of the first few courses of therapy; since the lymphokines produced by the T-cells stimulated by TF that is interferon, tumor necrosis factor, etc., exert their effect prior to the action of TF on immunoregulatory cells, and their effect on immunocyte interaction; e.g., B-cell/T-cell integration. (2) Placebo effect never lasts for six weeks. In all responders cited above, effects have lasted for at least 24 months, and in some cases 72 months. (3) Placebo effects occur in no more than $\frac{1}{3}$ of patients. Here marked improvement occurred in approximately 85%. The exacerbation of symptomatology in this disease following TF administration given monthly for six months by Dwyer et al. [123] was identical with that described in patients I reported in 122a. They selected 22 patients from amongst their 200 patients with FND. All 22 received TF one I. U. per month for four to six months. The exacerbation involved increase in their extreme fatigue, emotional ability, headaches, and vesiculations within various muscle groups, and an exacerbation of their impaired cerebration. By the end of the first month, five patients felt they had improved markedly. By the end of the third month, twelve individual patients had improved markedly with all the symptoms described above. In individual patients, headaches, tinnitus, and paresthesias disappeared after therapy. Although none of the patients felt cured at six months, 16% felt they had improved by 50%. It is also interesting that cutaneous anergy 89% pre-treatment was 38% post-treatment and that the absolute number of T-4 and T-8 cells each increased by 0.2×10^3 per cm. (Editorial note: First of all the nature of the donors was not cited. (1) Did the 16 who improved have household contact donors and the six who failed to improve did not? (2) It is very naive to expect one I.U. per month to produce cure or even sustained improvement in patients given only one unit a month for six months; relapse is sure to follow. We gave nine S.C. units every six weeks for 18 months in most patients. It took that time for complete normalization of tests and immunologic function. Those patients who felt they were normal and tried to resume their usual activities before such tests were normalized invariably relapsed. This is an example of trying to shoot an elephant with a pea-shooter, and it is surprising that the results were as good as stated. Perhaps the patients were only moderately affected.)

Yang and co-workers reported good results from semi-purified DLE derived from both human and porcine spleen lymphocyte extract hereafter termed $TF_{a.s.}$ in myasthenia gravis [124]. Another neurologic disease, perhaps due to aberrant immunologic response to measles virus, namely sub-acute sclerosing panencephalitis (SSP) has been treated with measles-specific DLE with halt of progression of the disease in a majority of recipients [125].

Failure of TF in multiple sclerosis was reported by Fog et al. [126]. However, these investigators used pooled cells from 100 random blood donors to make the DLE in Switzerland, after which it was administered by a neurologist in Copenhagen. No immunologic tests were performed on either donors or recipients. In contrast, Basten et al. [127] reported two years later in the same journal that in a double-blind study, DLE from pooled cells of carefully selected household contacts (herpes simplex positive) administered for 18 months slowed the rate of progression of the disease in patients in stages I and II, although it was not effective at the dose and frequency used in more seriously affected patients (stages III and IV); when the code was broken, it was obvious the non-responders in stages I and II had received the controlled preparation, namely herpes negative DLE. Recently, a Czechoslovakian group has used much larger doses of DLE and produced considerable clinical improvement in the majority of cases [128]. Guillain-Barre syndrome, another neurologic disease, presumably secondary to viral infection or vaccine and perhaps autoimmune, has also responded dramatically to DLE [34 a, 129 a, b, c, d].

The above data on multiple sclerosis indicate that TF made in one laboratory differs from TF made in another laboratory and that the two may differ in efficacy as much as a Rolls Royce does from a Model T Ford, though both are termed automobiles. Nonetheless, the "failures" of DLE-TF in one or another disease rarely mention whether or not the recipient was monitored before, during, and after therapy by tests of immunologic functions, and fail both to select appropriate recipients and to provide data necessary for optimal quantity and frequency of administration. Hence, most physicians are skeptical of the clinical efficacy of DLE-TF. The reasons for these failures are multiple: some are listed below under the subheading Donor Factors.

Five patients with Lyme Disease and with Polyradiculoneuropathy and three with Polyradiculoneuropathy, refractory to standard therapy, were given Czechoslovakian commercial suppressor factor TF derived from DLE prepared in the conventional fashion; all responded to a suppressor factor prepared from DLE and went on to complete recovery [128]; whereas non-specific DLE lacking suppressor factor had little effect [128]. All patients had low levels of suppressor T-cells.

2.2.8   Auto-immune diseases

Auto-immune diseases associated with decreased suppressor T-cells usually respond to DLyE. Response has been documented in juvenile [130 a] but not in adult [130 b] rheumatoid arthritis (however, in the adult arthritis study, random donors were used and the amount of DLE given was very small compared to our usual dosage). The juvenile arthritis cases were severe in that they were refractory to high dose steroids (60–80 milligrams daily) and immunosuppressant agents, e.g. Immuran 200 milligrams per day. Excellent results were obtained with DLE-TF in 3 cases with scleroderma [131], with complete recovery in 2 and considerable improvement in the third, in Wegener's granulomatosis [132], in systemic *lupus erythematosus* [133], in *myasthenia gravis* [124], and in auto-immune hypothyroidism [34 a]. In the lupus study, 13 of 34 patients treated with DLE (after 0.5 to 8.6 years of clinical symptoms) improved considerably, despite the fact that they received only two injections the first week and one injection weekly for one month, then one injection monthly for the following five months; it is surprising that such little DLE caused clinical improvement in so many; perhaps greater doses would have raised the percentage of responders greatly. It would also be important to ascertain whether those that did not improve had serum antibodies to RNA (since, as outlined below, TF is an oligoribonucleotide-peptide). It is also of interest that the patients who improved had a clear increase in monocyte chemotaxis and in phagocytosis of yeast. DLE has also produced dramatic results in auto-immune thrombocytopenic purpura [134]. It is also reported to be effective in preventing recurrent spontaneous abortion, associated with and presumably due to, antibodies to maternal tissue constituents [135], or perhaps by an effect on suppressor monocytes [136].

Several investigators found some patients with psoriasis had impaired CMI and good clinical response to TF [e.g., 137 a–d]. (Among European dermatologists, psoriasis is considered an auto-immune disease, perhaps due to an aberrant response to a virus or to an autoimmune response to cells altered by a virus [137 a-d]). Excellent results with TF, derived by injection of psoriatic scales into cows has been reported by two groups (e.g., complete, or almost complete clearing of all lesions). Forty cases of psoriasis were treated with DLE-TF$_{a.s.}$ for psoriatic scales. Thirty-eight (95%) showed dramatic improvement, i.e. disappearance or marked diminution in size of lesions [137 d].

Some forms of schizophrenia also appear to be auto-immune [138 a–d]. In 33 patients with severe chronic schizophrenia characterized by anxiety, hallucinations, depression, etc. (but not paranoia) control DLE originally emanating from cells of a random donor had no effect. Two thirds of these subjects had either complete disappearance or amelioration of symptoms with "educated" DLE, i.e. from a secondary donor pretreated with cells of primary donor, a household contact no longer able to donate because of illness. Nine additional patients did not have paranoia and responded in the same fashion, namely, no response to placebo DLE – good response to household contact DLE. It should be mentioned that a "huge" amount of DLE was given in one injection since DLE was not given directly to a the recipient but rather to a bovine primary recipient whose spleen served as the source of donor cells for the second recipient, namely, the patient. In the same fashion, the random DLE was given first to a cow whose spleen subsequently served as a source of donor cells for the secondary recipient, namely the patient. Only one injection was given [138 c].

In another paper when TF was given in addition to the usual tranquilizers (e.g., chlorpromazine), the majority of patients had marked improvement for an average duration of one month after each treatment. The author stated "It (TF) will eventually become a new way of therapy for mental diseases" [138 d].

Schizophrenia, or at least subset thereof, has been considered an auto-immune disease by ourselves and others [138 a–d]. We and others [138 a–d] have seen dramatic success with household contact TF in some patients with this "disease", in reality a syndrome, one subset of which is associated with immunologic aberrations [138 a, b]. We have successfully treated two of ten patients with severe "schizophrenia" of long duration (11 and 15 years, respectively); on therapy they both became completely normal. The one who had the disease for 15 years, had two Master of Arts degrees, one in computer sciences and one in fine arts, by age 20, and worked 8 hours daily making art by computer. After a viral illness, he refused to leave his own room, slept from 4 a.m. to 4 p.m., listened to rock music from 4 p.m. to 4 a. m. and spoke only a few words to his parents when they brought meals to his room, and also suffered hallucinations. The diagnosis by both his internist and psychiatrist was schizophrenia. He received immunotherapy for two years (all immune function tests were normal at 18 months; be received immunotherapy for another six months; and has now been off therapy for 30 months). He has been completely normal during these last 30 months, moving into his own apartment, flying from New York to San Francisco to see old friends, winning first place in an artist's exhibition sponsored by a local university, and interacting with people in social settings in a normal fashion [139].

2.2.8.1 Non-specific protective effects

The effects described below are not necessarily due to TF. They may be due to another moiety within the <6000 MW fraction. However, investigators have reported that "TF", especially DLE-TF$_{a.s.}$ has been very useful as an adjunct to cobalt[60] supra lethal radiation and/or chemotherapy in various tumors, especially when the TF was antigen-specific. The adverse side effects of the radiation and/or chemotherapy (e. g., nausea, anorexia, etc.) were markedly decreased in those given specific TF as compared to those receiving non-specific TF, which in turn were greater than those receiving saline placebo [140 a]. Experiments in mice show that administration of DLE before irradiation enable use of higher or repeated doses of ionizing radiation in instances of radiation induced hemopoietic and immune depression. The mechanism is via production of increased numbers of endogenous pluripotent spleen colony-forming units. Similar effects were observed when the DLE was administered after the irradiation. Thus DLE raised the survival time in direct proportion to the degree of elevation of colony-forming units [140 b].

As noted above, other investigators have seen marked improvement in some patients with schizophrenia when given immunotherapy, but in none was the improvement as dramatic as that in the patient described above.

2.3 *TF sources*

DLE containing TF can be derived from peripheral blood lymphocytes, bovine lymph nodes, spleen and placenta [76 e] of various species. It is present in all species thus far tested ranging from chicken [141], duck (it has been used to treat mammary gland benign hyperplasia with great success; complete disappearance of the lumps in 13 cases and nine marked diminution with only five cases showing no benefit) [142]; mouse [143 a, b, c], rat [144], rabbit [103], burro [145], cow [142 a], goat [147], horse (thus far only used in treating horse rheumatism) [148], dog [149 a, b], and infrahuman primates [34 a, 150 a–c], and many other species including man. Furthermore, it can cross species lines (e. g., cow to chicken [152], mouse [153], and man [e. g., 154 a–c], man to guinea pig [155], rat [156], and mouse [157], and rat, pig, duck, goose, etc. to man [e. g., 158 a–c] etc.) without adverse effect or loss of potency. It can be transferred without adverse effect from many other species both to man [e. g., 151] and to infrahuman primates [150 a–c], who could serve as test models (e. g., for $TF_{a.s.}$ simian AIDS.) As noted above, it can be prepared from peripheral blood lymphocytes obtained by [a] venipuncture (60 ml blood for the average condition), [b] by leukopheresis or lymphopheresis, and/or [c] by cell lines from a donor with known high cell-mediated immunity for a given antigen [159], by sensitizing cell lines with DLE containing TF of a known specificity in great amounts [160] and [d] from placenta *(vide infra).*

2.4   Reasons for therapeutic failures
2.4.1   *Donor factors*

1. Use of pooled donors (50–100) obtained from blood bank red-cell donors during a given day. If the recipient has an infection or a tumor that occurs only rarely in the general population, the pooled DLE will have little, if any, activity (see appendix). If the microorganism is one to which the majority of the population has immunity, the resultant DLE-TF will probably be effective; if not, the preparation will have little clinical value.
2. Use of a donor who [a] has little or no cell-mediated immunity (CMI) to the etiologic microbial agent or to the relevant tumor-cell antigen or [b] has a (broad spectrum) defect in CMI [161].
3. Viral infection of donor within four weeks prior to donation due in most instances to antigen-antibody complexes that inhibit the efferent arm of CMI.
4. Genetics of immune response in donor and recipient:
   TF (containing dialysates from mice that were either high or low responders to one of the antigens GAT^{10}, GLA^5, or ovalbumin) was assayed for its ability to transfer delayed hypersensitivity of appropriate specificity to murine recipients of either high or low responder phenotype. Dialysates from high responder strains contained TF that would transfer delayed hypersensitivity to both high and low responder recipients for that specificity. These transfers were not restricted by disparities at MHC or IgH loci. Identically prepared materials from low responder donors contained little or no TF activity and would not transfer delayed hypersensitivity to either high or low responder recipients. Thus, administration of TF transfers the high responder phenotype to low responder recip-

ients. The data also suggest that production of TF is regulated by Ir genes, but that the *immunologic activities* of TF are not [162].

2.4.2   Collection and/or storage

1. Too many granulocytes (>8%) in collected material plus no cooling of collection bag during collection. (Granulocyte enzymes destroy TF at temperatures as low as 6°C. As noted earlier, our pheresis unit provides us with leukocyte preparations of 92%–99% (average 95%) mononuclear cells [163] (see Appendix 1).
2. Use of granulocytes obtained from outdated blood of blood bags used to collect blood for red cell transfusions, a common practice in California.
3. Storage at refrigerator (4°–6°C) rather than freezer (−20°C) temperatures; (the peptide-nucleotide bond is split by proteases active at 4°C).

2.4.3   DLE administration

1. Inadequate amounts or low potency of the DLE-TF administered.
2. Recipient not monitored by immunologic tests to ascertain whether immunologic deficiency is corrected.
3. Insufficient frequency of administration to maintain immunologic homeostasis.

2.4.4   Recipient factors

1. Defective monocyte number or function in recipient: a small amount of monocytes (or monocyte supernatants) is necessary for optimal effect of DLE-TF [164].
2. Allergies to ragweed, pollens, etc.: If the patient has allergies and TF is given during the high pollen season, TF may not be effective. If given prior to pollen season, TF seems to diminish the severity of allergic symptoms (e.g., hay fever, allergic rhinitis) [6].
3. Chemical (enzymatic) hypersensitivity to foods or inhalants (e.g., petrochemical derivatives) [34a, 165].

4. Impaired endocrine function:

[a] Clinical hypothyroidism as gauged by hypersensitivity to cold, hypohydrosis and abnormally low first a.m. pulse and temperature (in some patients with one or another immunologic defect, thyroid function tests; e.g. free T3, free T4 and TSH may be normal, but the patient is clinically hypothyroid) [165–167].

[b] Adrenal cortical hypofunction or abnormal responsiveness to corticotropin releasing factor produced by hypothalamic and/or peripheral blood immune cells [165, 168, 169].

[c] Impaired ovarian function (in pre-menopausal females) [34a].

[d] Deficiencies in purine enzyme pathway [34a, 170, 171].

[e] Absent or dysfunctional thymus (e.g., thymic dysplasia) [170].

2.4.5   *Factors in either donor or recipient*

1. Marijuana use in donor or in recipient [172].
2. Patient encounters a virus not previously encountered by his donor [6]. One of our patients with recurrent viral infection that disappeared after maintenance of prophylaxis with DLE-TF from a household contact came in contact in London with a British family with an upper respiratory infection; he subsequently developed a severe viral infection, presumably due to a virus that the DLE-TF donor had never encountered. Another individual with similar symptoms, also doing very well on DLE-TF maintenance prophylaxis, developed severe URI while in Russia, presumably due to an organism that the donor had not previously encountered [34a, 122a].
3. Surgical anesthesia [34a, 165].
4. Severe painful stress (e.g., auto accident) [34a, 165].
5. Emotional stress (e.g., death of parent or spouse) [34a, 165].
6. Parasitic infection in either donor or recipient.
7. Genetics of both donor or recipient [162].

It should be noted that if the patient receiving DLE-TF has a viral infection at the time of, or shortly before, DLE-TF administration, the action of DLE-TF is blocked by an unknown mechanism, not only during the symptomatic phase, but also for five to seven days prior to the onset of symptoms and three to four weeks after the symptoms disappear [36]. It the patient has a bacterial infection, the action of

DLE-TF is blocked for the duration of symptoms only. In (1) through (5) above, the effect of TF is blocked for three to four weeks [6, 34a, 165].

2.4.6 *Potency*

As already mentioned, the use of potency assays for TF when the antigen from the etiologic organism is known and available has greatly increased the incidence of complete responses, and eradication of (e. g. Mycobacterium fortuitum, herpes zoster or simplex, systemic candidiasis, etc.). This is important since one donor with positive CMI for a given antigen may donate DLE that is 20-fold more potent than another with positive cell-mediated immunity to the same antigen. In instances where the etiologic agent is not known, others still rely on "International units" (amount of DLE derived from 5×10^8 lymphocytes) and we on South Carolina units (each about 40 I.U.). However, DLE from household contacts almost invariably has far greater potency than DLE from random donors [173].

3	**Frontiers in DLE-TF research**
3.1	Sources other than human blood cells
3.1.1	*Animal transfer factors*
3.1.1.1	In veterinary medicine

As noted earlier, antigen-specific TF from one species can transfer antigen-specific CMI to another species without significant loss of potency [152–158]. For example, bovine DLE made against the parasite coccidioides protects not only cows but also mice from an LD90 dose of this parasite; whereas, bovine DLE devoid of TF of this specificity has no protective effect [153] and antigen-specific bovine TF is effective in treatment of human herpes infections [174]. Bovine DLE containing TF specific for nematodes is effective in sheep infected with this parasite [175], with *Haemonchus contortus* infections [71d], and also with *Trichostrongylus axei* infections [71c], and bovine DLE, both from lymph nodes and colostrum, have been used for both prophylaxis and treatment of various viral and parasitic diseases of dogs (e.g., canine parvovirus), pigs (e.g., swine transmissible pharyngeolaryngeotracheitis) [176] and in chickens with infectious bursal disease, Newcastle's Disease, and other viral diseases [177, 152], such as chickens bred for the fast-food industry. Coccidioides destroys $ 250 million per year of prize cattle in Texas alone; bovine colostral DLE produced against this parasite could be produced in vast amounts, at low cost, and therefore has the potential for vast financial savings [178]; bovine Lymph Node Leukocyte Extract (BN-DLE) containing TF has been shown to dramatically protect cattle from infection with this organism [146], to prevent mastitis in cows, zero incidence in a treated group, 12% in a control group [179] and to prevent death from infection in newborn calves housed together; the treated and controlled untreated calves were housed together. Ten percent of the control group but none of the treated group died of infection [180]. Horse DLE has been shown to be very effective in treating rheumatism in horses [148]. Prophylactic use of DLE-TF$_{a.s.}$ for pathogenic *E. coli* and other pathogenic intestinal bacteria in man probably would prevent the Jack-in-the-Box Fast Food Restaurant syndrome – diarrhea and fever due to insufficient cooking (e. g., "rare" or "medium rare") of hamburgers.

3.1.1.2   In human medicine

As mentioned before, TF derived from infrahuman species has recently been used in therapeutic attempts in a variety of infectious and malignant diseases of man. Bovine DLE (B-DLE) has been given repeatedly to humans with no adverse reactions [e. g., 181]. Louie et al. eradicated cryptosporidiosis in humans with diarrhea due to this organism and with no known cause; e. g. AIDS: TF$_{a.s.}$ for cryptosporidiosis but not TF$_{a.s.}$ for coccidioides derived from BN-DLE eradicated the diarrhea and eliminated ova and parasites from the stools of those receiving the TF$_{a.s.}$ but had no effect on other patients [72a, 72b] receiving the control TF. McMeeking et al. administered the same BN-DLEs to patients with AIDS and cryptosporidiosis and diarrhea. Eight controls receiving BN-DLE-TF$_{a.s.}$ for coccidioides had no change in clinical status or in number of ova and parasites excreted in the stools in eight patients with AIDS and cryptosporidia (an organism that causes diarrhea and is found in only those humans with one or another immune deficiency); four of the eight responded in that the diarrhea disappeared, and ova and parasites were not present in the stool during therapy with bovine oral TF and for four weeks thereafter no adverse effects were encountered [72b]. Bovine TF has been administered by various routes and has been very useful in many other human disorders (e. g., human herpes infection) [73–75], and Jones et al. have successfully used oral bovine TF in the hyper IgE syndrome [154 b] (Job's syndrome) as have we in two patients (mother and daughter) [34 a]. In a 3-year-old child with periodic immune paralysis, every 28 days, duration 5 days, of high fever and marked granulocytosis, bacterial and viral cultures were persistently negative. After three months on immunotherapy, she had no further episodes for three years [34 a]. BN-DLE as well as porcine spleen DLE has also been repeatedly given to patients with malignancy without adverse effect [e. g., 107–108]. BN-DLE produced $TF_{a.s.}$ transfer of reactivity (e. g., to KLH) in individuals previously lacking such reactivity; more importantly, it had no adverse effects [154 a]; we have given colostral BN-DLE orally to one patient with severe FND for one year, apparently due to bovine herpes III; DLE to this bovine herpes was effective, whereas DLE to human herpes virus was ineffective; all previous medications including AZT had produced no improvement (several dozen had been tried over previous years) [182]. The success of oral bovine colostrum DLE induced $TF_{a.s.}$ reactivity in one of three calves given bovine DLE as fetuses [183]; indeed, Mohr had previously suggested that TF might be responsible for induction of CMI associated with ingestion of colostrum [184].

The potential for bovine colostrum-TF treatment of human diseases is fantastic since one can obtain so much more DLE at little cost. First, the absence of cells eliminates four steps in the preparation procedure; namely, isolating immunocytes, washing the immunocytes repeatedly, then rupturing their membranes by repeated freezing and thawing, and eventually spinning down the membranes so that a membrane-free supernate containing TF is obtained (in the colostrum, the TF is found free and in high concentration and there are few cells). Secondly, far more TF is obtained. Approximately 1000 x the amount of TF is present in one batch of bovine colostrum as is obtained in one lymphopheresis of a human [34 a]. At least in this country current blood bank regulations restrict immunocyte donation to 0.1% of total body lymphocytes every 6 weeks (10%–20% would be far more reasonable). This restriction to 0.1% seems especially ludicrous since serious adverse reactions to TF have never been reported, although some patients have developed complications of their particular disease (e. g., positive Coombs' test or microscopic hematuria in some patients with the Wiskott-Aldrich syndrome; however, administration of DLE from household contacts has reversed positive Coombs' tests and hematuria present before DLE-TF therapy in patients with the Wiskott-Aldrich syndrome [34a, 57]. Presumably the TF molecule is too small to be immunogenic despite repeated administration and, in addition, arises early, and has been remarkably conserved, during evolution. Hence, TF of a single specificity (e.g., KLH) may be identical in structure for any given specificity, or at least identical at the active site in humans, cows, mice, chickens, etc.

3.1.2   *Lymphoblastoid cell lines*

[a] Cells obtained from donor with high CMI to known antigen(s).
[b] Administration *in vitro* addition of potent TF of known specificity to immunologically virgin cloned single lymphocyte followed by clonal expansion [185].

3.1.3   *Placental sources*

Human placentas are already used for production of IgG and other materials. DLE derived from lymphocytes within the placenta has been successfully used in a variety of diseases of known origin [129b, 76e] and DLE from pooled human placentas might prove useful for therapy of organisms which are ubiquitous in nature and affect humans adversely. As cited above, it has already been successfully used for the treatment of infectious hepatitis [76e]. Indeed, DLE obtained from placentas of hepatitis B+ mothers or from animals (e.g., swine) deliberately given the hepatitis virus have proved useful in treatment of this disease [186]. DLE-TF obtained from spleens of hepatitis B+ donors whose spleens had been removed for portal hypertension have also been dramatically efficacious in treatment of hepatitis as compared to a control group who received DLE obtained from cells of spleens of subjects without hepatitis (160 cases had 93.7% clinical improvement or complete recovery by three months; whereas, HBVM negative leukocyte extract produced an improvement or recovery rate of 61.5%; 11½% of the first group relapsed in 7½ months and with diminution in size of liver and spleen in those patients in whom they were enlarged in 74% and 64% of cases, respectively) [76j]. Obviously some individuals will prefer the placental source and others will prefer spleen from immunized pigs or ducks, or even a human who has a good CMI to the relevant antigen.

Large volumes of antigen-specific TF can be produced by any of these three methods or once the structure of the various TFs of various specificities are known by genetic engineering techniques. With such large volumes of antigen-specific TFs, production costs will probably be no greater than costs of antibiotics specific for one or another bacterium.

3.1.4 *Tumor cell injection*

Injection of gastric cancer tissue and of lung cancer tissue into cows resulted in DLE-TF which, when administered to patients with gastric cancer [107 b] and non-small cell lung cancer [108 a, b] provided clinical benefit. Swine spleen TF was used in 29 patients with cancer of the colon; they were treated for three months, and the individuals who received it showed greater production of interferon and IL-2 and had a greater Ea and Et rosette formation rates than did the controls [107 a]. However, the beneficial effects would probably be far greater if the antigen used to induce DLE-TF in the recipient animal was the isolated tumor-specific antigen [188].

3.2 Prophylaxis

Opportunities for prophylaxis of various currently untreatable diseases are great. Especially exciting is the possibility of inexpensive therapy for a host of parasitic diseases, each effecting hundreds of millions of people in third world countries (e.g., schistosomiasis) [71b]. Currently DLE is being administered to approximately 6 000 000 people in China to prevent hepatitis [76 o]. As cited above, it has been shown to be curative in both acute hepatitis and chronic infectious hepatitis and in chronic active hepatitis as well; hence its prophylactic and therapeutic use will undoubtedly markedly reduce the incidence of hepatic cancer in this population.

Use of EBV specific TF may prevent Burkitt's lymphoma and/or nasopharyngeal carcinoma in individuals in populations at high risk. Similarly, its prophylactic use in individuals with a high familial incidence of breast cancer or colon cancer, if the characteristic chromosomal abnormality is detected in such asymptomatic individuals may well prevent occurrence of malignancy. When mass-production becomes feasible, antigen-specific TF will undoubtedly be inexpensive enough to be used, not only for therapy, but also for prophylaxis the parasitic diseases so common in third world countries.

3.3   Production by genetic engineering techniques

This will be feasible once the structure of TFs of various specificities is elucidated and could produce massive quantities of TF of differing specificities. For this large amounts of TF of a single specificity must be obtained and many laboratory are trying to do so. As yet, no one has purified TF of any specificity, in the DLE we obtain from 10^{10} mononuclear cells, the concentration of $TF_{a.s.}$ is one part per million. After a series of fractionation processes (e. g., Sephadex G25 permeation chromatography (fig. 13), Biogel P2, High Pressure Reverse Phase

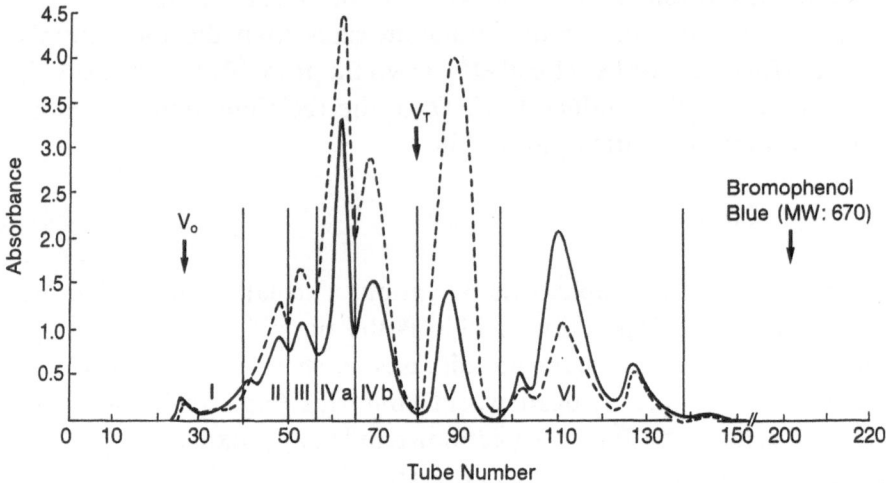

Figure 13
Sephadex G25 gel permeation chromatography containing PPD-positive TF and negative for coccidiomycoses antigen (cocci). Biological activity as measured by production of Leukocyte Migration Inhibition factor was confined to fraction IVB.

Liquid Chromatograph [HPLC] (fig. 14), boronate affinity chromatography, and isoelectric focusing [190]), we estimate the final concentration at approximately 12 parts per 100. Acrylamide gel electrophoresis showed six bands when stained with the usual stains for RNA and protein, but the biologically active material elutes from a position

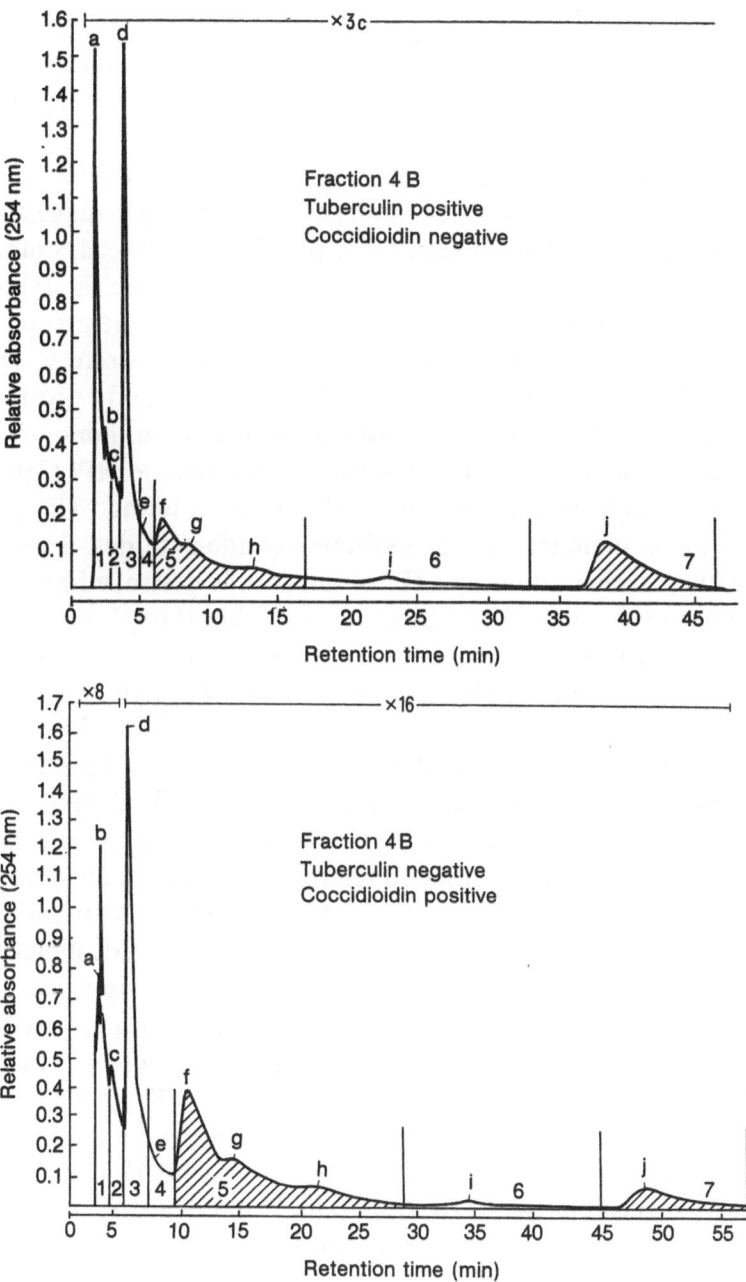

Figure 14

High pressure reverse phase liquid chromatography of Sephadex fraction IVB from two DLE preparations, one containing TF for tuberculin (PPD) and devoid of coccidian TF activity (top), and another devoid of TF for tuberculin but with biological activity for coccidioides (bottom). Note the strong similarity of patterns. In both preparations, biological activity was confined to peaks 5 and 7.

between the bands [190]. Nonetheless, we can arrive at a simplest case model based on enzyme inactivation experiments on DLE obtained from PBL of humans, burros, and cows; and bovine colostrum DLE [6, 191].

Results of enzyme inactivation experiments by ourselves [192] (Table 2) and others (e. g., Burger, et al. [193, 194]) strongly suggest that three different moieties exist with TF activity *in vitro* [195], as compared with our concept in 1981 when we knew of only two (see fig. 15) [192]. Two are present in HPLC peak 5: the first is probably the precursor of TF, hereafter termed TF_{pre}, and the second the secretory TF that is secreted, transported across the cell membrane, and exported, hereafter termed TF_{sec}. (This is the probable intercellular immune messenger [6].) Another moiety with TF activity is confined to HPLC peak 7; this appears to be membrane-bound TF, hereafter termed TF_{mem}. All three of these moieties are oligoribonucleotide-peptides, since biologic activity, as measured by LIF production, is destroyed by Pl nuclease and pronase, but not by DNA_{ase} (see Table 1) [194]. For the first two discovered, as mentioned above, the simplest case models are shown in Figure 15; the simplest case model for the secretory TF is shown in Figure 16.

TF_{sec} differs from TF_{pre} in that the latter has a phosphate on the 3' end. (This external phosphate appears to be the only difference between TF_{pre} and TF_{sec}.) TF_{mem} has no phosphate at its 2', 3' end, but it does have a phosphate sensitive to removal by bacterial alkaline phosphatase. This phosphate is required for activity. With no other site available, presumably the phosphate is on the peptide moiety, where it could possibly be attached to any of several amino acids.

The RNA data strongly suggest that TF_{pre} and TF_{sec} have internal purine residues, since activity was destroyed by $RNA_{ase}T1$ and RNA_{ase} U2, but not by $RNA_{ase}A$ [193]. In contrast, TF_{mem} has an internal pyrimidine residue, since activity was destroyed by RNase A. (In a sense, this is reminiscent of the situation with IL-1, which exists in three forms; namely, Il-1a, IL-1b, and IL-1 precursor; current evidence suggests that most of the membrane-associated IL-1 is the alpha form, and that only the beta form is secreted in extracellular fluid [196, 197]. In all three TFs (pre, sec, and mem), the N terminal end of the peptide is joined to the oligonucleotide, through, the 5' phosphate.

The peptide moieties in both TF_{pre} and TF_{mem} are free, since carboxypeptidase A destroyed activity. (Carboxypeptidase is an exonucleo-

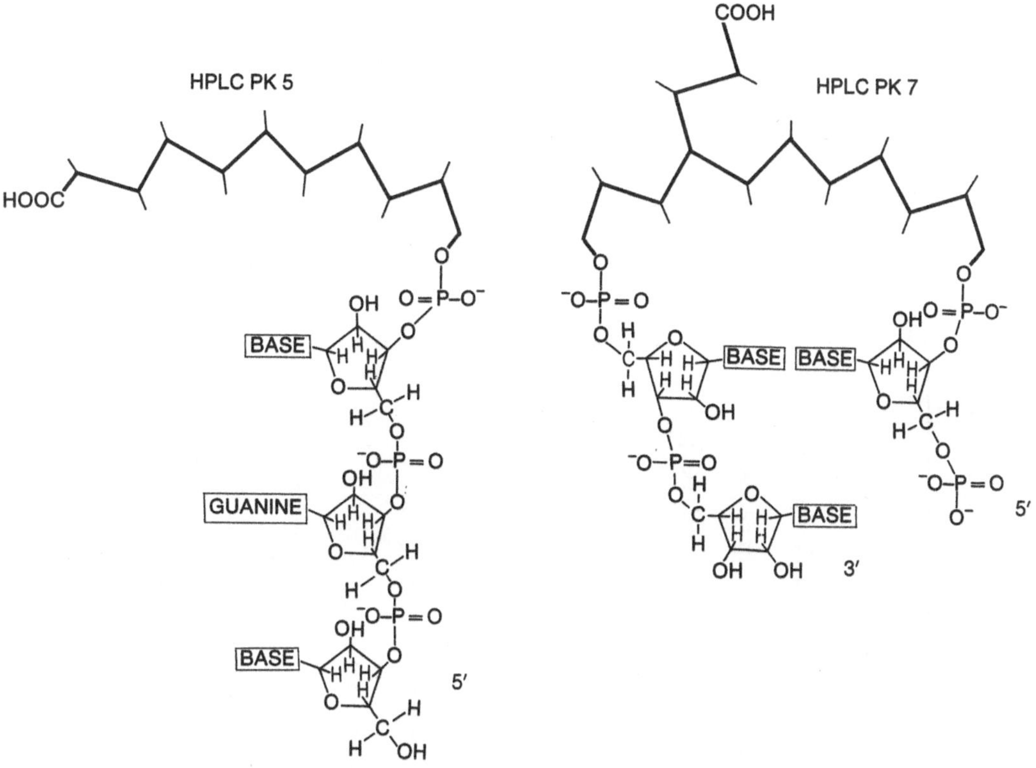

Figure 15
Simplest case models of TF-5 and TF-7 based on enzyme inactivation studies.

tide that hydrolyzes a peptide bond adjacent to the C-terminal end of a polypeptide). The amino terminal end of both TF_{pre} and TF_{mem} are blocked since leucine aminopeptidase (that hydrolyzes any peptide bond adjacent to a free amino group) did not destroy biologic activity. TF_{sec} and TF_{mem} activity were destroyed by snake-venom phosphodiesterase (SVP), indicating that the nucleotide's 3'end is free (i.e., not linked to peptide) and also not blocked at either the 2' or 3' position of the sugar residue. In contrast, TF_{pre} activity was not destroyed by SVP. However, TF_{pre} and TF_{sec} oligoribonucleotides lack free 5' ends since spleen phosphodiesterase (SP) also failed to destroy activity. Bacterial alkaline phosphatase (BAP) alone did not destroy the activity of TF_{pre} or TF_{sec}; however, BAP followed by SVP destroyed TF_{pre} activity and also, of course, TF_{sec} activity. This indicates that the 3' end of TF (pre, sec, or mem) is not blocked by a peptide but the 3' end of TF_{pre} is blocked by a phosphate. With regard to TF_{mem}, BP alone destroyed

Table 2
Enzymatic degradation studies of human TF activity in vitro (leukocyte migration inhibition assay)[c]

Enzyme incubation	Type of cleavage	HPLC Fraction 5	HPLC Fraction 7	Bovine TF[b]
RNase T1, 5 units, 1 hr. 37°C.	Endoribonuclease specific for Gp or Ip pApGp/CpUpGp	+	0	+
RNase A, 5 units, 1 hr. 37°C.	Endoribonuclease specific for pyrimidines, Cp and Up pApApGpCp/Up/Gp	0	+	0
RNase U2	Endoribonuclease specific for purines, Gp and Ap pAp/Ap/Gp/Cp/Up/Gp	+	0	+
P1 nuclease, 10 units, 5 hr. 37°C.	Endonuclease → 5'NMP pA/pA/gP/gC/pU/pG/p	+	+	+
Bacterial alkaline phosphatase, 25μg	Removes external 5'and 3' phosphate p/ApApGpCpUpG/p	0	+	N.T.
Spleen phosphodiesterase (phosphodiesterase II), 0.05 units, 12 hr. 37°C.	5'exonuclease → 3'NMP 5'HO Ap/Ap/Gp/Cp/Cp/Up/Gp3'	0	0	0
Bacterial alkaline phosphatase, then spleen phosphodiesterase	Nucleotide product + Pi	+	0	0
Snake venom phosphodiesterase (phosphodiesterase I), 1 μg, 1 hr. 37°C.	3'exnuclease → pA/pA/pG/pC/pU/pG OH 3'	+	0	+
DNase I, 200 units, 1 hr. 37°C.	Digests DNA to small oligonucleotides	0	0	0
Pronase, 1 P.U.K., 18 hr. 37°C.	General protease	+	+	+
Phospholipase A2, 10 units, 4 hr. 25°C.	Hydrolyzes fatty acyl ester at 2-positions	+	0	N.T.
Carboxypeptidase A_a, 5 units, 1 hr. 25°C.	Exopeptidase which hydrolyzes the peptide bone adjacent to the C-terminal end of a polypeptide	+	+	+
Leucine aminopeptidase, 5 units, 6 hr. 25°C.	Exopeptidase which hydrolyzes the peptide bond adjacent to a free amino group	0	0	0

(a) Pronase and carboxypeptidase A were independently confirmed to be devoid of ribonuclease activity.
(b) Bovine colostrum TF and TF liberated from antigen gave results very similar to those with Bovine TV.
(c) LIF activity was considered destroyed when the decrease in migration was <10%.
0 = No destruction of LIF activity
+ = Destruction of LIF activity
N.T. = Not tested
(Excerpted from Annu. Rev. Pharm. Tox. 1989. 29 : 475 with permission of the publisher)

activity, but SP did not. By analogy with the other two moieties, we suggest a phosphate somewhat on an amino acid residue sensitive to BAP. Thus TF_{mem} has an external phosphate that is required for its activity, whereas the TF_{pre} external phosphate is not required for activity [6]. Results identical to TF_{pre} and TF_{mem} from human DLE were obtained with TFs of burro DLE.

The pyrophosphate linkage proposed by Burger [194] is probably erroneous since no degradation of TF activity resulted on exposure to tobacco-acid pyrophosphatase [6]. The external phosphate is on the 3' end of TF_{pre} because its biologic activity is degraded by snake-venom phosphodiesterase I only if the phosphate is first removed by phosphatase. This external phosphate appears to be the only difference between TF_{pre} and TF_{mem}. Some confirmation of the proposed structures is provided by their affinity for 2', 3' cis-diols. If our models are correct, then TF_{sec} (fig. 16) and TF_{mem} should bind to boronate and TF_{pre} should not unless the 3' phosphate is removed, and indeed those were the results that we obtained. Antigen-liberated TF, TF obtained by incubation of lymphocytes at 37 °C, and bovine colostrum TF gave identical results in enzyme inactivation experiments.

3.4   Mechanisms of action

The mechanisms(s) whereby TF participates in the cell-mediated immune response are still unknown. (Indeed, the processes by which T-lymphocytes recognize and respond to antigenic stimulation are as yet poorly understood.) In simplistic terms, T-cell responses require specific antigen presentation by monocyte-macrophage cells or cells derived from them or, perhaps more importantly *in vivo,* by B-cells [198] in which the Ia-like antigens (products of the so-called immune response genes) play an important role [199]. However, Ia antigens are not present on the TF polypeptide [34a]. T-cell recognition of antigen involves membrane receptor sites. One hypothesis for the mechanism of action of TF is that TF forms a part of the T-lymphocyte receptor (T-AR) for antigen. If so, since T-cell activation is triggered by the binding of the Ia antigen determinants by monocytes and monocyte-derived cells, then obviously TF would be necessary for T-cell activation. This is supported by the fact that TF specific for PPD binds PPD but no other antigens such as candida and coccidiomycoses immitis [193]. However, additional data must be furnished so that the hypothe-

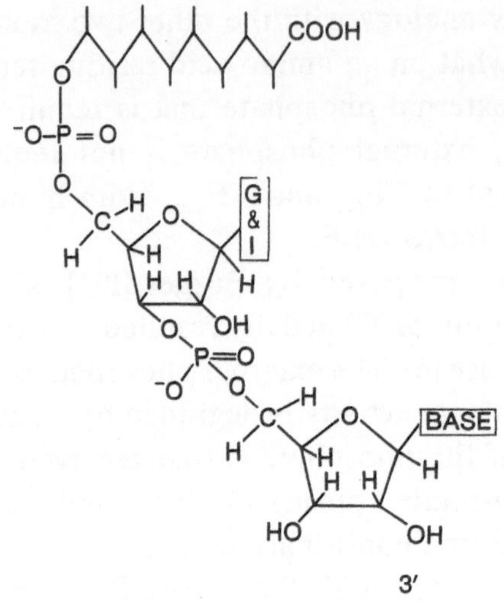

Figure 16
Simplest case model for secretory Transfer Factor (TFsec).

sis is compatible with, first, the activity of TF in the normal T cell-mediated immune response, and second, the ability of TF to transfer such immunity to a previously nonresponsive recipient in an antigen-specific fashion.

In the antigen-responsive subject, a small number of T-cells bearing receptors for a given antigen are continually present. These membrane receptor sites probably include the TF moiety. Specific antigen binding to the appropriate receptor probably initiates production and release of more TF, which then binds to immunologically uncommitted T-lymphocytes, thus rendering them antigen-sensitive and responsive. Similarly, in the transfer of immunity to the non-responsive host, the TF introduced to the subject presumably binds to the "immunologically virgin" cells. The binding of TF to membranes presumably results in the expression of the T cell-antigen receptor, perhaps by modification of existing membrane structure (since TF binding would require the presence of a receptor for TF, it is possible that this TF-binding site is capable of binding all TFs and that the resulting complex of antigen-specific TF and its membrane binding site forms the specific antigen receptor). However, *de novo* synthesis of the receptor or exposure of the relevant receptor by allosteric effects of the membrane proteins have not been excluded. Several additional hypotheses have been put forward, but the mechanism is probably so unusual that it has not yet been proposed.

If Kirkpatrick is indeed correct that there is no RNA, this would resemble the infectious but not contagious "slow virus" responsible for kuru and Creutzfeld-Jacob disease. Repeated sequence experiments find no DNA or RNA in this agent which can transmit the disease to primates [200]. Furthermore, it might provide evidence that the material is produced by mitochondrial genes and would fit with the finding of Cech listed below.

Recent findings of Cech [201] that DNA is present on the surface of 50% of T-lymphocytes in circulating peripheral blood [202] raise another intriguing possibility; namely, that the oligoribonucleotide portion of TF binds to complementary DNA on the cell surface and that both the DNA and the oligoribonucleotide bound to it are then internalized via the DNA receptor [203]. Furthermore, the TF might be cleaved, so that the peptide portion of TF remains at the cell surface and the TF peptide becomes part of the antigen receptor. DNA, acting as a ligase, could facilitate incorporation of the peptide into the antigen receptor.

A Japanese group has also found that oligonucleotide and peptides are present in DLE. Also, deoxyguanosine, which inhibits DNA synthesis because its catabolic product includes dGTP and an accumulation of dGTP inhibits DNA synthesis. Both lymphocytes and CEN cells [204].

Cech et al. [201] have shown that RNA enzymes ("ribozymes") cata lyze RNA splicing reactions like enzymes that act on other substances. The folded RNA, like a true enzyme, speeds up an otherwise slow reaction (in fact the rate of cell splicing is increased 10 billion times). Since RNA is an informational macromolecule, these findings may have relevance to the oligoribonucleotide portion of TF. Ribozymes do not merely accelerate the rate of the biochemical reaction, but show extraordinary specificity with respect to the substrate they act upon and the products they generate. McFarlane Burnett suggested decades ago [205] that the chief role of TF was to rapidly increase synthesis of more TF. Perhaps this ribozyme mechanism is involved. Most investigators in the TF area neglect the fact that induction of LIF secretion requires specific antigen and collaboration between T-lymphocytes and monocytes. Whether the two cell types are simultaneously involved or whether TF acts on one cell directly or acts indirectly on one cell population after the first cell population results in liberation of lymphokines that activate the second is unknown. DLE-TF had no effect on one recipient in whom no monocytes were detected in peripheral blood; when monocytes spontaneously reappeared about six months later, subsequent administration of DLE-TF produced improvement [188]. Thymic educated lymphocytes are also necessary since DLE has been ineffective in a patient with thymic dysplasia referred to above under Recipient Factors.

Further, patients with normal functions of individual immune cells, but a defect in cellular interaction (e. g., "acceptance" by T-cells of processed antigen ("epitope") presented by B-lymphocytes), TF of appropriate specificity will correct this as well. TF also causes an increase in natural killer cell activity. Current hot spots include preparation of TF from bovine sources since current policies permit only one-tenth of 1% of lymphocytes to be obtained by lymphopheresis and a thousand times as much can be obtained from one cow. Production by lymphoid cell lines also has great possibilities. Eventually, after purification, genetic engineering techniques will undoubtedly be used to synthesize peptides of differing composition, presumably the specificity resides herein and also the RNA, if present. Several methods exist for joining the two and RNA with short peptides attached are found in some viruses.

3.5   Purification and characterization

Future progress in this area depends on complete isolation and purification of TFs of different specificities. We believe that the RNA bases are responsible for activity and the peptides for antigen-specificity (if any of the 20 known amino acids can be at any of the 6–8 positions in the peptides, the number of different specificities can be in the billions). Thus far, two amino acids have not been found in these peptides [6]). Such delineation would make possible production of huge quantities of TFs of different specificities by solid phase synthesis of both peptides and nucleotides. This would also provide data helpful in understanding the mechanism of action of TF; many have been proposed (e. g., derepressor), but this author believes none of those thus far proposed is correct. It is conceivable that TF binds to the surface of virgin T-cells and by allosteric or other effect either uncovers the relevant receptor for the antigen in question, or fits into a "plastic" receptor itself to become the receptor for antigen. Possibilities as far-fetched as transport to microsomes or nucleoli by transport proteins, and subsequent synthesis of the TF constituents at these sites also warrant exploration.

4   Conclusion

Fundamental information regarding the nature of TF has accumulated slowly, because DLE contains 200 moieties rather than 1, as originally thought. Progress has also been hampered by those who refuse to believe in its clinical efficiency until the mechanism is known. However, penicillin was used in pneumococcal pneumonia for ten years with dramatic clinical results before the uncovering of its mechanism of action; namely, inhibition of replication of bacterial cell walls. Hopefully, in the next few years our understanding of the structure and mechanisms of TF will be greatly extended and TFs of various specificities will be produced by recombinant DNA methodology.

Although precise knowledge of its mechanism and/or structure is as yet unknown, DLE containing TF has become widely used in countries where labor is cheap since labor costs are by far the largest part of production costs. It is relatively inexpensive and there are no satisfactory alternatives in some diseases (e.g., various viral infections, etc.). In China (average $ 60 per month income), Czechoslovakia, East Germany, Poland, and Hungary, TF is widely used. The only high labor wage country where it is in use is Japan. The Japanese suddenly became interested in TF five years ago. In Czechoslovakia, two State Institutes have prepared a massive pool of DLE enriched in TF by Sephadex G25 gel filtration and have distributed it to every hospital in the country [207]. In Japan, the forty Red Cross Centers are providing DLE from pooled leukocytes or normal healthy donors to 400 hospitals for use in a wide variety of conditions [208]. In China, as already mentioned, porcine, bovine, goose, and/or duck DLE have been prepared in many centers and have been widely distributed for use in human diseases. Some of the disorders are listed in Table 2.

In view of the lack of any serious adverse side effects in humans receiving DLE-TF from infra-human species, it is likely that use of such TFs (especially bovine colostrum) will become standard therapy in any disease for which no current therapy exists, or when such therapy has toxic side effects. Bovine colostral DLE can be made in huge quantities at much lower cost and in much less time than is required for the production of human DLE-TF. Regulatory problems should be minimal in the U.S. since it has already been successfully used in many other countries, since it not only does not cause hepatitis, but is effective as hepatitis therapy, does not cause AIDS, and preliminary indications indicate that it may well be helpful in AIDS per se, or in some of the diseases afflicting AIDS patients. Furthermore, the FDA approved bovine TF for human use in 1985 and bovine colostrum use in 1980. In addition, two federal courts (one a Medicare court in a suburb of Washington and the other a health and human services court in San Francisco) ruled in 1987 that in diseases where no prescription medicine exists TF preparations ARE NOT experimental and furthermore ruled that insurance companies must reimburse the patients for the cost of TF preparation.

5   Acknowledgments

I am indebted to the Immunohematology Research Foundation and to the NeuroImmuno Therapeutics Research Foundation for their support of the original studies described in this paper. I would also like to thank Dr. Philip Klesius for his helpful discussions during preparation, to Haskell Fudenberg for editorial assistance, and to Carolyn Mando for her skill with the word processor.

6   Appendix

Sixty patients with a variety of supposedly non-treatable disorders of cognitive function and/or the central nervous system (CNS); e.g., Alzheimer's Disease (two subsets of four are immunologic), autism (one of three subsets are iummunologic), myalgic encephalomyelitis, amyotrophic lateral sclerosis (ALS), retinitis pigmentosa (the retina is at the end of the second cranial nerve), neurologic Behçet's Syndrome, and Creutzfeldt-Jakob Disease (two patients) received 281 batches of DLyE over a period ranging from three to five-years; the program was initiated and patients accrued during the 2½-year period, February, 1987, to August, 1989; we now have had a five-year trial period of observation. All patients received 12 to 18 South Carolina units of DLE initially every six weeks, then at longer intervals depending upon their immunologic status. Immunocytes (0.1% of total body pool) were obtained using the IBM-Kobe Cell Separator set at 4°C and set to obtain 5%, 12%, 15%, 25% and 35% granulocytes; the collection bag was placed on an ice tray. Immediately after cessation of the donation (2 to 2½ hours) a total white count and differential were performed and the cell suspension immediately frozen. The actual counts fell into five biologic bell curves (0% to 8%, 9% to 13%, 14% to 20%, 21% to 29%, and 30% to 40%). Each batch was evaluated for clinical response (1 to 4+) or non-response by criteria listed elsewhere by an investigator who was deliberately unaware of the donor and of the nature of each batch administered. Then, for statistical use, response was recorded as responder (1) or non-responder (0). For example, non-responders in A. D. and ALS had a gradual clinical decline over a period of six months; in Retinitis Pigmentosa, non-response was considered as loss of $\geq 3\%$ of computerized visual fields over twelve months. In autism, an increase of sleep from 0–1 hour to 1½–2½ hours/day, a quadrupling of attention span, a 40% to 60% diminution of repetitive motions, and a decrease of 50% in self-mutilation behavior was rated as 1+ = 2½ to 4 hours sleep span; attention span of ½ to 1½ hours; 2+ = 75% decrease in self-mutilation behavior, start socialization (eye contact and touch, etc.); 4+ = 8–10 hours sleep daily, no self-mutilatory behavior, no repetitive motions and enjoying being hugged and hugging.

Donors were usually household contacts; that is, parents, offspring, or spouse. Five patients received batches from several different household contacts, some received DLyE from random donors, and some from secondary donors (primary recipients). (See fig. 13 B).

Analysis

We tested batches of DLE initially to ascertain whether differences in the granulocyte percentages in the various batches were responsible for presence or absence of clinical improvement. Therefore, we prepared batches of 0% to 8% granulocytes, 9% to 19% granulocytes, 20% to 29% granulocytes (machine set for 25%), and 30% to 40%. A significant clinical response occurred in group 1 (granulocytes $\leq 19\%$) whereas those with granulocytes $\geq 20\%$ had significantly less benefit ($p < 0.05$). There was some suggestion that within the responder group batches derived from leukocyte preparations containing $\leq 8\%$ had a greater clinical response than batches derived from preparations containing 9% to 19%, but this was not statistically significant (p = 0.10) The model used for this analysis is the difference of two binomial proportions where the variance of a difference is modified to account for the intra-patient correlation between visits and which was specifically conceived for this study. (Recknor, Gross & Fudenberg in preparation.)

As shown in the Appendix (Table 3), the confidence intervals reflecting the differences in proportions excludes the value 0 for all combinations of the correlation coefficient as it varies between 0 and 1. We thus conclude the probability that a patient responds positively to a DLyE preparation derived from cell collections containing < 20% granulocytes is statistically significantly higher than the probability that a patient responds to DLyE derived from cell collections ≥ 20% granulocytes regardless of the value of the correlation coefficient. A more detailed version of the biometrical method used is in preparation for the Journal of Biometry.

Results of therapy with DLyE in one patient with ALS (TM) who used 23 batches of DLyE over a five-year period were evaluated separately. Donors included household contacts (wife and daughter), an intensive work/social contact (his administrative assistant for twelve years) random donors and his son, who had lived away from home for 3 years, preparations containing < 20% granulocytes. The best clinical results were obtained from his administrative assistant. When TM was accepted for therapy he could not roll over in bed and had severe bulbar symptoms (diagnosed as such at five separate medical schools). As described in the text of this review, after years of therapy he was working 40 hours a week and was functioning normally socially. The DLyE derived from three random donors were of no benefit; two batches derived from his son were of no benefit. To our surprise, one batch each from two technicians who drew and processed his blood, isolated the immune cells, and performed various laboratory tests upon them at each patient visit turned out to be donors as good as the wife and daughter in terms of clinical response. In one, the husband's DLE was also effective in TM.

In ten other patients in which the original donor was no longer available (because of death, divorce, or separation), sufficient DLE was available to administer two S.C. units to a secondary donor. DLE made from cells of secondary donors (33 batches) was effective in nine

Table 3
95% Confidence Intervals for p_1-p_2
<20% group
>20% group

rho	0.0	0.1	0.2	0.3	0.4	0.5	0.6	0.7	0.8	0.9
0.0	.21347	.21272	.21197	.21122	.21046	.20969	.20892	.20814	.20735	.20655
	.40323	.40397	.40472	.40547	.40624	.40699	.40777	.40855	.409344	.41015
0.1	.21027	.20955	.20883	.20809	.20736	.20662	.20587	.205112	.20434	.20356
	.40642	.40714	.40787	.40859	.40933	.41007	.4108	.41158	.41235	.41313
0.2	.20718	.20648	.20578	.20436	.20363	.20363	.20291	.20217	.20142	.20066
	.40952	.41021	.41092	.41163	.41234	.41306	.41379	.41453	.41527	.41603
0.3	.20412	.20349	.20281	.20213	.20143	.20073	.20002	.19931	.19856	.19784
	.41252	.41319	.41388	.41457	.41526	.41596	.41667	.41738	.41812	.41886
0.4	.20126	.20059	.19993	.19926	.19859	.19791	.19721	.19651	.19580	.19508
	.41543	.41609	.41676	.41743	.41811	.41879	.41948	.42018	.42089	.42161
0.5	.19842	.19775	.19713	.19647	.19582	.19515	.19448	.19379	.19309	.19239
	.41827	.41892	.41957	.42022	.42088	.42154	.42222	.42290	.42354	.42430
0.6	.19565	.19502	.19439	.19375	.19312	.19246	.19180	.19113	.19046	.18977
	.42104	.42167	.42230	.42294	.42358	.42424	.42489	.42556	.42624	.42693
0.7	.19295	.19234	.19172	.19109	.19047	.18983	.18919	.18853	.18787	.18719
	.42375	.42436	.42498	.42559	.42623	.42666	.427551	.42818	.42882	.42949
0.8	.19031	.18971	.18910	.18849	.18788	.18726	.18666	.18599	.18534	.18488
	.42639	.42699	.42758	.42819	.42881	.42944	.43007	.43071	.431336	.43202
0.9	.18773	.18714	.18655	.18595	.18535	.18474	.18412	.18349	.18286	.18221
	.42897	.42955	.43015	.43074	.43135	.43196	.43257	.43319	.43384	.43448

of eleven patients; indeed it appeared mored effective than cells from a primary donor. In addition, the secondary donor (primary recipient) usually noted a marked decrease in the incidence and severity of viral upper respiratory infections in the six to twelve months after receiving DLyE from the primary donor as compared to the previous year and as compared with persons in the same household.

Statistical procedure

If we let the vector of scores for the rth patient be $y_r = (y_1, y_2, ..., y_v)$ then

$\hat{P}_r = \sum\limits_{i=1}^{v} \frac{y_i}{V_r}$ is the estimator for P_r, the true probability that the patient

responds positively at any particular visit.
Now the variance of $\hat{P}_r$ is obtained for each patient by noting that

$$(1) \quad var \; (\hat{P}r) = \frac{P_r(1 - P_r)}{V_r} \left[1 + \frac{2p_r}{V_r(1 - P_r)} \left\{ V_r - \left(\frac{1 - p_r^{V_r}}{1 - p_r} \right) \right\} \right]$$

where p_r is the correlation coefficient for the rth patient.
In group 1 there are $n_1 = 50$ vectors of patient observations, and in group 2 there are $n_2 = 15$ vectors. If we let the indicator random variable y_{ijk} represent the response at the kth patient visit of the jth patient in the ith treatment group, then the overall $\hat{P}$ for each treatment group can be found by noting that

$$\hat{P}_i = \frac{\sum\limits_{j=1}^{n_j} \sum\limits_{k=1}^{V_{ij}} y_{ijk}}{\sum\limits_{j=1}^{n_j} V_{ij}} \quad , i = 1,2$$

We obtained $\hat{P}_1 = 0.6271186$ and $\hat{P}_2 = 0.368421$.
The overall variance of $\hat{P}$ for each treatment group was then obtained noting that

$$var \, (\hat{P}_i) = \frac{\sum\limits_{j=1}^{n_j} v_{ij}^2 \, var \left(\hat{P}_{ij} \right)}{\sum\limits_{j=1}^{n_j} (v_{ij})^2} \quad , i = 1,2.$$

where var $(\hat{P}_{ij})$ is given by (1) (with an additional subscript). Thus, one can obtain a $100(1 - \alpha)\%$ confidence interval for $(P_1 - P_2)$ as

$$(\hat{P}_1 - \hat{P}_2) + z_{\frac{\alpha}{2}} \sqrt{Var \, (\hat{P}_1) + Var \, (\hat{P}_2)}$$

where $z_{\frac{\alpha}{2}}$ is the upper $\frac{\alpha}{2}$ percentile of the standard normal distribution.

References

1 H. S. Lawrence: The cellular transfer of cutaneous hypersensitivity to tuberculin in man. Proc. Soc. Exp. Biol. Med., 71, 516 (1949).

2 A. Joffy: The Anatomy of the Lymphoid System, 3rd ed., Bristol, England (1955).

3 J. F. A. P. Miller: Immunologic significance of the thymus in adult mouse. Nature 195, 1318 (1962).

4 H. S. Lawrence: The transfer in humans of delayed skin sensitivity to streptococcal M substance and to tuberculin with disrupted leukocytes. J. Clin. Invest., 34, 219 (1955).

5 F. Karush and H. Eisen: Delayed hypersensitivity is due to an antibody of high afinity. Science 136 page 103–1034 (1962).

6 H. H. Fudenberg and H. L. Fudenberg: Transfer Factor: Past, Present, and Future in Annual Review of Pharmacology and Toxicology, p. 475–516, ed. E. Jucker, Birkhäuser Verlag; Basel, Switzerland (1989).

7a A. S. Levin, L. E. Spitler, D. P. Stites, and H. H. Fudenberg: Wiskott-Aldrich Syndrome, a genetically determined cellular immunologic deficiency: clinical and laboratory responses the therapy with transfer factor. Proc. Natl. Acad. Sci., USA 67, 821 (1970).

7b L. E. Spitler, A. S. Levin, D. P. Stites, H. H. Fudenberg, B. Pirofsky, C. S. August, E. R. Stiehm, W. H. Hitzig, R. A. Gatti: The Wiskott-Aldrich syndrome. Results of transfer factor therapy. Jour. Clin. Invest., 51, 3216–24 (1972).

8 H. H. Fudenberg, C. L. Smith: Immunomodulation and immunotherapy: an overview of biologic and synthetic agents and their effects on the human immune system. EOS Riv. Immunol. Immunopharmacol., 1, 3–11.

9 G. B. Wilson and H. H. Fudenberg: Is controversy about "transfer factor" nearing an end? Immunol. Today, 4, 157 (1983).

10 R. Ashorn, K. Krohn: Personal communication (1976).

11a G. B. Wilson, H. T. Jonsson, Jr., P. V. Halushka, B. P. Garner, M. N. Berkaw, et. al.: Contribution of prostaglandins to the biological activity of dialyzable leukocyte extracts containing transfer factor activity in Immune Regulators in Transfer Factor, p. 137, ed. A. Khan, C. H. Kirkpatrick, N. O. Hill. Academic Press New York (1979).

11b G. B. Wilson, T. M. Welch, D. R. Knapp, A. Horsmanheimo, and II. H. Fudenberg: Characterization of Tx, an active subfraction of human dialyzable transfer factor. I. Identification of the major component of TF, a precursor of Tx, as hypoxanthine. Clin. Immunol. Immunopathol. 8, 551 (1977).

11c D. R. Burger, A. A. Vandenbark, D. Daves, W. A. Anderson, Jr., R. M. Vetto, P. Finke: Nicotinamide suppression of lymphocyte transformation with a component identified in human transfer factor. J. Immun. 117, 797–801 (1976).

12 H. H. Fudenberg: Dialyzable transfer factor in the treatment of osteosarcoma: an analytical review. Ann. NY Acad. Sci., 277, 245–58 (1976).

13 V. E. M. Rosso, D. S. Secondo, P. Pontecucchi, G. Piccolo, et al.: Purification of an immunosuppressive factor from dialyzable leukocyte extracts in Recent Advances of Transfer Factor and Dialyzable Leukocyte Extracts, p. 73–9, ed. T. Fujisaw et al., Maruzen Co. Ltd., Japan (1992).

14 G. B. Wilson, G. V. Paddock, and H. H. Fudenberg: Bovine "transfer factor": an oligoribonucleotide which initiates antigen-specific lymphocyte responsiveness, Thymus, 4, 335 (1982).

15a C. H. Kirkpatrick: Purification and composition of transfer factors. Molecular Immunology, 29, 167 (1992).

15b S. J. Rozzo, J. Boymel, C. H. Kirkpatrick: Composition and purification of transfer factors in Recent Advances of Transfer Factor and Dialyzable Leukocyte Extracts, p. 11–22, et T. Fujisaw et al., Maruzen Co. Ltd., Japan (1992).

15c C. H. Kirkpatrick: Personal communication (1992).

16a G. Metzner: personal communication (1993).

16b I. Schröder, H. Werner, H. Schiller, A. Matz, J. Rovensky, G. Vietinghoff: On the characterization of the biological activity of DLE fractions. Comparison of transfer factor preparations of different origin in Recent Advances in Transfer Factor and Dialyzable Leucocyte Extracts, p. 51–6, ed T. Fujisawa, S. Sasakawa, Y. Iikura, F. Komatsu, Y. Yamaguchi. Maruzen Co., Ltd.; Tokyo, Japan (1992).

16c Z. Wan, Maojifang, Wanghua, A. Yang, F. Guo: Antigen-dependent activities and physico-chemical characterization of specific goat's transfer factor to human gastric adenocarcinoma in Research and Application of Transfer Factor and DLE, p. 17–24, ed. Huo Bao-lai, Wang Ru-zhang, Zou Zhao-fen. Xueyuan Press; Beijing, China (1989).

16d Recent Advances in Transfer Factor and Dialyzable Leucocyte Extracts, ed. T. Fujisawa, S. Sasakawa, Y. Iikura, F. Komatsu, Y. Yamaguchi. Maruzen Co., Ltd.; Tokyo, Japan (1992).

16e H. H. Fudenberg, R. Keller, G. B. Wilson: unpublished observations (1980).

17 H. H. Fudenberg, H. L. Fudenberg: Transfer Factor: Past, Present, and Future, p. 551–598, in Research and Applications of Transfer Factor and DLE, ed. B. Huo, R. Wang, Z. Zou, Beijing, China, pub. Xue Yuan Press (1989).

18a D. Viza, J. M. Vich, J. Phillips, F. Rosenfeld: Orally administered specific transfer factor for the treatment of herpes infections. Lymphok. Res., 4, 27–30 (1985).

18b W. S. Jeter, R. Kibler, C. A. L. Stephens: Oral administration of dialyzable transfer factor to tuberculin to human volunteers. J. Reticulo Endothel. Soc., 22, 46a (1977).

18c O. Tatsuzawa, M. Nagata, Y. Wado, T. Satoh, Y. Koike, K. Nihei, N. Wada: Clinical application of a transfer factor suppository in Recent Advances in Transfer Factor and Dialyzable Leucocyte Extracts, p. 243–6, ed. T. Fujisawa, S. Sasakawa, Y. Iikura, F. Komatsu, Y. Yamaguchi, Maruzen Co., Ltd.; Tokyo, Japan (1992).

18d A. N. Matz, H. Werner, S. N. Skopinskaya, N. P Perepechkina, O. V. Perelygina, N. A. Pereverzev: Amplification of the transfer factor activity of lymphocytic ultrafiltrate incorporated into liposomes in Recent Advances in Transfer Factor and Dialyzable Leucocyte Extracts, p. 57–66, ed. T. Fujisawa, S. Sasakawa, Y. Iikura, F. Komatsu, Y. Yamaguchi. Maruzen Co., Ltd., Tokyo, Japan (1992).

19 G. S. Gordon, personal communication (1976).

20 G. B. Wilson and H. H. Fudenberg: Leukocyte migration inhibition as a method for assaying transfer activities in Lymphokines, vol. IV, p. 107, ed. E. Pick and M. Landy. Academic Press; New York (1981).

21 Discussion in Immune Regulators in Transfer Factor, ed. A. Khan, C. H. Kirkpatrick, N. O. Hill. Academic Press; New York (1976).

22 P. M. Hoffman, L. E. Spitler, M. Hsu, and H. H. Fudenberg: Leukocyte migration-inhibition in agarose. Cell Immunol., 18, 21 (1975).

23 H. H. Fudenberg, G. B. Wilson, and K. Y. Tsang: Evaluation of potency and predictability of clinical response to DLE containing transfer factor in Immunomodulation and Thermotherapy, p. 141, ed. H. H. Fudenberg and P. Pontiggia. Acta Medica; Rome, Italy (1983).

24 J. Koistininen, J. Leikola: Personal communication (1976).

25 G. B. Wilson, H. H. Fudenberg: Unpublished observations (1976).
26 H. H. Fudenberg, G. B. Wilson, R. H. Keller, J. F. Metcalf, E. E. Paulling, et al.: Clinical applications of the leucocyte migration inhibition assay – new methods for determining transfer factor potency and for predicting clinical response in Immunobiology of Transfer Factor, p. 293–310, ed. C. H. Kirkpatrick, H. S. Lawrence. D. R. Burger. Academic Press; New York (1983).
27a G. B. Wilson, H. H. Fudenberg, M. Horsmanheimo: Effects of Dialyzable Leukocyte Extracts (DLE) with Transfer Factor (TF) activity on leukocyte migration in vitro. I. Antigen-dependent inhibition and antigen-independent inhibition and enhancement of migration. J. Lab. Clin. Med., *93*, 800 (1979).
27b G. B. Wilson and H. H. Fudenberg: Effects of dialyzable leukocyte extracts with transfer factor activity on leukocyte migration in vitro. II. Separation and partial characterization of the components in DLE producing antigen-dependent and antigen-independent effects. J. Lab. Clin. Med. *93*, 819 (1979).
28 H. H. Fudenberg, J. M. Goust: Unpublished observations (1984).
29a T. M. Welch, R. Triglia, L. E. Spitler, H. H. Fudenberg: Preliminary studies on human "transfer factor" activity in guinea pigs: systemic transfer of cutaneous delayed-type hypersensitivity to PPD and SKSD. Clin. Immunol. Immunopathol., *5*, 407 (1976).
29b E. W. Ramsey, L. J. Brandes, G. J. Goldenberg: The effect of skin testing on cellular immunity as measured in vitro by leukocyte migration inhibition. Cell. Immunol. *30*, 156 (1977).
30 M. P. Arala-Chaves and H. H. Fudenberg: Specificity of transfer factor. Nature, *262*, 1555 (1976).
31a L. Cohen, R. S. Holzman, F. T. Valentine, H. D. Lawrence: Requirement of precommitted cells as targets for the augmentation of lymphocyte proliferation by leukocyte dialysates, J. Exp. Med., *143*, 791 (1976).
31b M. P. Arala-Chaves, H. H. Fudenberg, unpublished observations (1976).
32 M. P. Arala-Chaves, A. Silva, M. T. Porto, A. Picoto, M. T. F. Ramos, H. H. Fudenberg: In vitro and in vivo studies of the target cell for dialyzable leukocyte extracts. Evidence for recipient specificity. Clin. Immunol. Immunopathol., *8*, 430 (1977).
33a A. A. Gottlieb, J. L. Farmer, E. Benes, A. Montgomery, C. DelSignore, R. Smith, D. Bertucci, S. Sinha: Augmentation of antigen-induced Interleukin-2 receptor expression and gamma-interferon production by IMREG-1, a leukocyte derived immunomodulator in Clinical Immunology, p. 375, ed. W. Pruzanski, M. Seligmann. Elsevier; New York Amsterdam London (1987).
33b S. K. Singh, R. C. Sizemore, A. A. Gottlieb: Immunomodulatory components present in IMREG-1, an experimental immunosupportive biologic. Biotechnology, *6*, 810–15.
33c A. A. Gottlieb, M. S. Gottlieb: Clinical and biological effects of IMREG-1 and IMREG-2, two immunologically active components of leukocyte dialysates in Recent Advances in Transfer Factor and Dialyzable Leucocyte Extracts, p. 3–10, ed. T. Fujisawa, S. Sasakawa, Y. Iikura, F. Komatsu, Y. Yamaguchi, Maruzen Co., Ltd.; Tokyo, Japan (1992).
34a H. H. Fudenberg: Unpublished observations.
34b Peng, Li-yi, Yang Dao-li, QiFa-lian, Jia Bo-sen, Wang Bao-cheng Du Gung-zu: Efficiency and immunological function observation on 100 cases malignant tumor treater with dialyzable placenta extracts in Recent Advances in Transfer Factor and Dialyzable Leucocyte Extracts, p. 354–5, ed. T. Fujisawa, S. Sasakawa, Y. Iikura, F. Komatsu, Y. Yamaguchi, Maruzen Co., Ltd.; Tokyo, Japan (1992).

34c H. H. Fudenberg, H. L. Fudenberg: Unpublished observations (1987).

35 A. S. Levin, V. S. Byers, H. H. Fudenberg, J. Wybran, A. J. Hackett, et al.: Osteogenic sarcoma: Immunologic parameters before and during immunotherapy with tumorspecific transfer factor. J. Clin. Invest.; 55, 487 (1975).

36 J. Wybran, M. C. Carr, and H. H. Fudenberg: The human rosette-forming cell as a marker of the population of thymus-derived cells. J. Clin. Invest., 51, 2537 (1972).

37 J. Wybran, A. S. Levin, L. E. Spitler, and H. H. Fudenberg: Rosette-forming cells, immunologic deficiency diseases and transfer factor. New Eng. J. Med., 288, 710 (1973).

38a S. Horowitz, T. Groshong, R. Albrecht, R. Hong: The "active" rosette test in immunodeficiency diseases. Clin. Immunol. Immunopathol., 4, 405 (1975).

38b X. Jiang, W. Zhu: In vitro experimental study on the activating effect of sheep spleen transfer factor on E receptor of human T lymphocytes in Research and Application of Transfer Factor and DLE, p. 32–36, ed. Huo Bao-lai, Wang Ru-zhang. Zou Zhaofen. Xueyuan Press; Beijing, China (1988).

39a K. Nekam, L. Kalmar, P. Gergely, G. Kelemen, B. Fakete, and I. Lang: In vitro effect of transfer factor on active rosettes and leukocyte migration of patients with cancer. Clin. Exp. Immunol., 27, 416 (1977).

39b I. L. Sargent, R. S. Myer, and H. Valdimarsson: Effects of transfer factor (TF) and thymosin on the revovery of E-rosetting capacity in trypsinised lymphocytes in Immune Regulators in Transfer Factor, p. 172, ed. A. Khan, C. H. Kirkpatrick, N. O. Hill. Academic Press; New York (1979).

39c K. Nekam, H. H. Fudenberg: Unpublished observations (1976).

39d X. Guo, Y. Li, Q. Meng: Study of production and Character of transfer factor of normal swine in Research and Application of Transfer Factor and DLE, p. 49–54, ed. Huo Bao-lai, Wang Ru-zhang, Zou Zhao-fen. Xueyuan Press; Beijing, China (1988).

40 J. M. Goust and H. H. Fudenberg: T-cell binding to B-lymphoid cell lines in humans: A marker for T-B cell-interaction. J. Immunol. Methods, 59, 29 (1983).

41 H. H. Fudenberg: In preparation (1993).

42 H. H. Fudenberg: Transfer factor: update (invited mini review) Proc. Soc. Exp. Med. Biol. 178, 327 (1985).

43 P. Dorfling, I. Schroder: Effect of the dialyzable leukocyte extract and its different fractions on the production of H_2O_2 and IL-1 by macrophages, p. 141–45 in Leukocyte Dialysates and Transfer Factor, ed. V. Mayer, J. Borvak. Inst. Virol., Slovak Acad. Sci.; Bratislava, Czecheslovakia (1987).

44 K. Nekam, H. H. Fudenberg, B. Mandi, I. Lang, P. Gergely, G. Petranyi: Resynthesis of trypsinized sheep red blood cell receptors on human lymphocytes: comparison of the effects of immunopotentiators of biological and synthetic origin in vitro. Immunopharmacology 3, 31–9.

45 K. Nekam, I. Lang, K. Torak, L. Kalmar, P. Gergely, and G. Petranyi: Effects of therapy with dialyzable leukocyte extracts containing transfer factor activity on antibody-dependent cytotoxic activity in humans. Clin. Immunol. Immunopathol., 13, 407 (1979).

46 A. Uotila, K. Krohn, K. M. Marnela, and J. Antonen: Mechanism of the in vitro augmentation of lymphocyte transformation by transfer factor and by other cellular Dialysates in Immunobiology of Transfer Factor, pp. 293–310. Eds. C. H. Kirkpatrick and H. S. Lawrence. Academic Press; New York (1983).

47 B. Dupont, M. Ballow, J. A. Hansen, C. Quick, E. J. Yunis, and R. A. Good: Effect of transfer factor therapy on mixed lymphocyte culture reactivity. Proc. Natl. Acad. Sci. USA 71, 867 (1974).

48 J. I. Gallin and C. H. Kirkpatrick: Chemotactic activity in dialyzable transfer factor. Proc. Natl. Acad. Sci. USA, 71, 498 (1974).

49 I. Lang, K. Nekam, P. Gergely, and G. Petranyi: Effect of in vivo and in vitro treatment with dialyzable leukocyte extracts containing transfer factor activity on human natural killer cell activity. Clin. Immunol. Immunopathol., 25, 139 (1982).

50 H. S. Lawrence: Transfer factor. Adv. Immunol., 11, 195 (1969).

51 K. Nekam, A. Perl, P. Gergely, I. Lang, R. Gonzales-Cabello, and J. Feher: Effects of dialyzable leukocyte extracts on lectin dependent cell mediated cytotoxicity in vitro in Leukocyte Dialysates and Transfer Factor, pp. 171–5, ed. V. Mayer and J. Borvak. Instit. Virol., Slovak Acad. Sci.; Bratislava, Czechoslovakia (1987).

52 V. S. Byers, A., S. Levin, A. J. Hackett, and H. H. Fudenberg: Tumor-specific cell-mediated immunity in household contacts of cancer patients. J. Clin. Invest., 55, 500 (1975).

53 H. H. Fudenberg: Transfer factor in immunodeficiencies: One man's one-eyed perspective in Progress in Immunology II, Vol. 5, p. 215–21, ed. L. Brent, J. Holborrow, North-Holland; Amsterdam (1974).

54a H. H. Fudenberg, A. S. Levin, L. E. Spitler, J. Wybran, and V. Byers: The therapeutic uses of transfer factor. Hospital Practice, 9, 95–104 (1974).

54b H. H. Fudenberg, J. Wybran: Experimental Immunotherapy in Basic and Clinical Immunology, p. 722–36, ed. H. H. Fudenberg, D. P. Stites, J. L. Caldwell, J. V. Wells), Third Edition. Lange Medical Publications; Los Altos, California (1980).

54c K. Y. Tsang, H. H. Fudenberg: Transfer factor and other T cell derived factor (non-LKs). Springer Seminars in Immunopathology, Vol. 8, No. 4 (1986).

54d H. H. Fudenberg: Transfer factor: past, present and future. Plenary Lecture V. Intl. Symposium on Transfer Transfer. Bratislava, Czecheslovakia (1986).

55 C. H. Kirkpatrick and L. E. Greenberg: Treatment of chronic mucocutaneous candidiasis with transfer factor in Immune Regulators in Transfer Factor; ed. A. Khan, C. H. Kirkpatrick, N. O. Hill. Academic Press; New York (1979).

56 B. H. Littman, R. E. Rocklin, R. Parkman, and J. R. David; Transfer factor treatment of chronic mucocutaneous candidiasis: Requirement for donor reactivity to candida antigen. Clin. Immunol. Immunopathol., 9, 97 (1978).

57a L. E. Spitler, A. S. Levin, H. H. Fudenberg: Transfer Factor II: Results of therapy, p. 449–56, in Primary Immunodeficiency Diseases in Man, ed. D. Bergsma, R. A. Good, J. Finstad, N. W. Paul. Nat. Foundation Press; White Plains, NY (1975).

57b R. Conte, M. Masi, G. Pizza, R. Ricci et al.: Il Transfer Factor Nel Trattamento di Quadri Clinici Diversa: Candidiasis Mucocutanea Cronica, infectioni gravi, sindrome di Behçet. La Trasfusione del Sangue, 28, 386–96 (1983).

57c H. Valdimarsson, J. M. Higgs, T. S. Wells, M. Yamamara, J. R. Hobbs, and P. J. L. Holt: Immune abnormalities associated with chronic mucocutaneous candidiasis. Cell. Immunol., 6, 348 (1973).

59 W. M. Lee, H. P. Holley, J. Stewart, and G. M. P. Galbraith: Refractory esophageal candidiasis associated with a plasma inhibitor of T-lymphocyte function: Response to plasma exchange. Am. J. Med. Sci., 292, 47 (1986).

60 A. Catanzero and L. E. Spitler: Clinical and immunologic results of TF therapy in coccidiomycosis, p. 477–94, in Transfer Factor: Basic Properties

and Clinical Applications, ed. M. S. Asher, A. A. Gottlieb, C. H. Kirkpatrick. Academic Press; New York (1976).

61 B. Myrvang, T. Godal, D. S. Ridley, S. S. Froland, and Y. K. Song: Immune responsiveness to Mycobacterium leprae and other mycobacterial antigens through out the clinical and histopathological spectrum of leprosy. Clin. Exp. Immunol., *14*, 541 (1973).

62 W. E. Bullock, J. P. Fields, M. W. Bandvias: An evaluation of transfer factor as immunotherapy for patients with lepromatous leprosy. New Eng. J. Med., 287, 10 53 (1972).

63a R. C. Hastings, M. J. Morales, E. J. Shannon, and R. R. Jacobson: Preliminary results in the safety and efficacy of transfer factor in leprosy in Transfer Factor: Basic Properties and Clinical Applications, p. 465–76, ed. M. S. Asher, A. A. Gottlieb, C. H. Kirkpatrick. Academic Press; New York (1976).

63b X. Dang, Z. Jin: Study on the treatment of leprosy with transfer factor in Research and Application of Transfer Factor and DLE, p. 411–23, ed. Huo Bao-lai, Wang Ru-zhang, Zou Zhao-fen. Xueyuan Press; Beijing, China (1989), p. 325–9.

64 P. G. Lesser, L. Margarido, W. Bolda, S. G. Sartori, W. A. Hares, C. A. Freire, R. Fleury, M. R. Montenegro, W. Leser, C. K. Naspitz: Cell mediated immunity in patients with Virchowian Hanseniasis before and after treatment with transfer factor, p. 3–27, pub. Hansenol. Int. J., 5(1), 3–27 (1980).

65a M. Horsmanheimo and H. H. Fudenberg: unpublished observations (1981).

65b J. Pekarek, K. Cech, K. Barnet: The clinical use of specific transfer factors in Recent Advances in Transfer Factor and Dialyzable Leucocyte Extracts; p. 256–63, ed. T. Fujisawa, S. Sasakawa, Y. Iikura, F. Konatsu, Y. Yamaguchi. Maruzen Co., Ltd.; Tokyo, Japan (1992).

66 G. B. Wilson, J. F. Metcalf, Jr., and H. H. Fudenberg: Treatment of Mycobacterium-fortuitum pulmonary infection with "transfer factor" (TF): New methodology for evaluating TF potency and predicting clinical response. Clin. Immunol. Immunopathol., *23*, 478 (1982).

67 J. F. Metcalf, J. F. John, Jr., G. B. Wilson, H. H. Fudenberg, and R. A. Harley: Mycobacterium fortuitum pulmonary infection associated with an antigen-selective defect in cellular immunity. Am. J. Med., 71, 485 (1981).

68 M. K. Sharma, F. Anaraki, and F. Ala: Preliminary results of transfer factor therapy of persistent cutaneous leishmania infection. Clin. Immunol. Immunopathol., *12*, 183 (1979).

69 M. Sharma, R. Firouz, and F. Ala: Transfer factor therapy in human cutaneous leishmania infection (CLI): A double-blind clinical trial in Immune Regulators in Transfer Factor, p. 563–70, ed. A. Khan, C. H. Kirkpatrick, N. O. Hill. Academic Press; New York (1979).

70 O. Delgado, E. L. Romano, E. Belfort, F. Pifano, J. V. Scorza, and Z. Rojas: Dialyzable leukocyte extract therapy in immunodepressed patients with cutaneous leishmaniasis. Clin. Immunol. Immunopathol., *19*, 351 (1981).

71a S. E. Maddison, M. D. Hicklin, B. P. Conway, I. J. Cagan: Transfer factor: Delayed hypersensitivity to schistosomiasis and tuberculin in Macaca Mulatta. Science *178*, 757–8.

71b S. E. Maddison, M. D. Hicklin, I. G. Keegan: Schistosoma mansoni: reduction in clinical manifestations and in worm burdens conferred by serum and transfer factor from immune or normal rhesus monkeys. Expl. Parasit., *39*, 29–39 (1976).

71c J. G. Ross, W. G. Halliday: Investigations of transfer factor activity in the transfer of immunity to Trichostrongylus acei infections in sheep. Res. Vet. Sci., *26*, 41–6 (1979).

71d J. G. Ross, J.L. Duncan, W. G. Halliday/ Investigation of Haemonchus contortus infections in sheep: comparison of irradiated larvae and transfer factor treatment. Res. Vet. Sci., 27, 258–9 (1979).

72a E.Louie, W. S. Borkowsky, P. H. Klesius, T. B. Haynes, S. Gordon, et al.: Treatment of Cryptosporidiosis with oral bovine transfer factor. Clin. Immunol. Immunopathol., 44(3), 329 (1987).

72b A. McMeeking, W. Borkowski, P. H. Klesius, S. Bonk, R. S. Holzman, H. S. Lawrence: A controlled trial of bovine dialyzable leukocyte extract for cryptosporidiosis in patients with AIDS. J. Infect Dis., 161, 108–12 (1990).

73 R. W. Steele, M. G. Myers, and M. M. Vincent: Transfer factor for the prevention of varicella zoster infection in childhood leukemia. New Engl. J. Med., 303, 355 (1980).

74a H. H. Fudenberg: Ophthalmologic Herpes Zoster: Complete remission in six hours with dialyzable transfer factor. J. Clin. Lab. Immunol., 18, 49 (1985).

74b D. Viza, J. M. Vich, J. Phillips, F. Rosenfeld: Orally administered specific transfer factor for the treatment of herpes infections. Lymphok. Res., 4, 27–30 (1985).

75a D. Viza, J. M. Vich, J. Phillips, F. Rosenfeld, D. A. L. Davies: Specific transfer fact or protects mice against lethal challenge with herpes simples virus. Cell. Immun., 100, 555–62 (1986).

75b D. Viza, J. M. Vich, J. Phillips, D. A. L. Davies: Use of specific transfer factor for the prevention or the treatment of herpes infections in mice and in man. J. Exp. Path., 3, 407–420 (1987).

75c V. Mayer, S. Necas, J. Borvak, M. Horvathova: Marked therapeutic effect of human leucocyte ultrafiltrate in herpes zoster: association with cell-mediated immune response induction in Recent Advances in Transfer Factor and Dialyzable Leucocyte Extracts, p. 231–7, ed. T. Fujisawa, S. Sasakawa, Y. Iikura, F. Komatsu, Y. Yamaguchi. Maruzen Co., Ltd., Tokyo, Japan (1992).

75d H. Qi, X. Zhu, C. Uy, Z. Wan, C. Su: HSV-1 specific transfer factor for the treatment of herpes simplex keratitis in Recent Advances in Transfer Factor and Dialyzable Leucocyte Extracts, p. 227–30, ed. T. Fujisawa, S. Sasakawa, Y. Iikura, F. Komatsu, Y. Yamaguchi. Maruzen Co., Ltd.; Tokyo, Japan (1992).

75e R. Cabeza-Quiroga, S. Estrada-Parra, L. Padierna-Olivos, R. Ysla-Garcia: Effects of DLE in patients with herpes in Research and Application of Transfer Factor and DLE, p. 292–305, ed. Huo Bao-lai, Wang Ru-zhang, Zou Zhao-fen. Xueyuan Press; Beijing, China (1989).

76a Z. Li: Studies of Hepatitis B virus specific DLE in Research and Application of Transfer Factor and DLE, p. 214–24, ed. Huo Bao-lai, Wang Ru-zhang, Zou Zhaofen. Xueyuan Press; Beijing, China (1989).

76b Zhang Guang-Shu, Hou Xian-Rong, Zhao Hui-Chuan, Du Qing-Ling, Wang Gen-Ting, Lin Gua-Xian: Evaluation of the effects of acute hepatitis B treated with specific placenta transfer factor in Recent Advances in Transfer Factor and Dialyzable Leucocyte Extracts, p. 217–21, ed. T. Fujisawa, S. Sasakawa, Y. Iikura, F. Komatsu, Y. Yamaguchi. Maruzen Co., Ltd.; Tokyo, Japan (1992).

76c G. Metzner, M. Reinhardt, H. M. R. K. Muschner, W. Franke: Effect of DLE in patients suffered from chronic active chronic persistent HBs-antigen-positive hepatitis in Recent Advances in Transfer Factor and Dialyzable Leucocyte Extracts, p. 204–12, ed. T. Fujisawa, S. Sasakawa, Y. Iikura, F. Komatsu, Y. Yamaguchi. Maruzen Co., Ltd.; Tokyo, Japan (1992).

76d Wu Jing-xin, Liu Ju-xiang: Treatment of hepatitis B with bovine spleen transfer factor in Recent Advances in Transfer Factor and Dialyzable Leucocyte Extracts, p. 213–6, ed. T. Fujisawa, S. Sasakawa, Y. Iikura, F. Komatsu, Y. Yamaguchi, Maruzen Co., Ltd.; Tokyo, Japan (1992).

76e G. Zhang, Z. Li, X. Y. Wang: Survey on the treatment of 200 CAH cases with specific transfer factor extracted from HBVM positive placenta in Research and Application of Transfer Factor and DLE, p. 411–23, ed. Huo Bao-lai, Wang Ruzhang, Zou Zhao-fen. Xueyuan Press; Beijing, China (1989).

76f Z. Li: Clinical application of transfer factor in China in Research and Applications of Transfer Factor and DLE, p. 478–90, ed. Huo Bao-lai, Wang Ru-zhang, Zou Zhao-fen. Xueyuan Press; Beijing, China (1989).

76g G. Mazzella, M. Ronchi, N.Villanova, A. A. Mohamed, G. Pizza, C. De-Vinci, D. Viza, E. Roda, L. Barbara: Treatment of chronic B-virus hepatitis with specific transfer factor. J. Exp. Pathol., *3*, 421–3 (1987).

76h K. Sumiyama, M. Kobayashi, M. Koike: Combined therapy with transfer factor and large dose SNMC in juvenile chronic hepatitis Type B (HBe Ag positive) in Recent Advances in Transfer Factor and Dialyzable Leucocyte Extracts, p. 197–203, ed. T. Fujisawa, S. Sasakawa, Y. Iikura, F. Komatsu, Y. Yamaguchi. Maruzen Co., Ltd.; Tokyo, Japan (1992).

76i B. Huo, J. Wu: Clinical observation on the effects of dialyzable leukocyte extracts in Recent Advances in Transfer Factor and Dialyzable Leucocyte Extracts, p. 304–10, ed. T. Fujisawa, S. Sasakawa, Y. Iikura, F. Komatsu, Y. Yamaguchi, Maruzen Co., Ltd.; Tokyo, Japan (1992).

76j G. Zhang, Z. Li, X. Wang: Treatment of chronic hepatitis B with specific transfer factor extracted from HBVM positive spleen in Research and Application of Transfer Factor and DLE, p. 243–52, ed. Huo Bao-lai, Wang Ru-zhang, Zou Zhao-fen. Xueyuan Press; Beijing, China (1989).

76k S. Matsumato, Y. Takasachi, Y. Sakiyama: Treatment of chronic hepatitis B with high dose of specific dialyzable leukocyte extracts in Recent Advances in Transfer Factor and Dialyzable Leucocyte Extracts, p. 30–9, ed. T. Fujisawa, S. Sasakawa, Y. Iikura, F. Komatsu, Y. Yamaguchi, Maruzen Co., Ltd., Tokyo, Japan (1992).

76m S. T. Schulman, J. M. Hutto, E. M. Ayoub: A double-blind of evaluation of transfer factor of HBsAg-positive chronic aggressive hepatitis: preliminary report of efficacy Cell Immunol., *43*, 352 (1979).

76n p. 27 China #

76o Z. Li: Personal communication (1990).

76p G. Pizza, D. Viza, A. Roda, R. Aldini, E. Roda, L. Barbara: Transfer Factor for the treatment of chronic active hepatitis. N. Eng. J. Med., *300*, 1332 (1979).

76q E. Roda. D. Viza, G. Pizza, L. Mastroroberto, J. Phillips, C. De Vinci, L. Barbara: Transfer Factor for the treatment of HBsAg-positive chronic active hepatitis. P. Soc. Exp. Med., *178*, 468-475 (1985).

77a C. U. Kyong, G. B. Wilson, H. H. Fudenberg, J. M. Goust, P. Richardson, J. Eckerd: Chorioretinitis with a combined defect in T and B lymphocytes and granulocytes: A new syndrome successfully treated with dialyzable leukocyte extracts (Transfer Factor). Am. J. Med., *68*, 955 (1980).

77b J. Prochazkova, E. Parizkova, J. Horacek, O. Pozler, V. Chylkova, et al.: Clinical and immunological improvement in infants with HCMV infection treated with dialyzable leukocyte extract, p. 403–411 in Leukocyte Dialysates and Transfer Fact or, ed. V. Mayer, J. Borvak, Inst. Virol. Slovak Acad. Sci.; Bratislava, Czechoslovakia (1987).

77c Discussion in Recent Advances in Transfer Factor and Dialyzable Leucocyte Extracts, ed. T. Fujisawa, S. Sasakawa, Y. Iikura, F. Komatsu, Y. Yamaguchi. Maruzen Co., Ltd., Tokyo, Japan (1992).

77d F. K. Nkrumah, G. Pizza, D. Viza, J. Phillips, C. DeVinci, P. H. Levine: Regression of progressive lymphoadenopathy in a young child with acute cytomegalovirus (CMV) infection following administration of transfer factor with specific anti-CMV activity. Lymphokine Res., *4*, 237–241 (1985).

77e J. F. Jones, L. L. Minnich, W. S. Jeter, R. F. Pritchett, V. A. Fulginiti, R. J. Wedgwood: Treatment of childhood combined Epstein-Barr virus/cytomegalovirus infection with oral bovine transfer factor. Lancet, *18; 2* (8238), 122–4 (1981).

78a D. Viza, C. Boucheix, J. P. Cesarini, D. V. Ablashi, G. Armstrong, P. Levine, G. Pizza: Characterization of a human lymphoblastoid cell line, LDV/7, used to replicate transfer factor and immune RNA. Bio. Cell, *46*, 1–10 (1982).

78b J. F. Jones, G. Pizza, C. DeVinci: Infectious mononucleosis: immunotherapy woth EBV-specific transfer factor. J. Exp. Pathol., *3*, 399–406 (1987).

78c C. De Yuan, X. Ming-Rong, L. Hua-Ran, W. Huy-Min, et al.: The development of specific transfer factor for EB virus in Recent Advances in Transfer Factor and Dialyzable Leucocyte Extracts, p. 247–52, ed. T. Fujisawa, S. Sasakawa, Y. Iikura, F.Komatsu, Y. Yamaguchi, Maruzen Co., Ltd.; Tokyo, Japan (1992).

79a D. Viza, A. Lefesvre, M. Patrasco, J. Phillips, N. Hebbrecht, G.Laumond, J. M. Vich: A preliminary report on three AIDS patients treated with anti-HIV specific transfer factor. J. Exp. Path., *3*, 653–9 (1987).

79b D. Viza, J. M. Vich, A. Minarro, D. V. Albashi, S. Z. Salahuddin: Soluble extracts from a lymphoblastoid cell line modulate SAIDS evolution. J. Virol. Met., *21*, 241–253 (1988).

79c J. Borvák, H. Schmidtmayerová: Inhibition of HIV-1 reverse transcriptase activity by HPLC fractions of lysed leukocyte ultrafiltrate in Recent Advances in Transfer Factor and Dialyzable Leucocyte Extracts, p. 87–94, ed. T. Fujisawa, S. Sasakawa, Y. Iikura, F. Komatsu, Y. Yamaguchi, Maruzen Co., Ltd.; Tokyo, Japan (1992).

80 R. E. Wolf, H. H. Fudenberg, T. M. Welch, L. E. Spitler, and M. Ziff: Treatment of Behçet's syndrome with transfer factor. J. Am. Med. Assoc., *238*, 869 (1977).

81 K. Freiburger and H. H. Fudenberg: Behçet's Disease: Pitfalls in therapy and diagnosis. Hosp. Pract., *15*, 40 (1980).

82 L. R. Heim: Atopic dermatitis, specific virus infections, and Behçet's syndrome: transfer factor therapy in Immune Regulators in Transfer Factor, p. 531–6, ed. A. Khan, C. H. Kirkpatrick, N. O. Hill. Academic Press; New York (1979).

83 J. J. Hooks: Possibility of a viral etiology in recurrent aphthous ulcers and Behçet's syndrome. J. Oral Pathol., *7*, 353 (1978).

84 T. Lehner: Immunologic aspects of recurrent oral ulceration and Behçet's syndrome. J. Oral Pathol. *7*, 424 (1978).

85 G. M. P. Galbraith, H. H. Fudenberg: Transfer factor in Dermatologic Immunology and Allergy, p. 889–98, ed. J. Stone. Mosby; St. Louis, Mo (1985).

86a G. M. P. Galbraith, H. H. Fudenberg: Unpublished observations (1987).

86b H. H. Fudenberg: In preparation.

87 A. Rook: Common baldness and alopecia areata in Recent Advances in Dermatology, ed. A. Rook, pp. 223–47. Churchill Livingstone; New York (1977).

88 G. M. P. Galbraith, B. H. Thiers, D. B. Vasily, and H. H. Fudenberg: Immunological profiles in alopecia areata. Br. J. Dermatol., 110, 163 (1984).

89a F. Fomatsu: Effects of DLE and inosine fraction of DLE on lymphocytes in Research and Application of Transfer Factor and DLE, p. 14–16, ed. Huo Bao-lai, Wang Ru-zhang, Zou Zhao-fen. Xueyuan Press; Beijing, China (1989).

89b K. Barnet, V. Hribalová, J. Pekárek, K. Cech: The effect of DLE and isoprinosine and guinea pig thymocytes in the comitogentic test in Research and Application of Transfer Factor and DLE, p. 86–94, ed. Huo Bao-lai, Wang Ru-zhang, Zou Zhao-fen. Xueyuan Press; Beijing, China (1989).

89c H. H. Fudenberg, A. Tsang: In preparation.

90 R. E. Wolff, H. H. Fudenberg, and J. N. Gilliam: Transfer factor therapy in a case of pemphigus vegetans associated with chronic mucocutaneous candidiasis. Clin. Immunol. Immunopathol., 10, 292 (1978).

91 H. H. Fudenberg, A. J. Strelkauskas, J. M. Goust, D. Osborne, D. Fort, and D. Vasily: "Discoid" lupus erythematosis: Dramatic clinical and immunological response to dialyzable leukocyte extract (Transfer Factor). Trans. Assoc. Am. Physicians, 94, 279 (1981).

92 D. B. Vasily, F. Miller, H. H. Fudenberg, J. M. Goust, and G. B. Wilson: Epidermodysplasia verriciformis: response to therapy with dialyzable leukocyte extract (transfer factor) derived from household contacts. J. Clin. Lab. Immunol., 14, 49 (1984).

93 Deleted in proof.

94 Deleted in proof.

95 J. M. Dwyer, E.Topper, and R. Sherwin: The prevention of diabetes in BB rats by the administration of transfer factor in 5th International Symposium on Transfer Factor, ed. V. Mayer, J. Borvak, pp. 275–84. Inst. Virol. Slovak Acad. Sci.; Bratislava, Czechoslovakia (1987).

96 W. H. Clark, M. J. Mastrangelo, A. M. Ainsworth, D. Berd, R. E. Bellet, and E. A. Bernardino: Current concepts of the biology of human cutaneous malignant melanoma. Adv. Cancer Res. 24, 267 (1977).

97 R. M. Bukowski, S. Deodhar, J. S. Hewlett, and R. Greenstreet: Randomized controlled trial of transfer factor in stage II malignant melanoma. Cancer, 51, 269 (1983).

98 R. M. Bukowski, J. S. Hewlett, and S. H. Deodhar: Immunotherapy of stage II malignant melanoma and renal cell carcinoma with transfer factor in clinical results in Immune Regulators in Transfer Factor, p. 581–90, ed. by A. Khan, C. H. Kirkpatrick, N. O. Hill. Academic Press; New York (1987).

99 R. M. Vetto, D. R. Burger, J. E. Nolte, A. A. Vandenbark: Transfer factor immunotherapy in cancer in Transfer Factor: Basic Properties and Clinical Applications, p. 523–36, ed. M. S. Asher, A. A. Gottlieb, C. H. Kirkpatrick. Academic Press; New York (1976).

100 V. S. Byers, A. S. Levin, A. J. Hackett, H. H. Fudenberg: Tumor-specific cell mediated immunity in household contacts of cancer patients. J. Clin. Invest., 55, 500 (1975).

101 A. Levin, V. Byers, H. H. Fudenberg: unpublished observations (1982).

102 H. H. Fudenberg, K. Y. Tsang: In utero osteosarcoma tolerized hamsters: a model for human cancer and immunocyte differentiation, p. 23–43, in Theories and Models in Cellular Transformation, ed. L. Saanti, L. Zardi. Academic Press; London, England (1985) (Proceedings Scientific Celebration: A. Nobel's 150th birthday).

103 K. Y. Tsang, H. H. Fudenberg, and J. F. Pan: Transfer of osteosarcoma specific cell-mediated immunity in hamsters by rabbit dialyzable leukocyte extracts. Cell Immunol., 90, 295 (1985).

104 F. Corrado, G. Pizza, G. Severini, C. DeVinci, S. Casanova, D. Menniti, G. Corrado, P. Mauer: Immunochirurgia del tumori vescicali in Chirurgia e Immunitá, p. 317–27, ed. G. Balbo, E. C. Farina. Edizioni Masson; Milano, Italy (1988).

105 G. Pizza, G. Corrado, C. DeVinci, V. Fornarola, F. Corrado: Prospettive del trattamento immunologico del carcinoma renale in E Tumori Urolog-

ici: Recenti Progressi e Nuovi Obbiettivi Della Ricerca, p. 223–32, ed. F. Corrado, et al. Monduzzi Editore; Bologna, Italy (1992).

106   F. K. Nkruman, G.Pizza, J. Neequaye, D. Viza, C. DeVinci, P. H. Levine: Transfer factor in prevention of Burkitt's lymphoma relapses. J. Exp. Pathol., *3*, 463–69 (1987).

107a   W. Wei-zhong, S. Rong-wu, K. Xi-xiong, B. Li-qi, Y. De-fa, W. Wei, J. Hui-rong. W. Biao, Z. Ji-sheng: The effects of swine spleen transfer factor on the subset of T-lymphocyte and cell factor in the patients with cancer of large intestine in Recent Advances in Transfer Factor and Dialyzable Leucocyte Extracts, p. 360–6, ed. T. Fujisawa, S. Sasakawa, Y. Iikura, F. Komatsu, Y. Yamaguchi. Maruzen Co., Ltd.; Tokyo, Japan (1992).

107b   He Guangfa, Mu Yuande: Production of transfer factor from human leucocytes and its Clinical Application in Research and Application of Transfer Factor and DLE, p. 446–7, ed. Huo Bao-lai, Wang Ru-zhang, Zou Zhao-fen. Xueyuan Press; Beijing, China (1989).

108a   B. Massayuki, T. Fujisawa, Y. Yamaguchi, H. Kimura, M. Shiba, C. Kadayama, T. Yusa: Postsurfical Adjuvant immunotherapy for non-small cell lung carcinomas in Recent Advances in Transfer Factor and Dialyzable Leucocyte Extracts, p. 367–374, ed. T. Fujisawa, S. Sasakawa, Y. Iikura, F. Komatsu, Y. Yamaguchi. Maruzen Co., Ltd.; Tokyo, Japan (1992).

108b   L. Busutti, A. Blotta, M. Mastrorilli, G. Savorani, G. Pizza, C. DeVinci: Transfer factor adjuvant therapy in non small-cell lung carcinoma (NSCLC) after surgery and radiotherapy. J. Exp. Pathol., *3*, 565–8 (1987).

108c   T. Jujisawa, Y. Yamaguchi, H. Kimura: Randomized controlled study of leucocyte dialysate and N-CWS as an adjunct to surgical treatment for primary non-small cell carcinoma of the lung in Research and Application of Transfer Factor and DLE, p. 389–98, ed. Huo Bao-lai, Wang Ru-zhang, Zou Zhao-fen. Xueyuan Press; Beijing, China (1989).

109a   T. Fikuvoa, H. Mareckova, O. Krystûkova, K. Cech, J. Pekárek: DLE in immunosuppressed patients in Recent Advances in Transfer Factor and Dialyzable Leucocyte Extracts, p. 315–22, ed. T. Fujisawa, S. Sasakawa, Y. Iikura, F. Komatsu, Y. Yamaguchi. Maruzen Co., Ltd.; Tokyo, Japan (1992).

109b   Y Lian, Q. Bian, L. Wang, D. Chen, Z. Li: Short-term observation on administering BTF combined with 60Co radiotherapy for nasopharygeal carcinoma in Research and Application of Transfer Factor and DLE, p. 319–24, ed. Huo Bao-lai, Wang Ruzhang, Zou Zhao-fen. Xueyuan Press; Beijing, China (1989).

109c   O. Sibl, J. Pekárek, K. Cech, J. Svejcar: The adjuvant therapy of the nasopharyngeal tumor with transfer factor in Research and Application of Transfer Factor and DLE, p. 403–10, ed. Huo Bao-lai, Wang Ru-zhang, Zou Zhao-fen. Xueyuan Press; Beijing, China (1989).

110a   S. K. Morrison, H. H. Fudenberg, and D. B. Vasily: Ten year survival of a patient with hypernephroma and pulmonary metastases, in preparation (1993).

110b   F. Corrado, G. Pizza, C. DeVinci, G. Corrado: Il trattamento con transfer factor delle metastasi ossee da adenocarcinoma della prostata, p. 1233–5, in Le Metastasi, ed. F. Saccani et al. Monduzzi Editore; Bologna, Italy (1987).

111a   H. H. Fudenberg, H. D. Whitten, P. Arnaud, N. Khansari: Hypothesis: Is Alzheimer's Disease an immunological Disorder? Clin. Immuno. and Immunopath., *32*, 127–31 (1984).

111b   H. H. Fudenberg, H. D. Whitten, P. Arnaud, N. Khansari, K. Y. Tsang, C. G. Hames: Immune diagnosis of subset of Alzheimer's disease with preliminary implications for immunotherapy. Biomed. Pharmacol., *38*, 290–7 (1984).

111c H. H. Fudenberg, V. J. Singh: Implications of Immunomodulant therapy in Alzheimer's Disease. p. 21–42, in Progress in Drug Research, ed. E. Jukker. Birkhäuser Verlag, Basel, Switzerland (1988).

112 H. H. Fudenberg: Hetergeneity of Alzheimer's Disease in Proceedings of International Symposium of Neurologic Disorders. Molecular Chemistry, in press (1993).

113 H. H. Fudenberg, M. Coleman, R. Rosberger, H. L. Fudenberg: Immunotherapy of severe infantile onset autism. (Abstract). Clin. Res., 37, 556a (1989).

114a H. H. Fudenberg and V. J. Singh: Immunodiagnosis and immunotherapy in autistic children. Ann. N.Y. Acad. Sci., 540, 602–4 (1988).

114b H. H. Fudenberg, M. Coleman, D. Rosberger: In preparation (1993).

115 H. H. Fudenberg: Immunotherapy and immunodiagnosis of central nervous system disease subsets. In preparation (1993).

116a G. M. P. Galbraith and H. H. Fudenberg: One subset of patients with retinitis pigmentosa has immunologic defects. Clin. Immunol. Immunopathol., 31, 254 (1984).

116b G. M. P. Galbraith, D. Emmerson, H. H. Fudenberg, C. J. Gibbs, and D. C. Gadjusek: Antibodies to neurofilament protein in retinitis pigmentosa. J. Clin Invest., 78, 865 (1986).

117 S. Bahmanyar, M. C. Moreau-Dubois, P. Brown, F. Cathala, and D. C. Gadjusek: Serum antibodies to neurofilament antigens in patiens with neurological and other diseases and in healthy controls. J. Neuroimmunol., 5(2), 191 (1983).

118 V. K. Singh, R. P. Warren, J. D. Odell, W. L. Warren, P. Cole: Antibodies to Myelin basic protein in children with austic behavior. Brain Behav. and Immun., 7, 97–103 (1993).

119 J. Fleishman: Personal communication (1987).

120 J. F. Jones, S. E. Straus: Chronic Epstein-Barr virus infection. Ann. Rev. Med., 38, 195–209 (1987).

121a G. Parish, D. Bell, B. Hyde, H. Rubinstein: The disease of a thousand names in The Clinical and Scientific Basis of Myalgic Encephalomyeltis Chronic Fatigue Syndrome, p. 3–4, ed. B. M. Hyde, J. Goldstine, P. Levine. The Nightingale Research Foundation; Ottawa, Ontario, Canada (1992).

121b H. Rubinstein: "Spasmophilia" and/or "Myalgic Encephalomyelitis"? in The Clinical and Scientific Basis of Myalgic Encephalomyeltis Chronic Fatigue Syndrome, p. 100–3, ed. B. M. Hyde, J. Goldstine, P. Levine. The Nightingale Research Foundation; Ottawa, Ontario, Canada (1992).

122a H. H. Fudenberg: Florence Nightingale Disease: a five year analysis of 50 patients with special emphasis on results of immunotherapy in Clinical and Scientific Basis of Myalgic Enkephalitis/Chronic Fatigue, p. 651–653, ed. B. Hyde, Ottawa U. Press; Ottawa, Canada, and Ogdensburg, NY (1992).

122b B. M. Hyde: Personal communication (1992).

122c H. H. Fudenberg: Cox constellation complex. In preparation (1993).

123 J. M. Dwyer, A. Lloyd, D. Wakefield: Transfer factor for chronic fatigue syndrome in Recent Advances in Transfer Factor and Dialyzable Leucocyte Extracts, p. 288–91, ed. T. Fujisawa, S. Sasakawa, Y. Iikura, F. Komatsu, Y. Yamaguchi, Maruzen Co., Ltd.; Tokyo, Japan (1992).

124 B. Yang, Z. Li, Z. Cui, Y. Luo: Mechanisms of development of myasthenia gravis and the treatment effects of transfer factor. Int. J. Immunopharmacol. (1989).

125 K. Takenouchi, S. Sasakawa: Effects of dialyzable leukocyte extracts (DLE) in survival curves of subacute sclerosing panencephalitis (SSPE) patients in Recent Advances in Transfer Factor and Dialyzable Leucocyte

Extracts, p. 238–242, ed. T. Fujisawa, S. Sasakawa, Y. Iikura, F. Komatsu, Y. Yamaguchi. Maruzen Co., Ltd., Tokyo, Japan (1992).

126 T. Fog, L. Pedersen, N. E. Raun, S. Kam-Hansen, E. Mellerup, et al.: Long-term transfer factor treatment of multiple sclerosis. Lancet, *i*(8069), 851 (1979).

127 A. Basten, J. D. Pollard, G. J. Stewart, J. A. Frith, J. G. Mcleod et al.: Transfer factor in treatment of multiple sclerosis. Lancet, *2*, 9341 (1980).

128 J. Pekárek, K. Cech, O. Nevsímal, K. Barnet, S. Doutlík, O. Cervenková: The use of DLE-TF fraction with the suppressive effect in some autoaggressive diseases in Recent Advances in Transfer Factor and Dialyzable Leucocyte Extracts, p. 326–332, ed. T. Fujisawa, S. Sasakawa, Y. Iikura, F. Komatsu, Y. Yamaguchi. Maruzen Co., Ltd.; Tokyo, Japan (1992).

129a H. H. Fudenberg, E. L. Hogan, J. M. Goust, S. W. Brostoff: Guillain-Barre syndrome, cellular immune deficiency and lymphoma: A case report. Eur. Rev. Med. Pharmacol. Sci., *3*, 1–7 (1981).

129b F. Yizhen, S. Xiurong, H. Hongzhen, W. Shirong: Effects and immunological analysis of transfer factor (TF) and placental factor (PF) on Guillain-Barre's syndromes (BGS) in children in Recent Advances in Transfer Factor and Dialyzable Leucocyte Extracts, p. 335–338, ed. T. Fujisawa, S. Sasakawa, Y. Iikura, F. Komatsu, Y. Yamaguchi. Maruzen Co., Ltd.; Tokyo, Japan (1992).

129c L. Baoqun, X. Jianyang, Chengguanliang: Transfer factor and thymosin in the treatment Guillain-Barre's syndrome in Recent Advances in Transfer Factor and Dialyzable Leucocyte Extracts, p. 339–342, ed. T. Fujisawa, S. Sasakawa, Y. Iikura, F. Komatsu, Y. Yamaguchi. Maruzen Co., Ltd.; Tokyo, Japan (1992).

129d B. Liu, K. Diao, J. Guo, Z. Fan: Acute infectious polyneuritis treated with transfer factor in Research and Application of Transfer Factor and DLE, p. 432–6, ed. Huo Bao-lai, Wang Ru-zhang, Zou Zhao-fen. Xueyuan Press; Beijing, China (1989).

130a J. Rovensky, I. Rybar, M. Orlovska, L. Rauova, J. Pekárek: DLE in the therapy of juvenile chronic arthritis in Recent Advances in Transfer Factor and Dialyzable Leucocyte Extracts, p. 323–5, ed. T. Fujisawa, S. Sasakawa, Y. Iikura, F. Komatsu, Y. Yamaguchi. Maruzen Co., Ltd.; Tokyo, Japan (1992).

130b L. Spitler, M. Ziff, H. H. Fudenberg: Unpublished observations (1972).

131 Xiao Xiuxin: Observation of curative effect curing scleroderma with transfer factor of health person in Recent Advances in Transfer Factor and Dialyzable Leucocyte Extracts, p. 437–9, ed. T. Fujisawa, S. Sasakawa, Y. Iikura, F. Komatsu, Y. Yamaguchi. Maruzen Co., Ltd.; Tokyo, Japan (1992).

132 J. Rovensky, I. Mucska, R. Redhammer, J. Pekárek, P. Pruzinec: Wegener's granulomatosis: some comments on the diagnosis and therapy in Recent Advances in Transfer Factor and Dialyzable Leucocyte Extracts, p. 349–353, ed. T. Fujisawa, S. Sasakawa, Y. Iikura, F. Komatsu, Y. Yamaguchi. Maruzen Co., Ltd.; Tokyo, Japan (1992).

133 I. Sonkoly, I. Schroder, E. Bodolay, K. Lukacs and GY. Szegedi: Treatment of SLE with Transfer Factor Research and Application of Transfer Factor and DLE, page 430, Xueyuan Press, Beijing (1989).

134 W. Borkowski, S. Karpatkin: Leukocyte migration and inhibition of buffy coat from patients with autoimmune TP when exposed to normal placed: modulation by TF. Blood, *63*, 83–87 (1984).

135 M. Karl, N. Domke, W. Franke, and G. Metzner: Immunotherapy of women with recurrent spontaneous abortions by human large pool dialyzable leukocyte extract (DLE) in Recent Advances in Transfer Factor and Dialyzable Leucocyte Extracts, p. 311–314, ed. T. Fujisawa, S. Sasakawa,

Y. Iikura, F. Komatsu, Y. Yamaguchi, Maruzen Co., Ltd.; Tokyo, Japan (1992).

136   N. Khansari, H. H. Fudenberg: Functional heterogeneity of human cord blood monocytes. J. Immunol., *19*, 337–42 (1984).

137a   J. Rovensky, I. Schroder, J. Pekárek, J. Svejcar, F. Vlcek: Transfer factor treatment in patients with psoriasis, p. 605–32, in Immune Regulators in Transfer Factor, ed. A. Khan, C. H. Kirkpatrick, N. O. Hill, Academic Press, NY (1979).

137b   R. S. Schwartz and W. S. Jeter: Oral administration of human dialyzable transfer factor in a patient with psoriasis. Arch. Dermatol. *117*, 3 (1981).

137c   F. Vlcek, J. Rovensky, T. Urbanek, V. Svec, J. Lukac, et al.: Immunomodulatory therapy with dialyzable leukocyte extract (DLE) in psoriasis in Leukocyte Dialysates and Transfer Factor, p. 565–70, ed. V. Mayer, J. Borvak, Inst. Virol. Slovak Acad. Sci.; Bratislava, Czechoslavakia (1987).

137d   D. Yan, Y. Xie, L. Pen, F. Qi, R. Zhong: The effect of DLE induced by psoriasis scale on psoriasis patients and their immunological function in Research and Application of Transfer Factor and DLE, p. 253–8, ed. Huo Bao-lai, Wang Ru-zhang, Zou Zhao-fen. Xueyuan Press; Beijing, China (1989).

138a   H. H. Fudenberg, H. D. Whitten, E. Merler, O. Farmati: Is Schizophrenia an autoimmune receptor disorder? Med. Hypoth. *12*, 85–92 (1983).

138b   H. H. Fudenberg, H. D. Whitten, Y. K. Chou, P. Arnaud, A. A. Shums, N. K. Khansari: Sigma receptors and autoimmune mechanisms in schizophrenia: preliminary findings and hypotheses. Biomedicine and Pharmacotherapy, *38*, 285–90 (1984).

138c   L. E. DeLisi, R. J. Weber, C. B. Pert: Are there antibodies against brain in sera from schizophrenic patients? Biol. Psychiatry, *20*, 94–119 (1985).

138d   D. Xie, T. Wang, B. Huo, X. Du: Clinical observation on 37 cases of schizophrenia treated with transfer factor from bovine spleen in Research and Application of Transfer Factor and DLE, p. 354–6, ed. Huo Bao-lai, Wang Ru-zhang, Zou Zhao-fen. Xueyuan Press; Beijing, China (1989).

138e   Y. Han, J. Liu, B. Huo, E. Wu: A control study of transfer factor and Chlorpromazine in the Treatment of Schizophrenics in Research and Application of Transfer Factor and DLE, p. 347–54, ed. Huo Bao-lai, Wang Ru-zhang, Zou Zhao-fen. Xueyuan Press; Beijing, China (1989).

139   H. H. Fudenberg, M. Waisten: Dramatic results of immunotherapy in a severe schizophrenic. In preparation.

140a   V. Kofranek, K. Barnet, J. Pekárek, K. Cech: Radioprotective effects of DLE in Research and Application of Transfer Factor and DLE, p. 306–13, ed. Huo Bao-lai, Wang Ru-zhang, Zou Zhao-fen. Xueyuan Press; Beijing, China (1989).

140b   V. Kofranek, K. Barnet, J. Pekárek, K. Cech: The radioprotective effects of DLE-TF on BM cells in mice in Recent Advances in Transfer Factor and Dialyzable Leucocyte Extracts, p. 140–4, ed. T. Fujisawa, S. Sasakawa, Y. Iikura, F. Komatsu, Y. Yamaguchi, Maruzen Co., Ltd.; Tokyo, Japan (1992).

141   J. J. Giambrone, P. H. Klesius, and H. H. Fudenberg: Adoptive transfer of delayed wattle reactivity in chickens with a dialyzable leukocyte extract containing transfer factor. Poultry Sci., *62*(5), 767 (1983).

142   Liu Kui, Liu Wen: Clinical application of transfer factor of tun duck blood in Recent Advances in Transfer Factor and Dialyzable Leucocyte Extracts, p. 253–55, ed. T. Fujisawa, S. Sasakawa, Y. Iikura, F. Komatsu, Y. Yamaguchi. Maruzen Co., Ltd.; Tokyo, Japan (1992).

143a   R. Moulias: Use of murine transfer factor in AIDS. Instit. Virol., Slovak Acad. Sci.; Bratislava, Czechoslovakia (1988).

143b N. Bhardwaj, E. Brummer, L. G. Foster, H. S. Lawrence: Transfer of DTH to SK-SK and tetanus toxoid in BALB/c mice by TFd prepared from purified subpopulations of murine lymphocytes in Immune Regulators in Transfer Factor, p. 285, ed. Khan, et al. Academic Press; New York (1979).

143c P. Rifkind, J. A. Frey, E. A. Petersen, M. Dinowitz: Transfer of delayed hypersensitivity of mice to microbial antigens with dialyzable transfer factor. Infect. Immun. 16, 258–62 (1977).

144 E. M. Liburd, H. R. Pabst, and W. D. Armstrong: Transfer factor in rat coccidiosis. Cell. Immunol., 5, 487 (1972).

145 G. B. Wilson, M. L. Morin, L. D. Stuart, A. M. Williams, et al.: Transfer of cell-mediated immunity in vitro to human lymphocytes using dialyzable leukocyte extracts from immune burros in Immunobiology of Transfer Factor, p. ????, ed. C. H. Kirkpatrick, H. S. Lawrence, D. R. Burger. Academic Press; New York (1983).

146a P. H. Klesius and H. H. Fudenberg: Bovine transfer factor: in vivo transfer of cell-mediated immunity to cattle with alcohol precipitates. Clin. Immunol. Immunopathol., 8, 238 (1977).

147 Haiyan Qi, Zhifang Wan, Chengzhi Su: HSV-1 specific transfer factor in goat leukocyte dialysates: Purification and biochemical characterization in Recent Advances in Transfer Factor and Dialyzable Leucocyte Extracts, p. 145–9, ed. T. Fujisawa, S. Sasakawa, Y. Iikura, F.Komatsu, Y. Yamaguchi, Maruzen Co., Ltd.; Tokyo, Japan (1992).

148 Guo Xiu Li, Li Xin Min, Meng Qing Jun: Experiment and study for treatment of rheumatism using transfer factor of horse in Research and Application of Transfer Factor and DLE, p. 520–5, ed. Huo Bao-lai, Wang Ru-zhang, Zou Zhao-fen. Xueyuan Press; Beijing, China (1989).

149a M. R. Simon, J. Silva, D. Freier, J. Brunner, R. Williams: Tuberculin specific transfer factor in dogs. Infect. Immun., 18, 73–7 (1977).

149b M. Shifrine, J. Thilsted, D. Pappagionis: Canine transfer factor in Transfer Factor: Basic Properties and Clinical Applications, p. 349, ed. Ascher, et al. Academic Press; New York (1976).

150a P. Baram, W. Condoulis: Studies on Rhesus monkey, non-dialyzable and dialyzable. Transplantn. Proc. 6, 209–15 (1974).

150b M. R. Mazaheri, A. J. Zuckerman, A. S. Hamblin, D. Dumonde: Specificity determinants of dialyzable transfer factor (DTF) in the rhesus monkey model in Immune Regulators in Transfer Factor, p. 65, ed. Khan, et al. Academic Press, New York (1979).

150c J. W. Eichberg, R. W. Steele, S. S. Kalter, W. T. Kniker, R. L. Heberling, J. J. Eller, A. R. Rodriguez: Cellular immunity in gnotobiotic primates induced by transfer factor. Cell Immun., 26, 114–9 (1976).

151 P. H. Klesius, H. H. Fudenberg, C. L. Smith: Review: Comparitive studies on dialyzable leukocyte extracts containing transfer factor. Comp. Immun. Microbiol. Infec. Dis., 3, 247–260 (1981).

152 G. B. Wilson, J. D. Fort: Interspecies transfers of cell-mediated immunity using specific immunity inducers with potency-prevention in selected diseases in Leukocyte Dialysates and Transfer Factor, p. 333–358, ed. V. Mayer, J. Borvak, Inst. Virol., Slovak Acad. Sci.: Bratislavia, Czecheslovakia (1983).

153 P. H. Klesius, D. F. Qualls, A. L. Alston, and H. H. Fudenberg: Effects of bovine transfer factor (TF) in mouse coccidiosis (Eimeria ferrisi). Clin. Immunol. Immunopathol., 10, 214 (1978).

154a D. R. Burger, P. H. Klesius, A. A. Vandenbark, R. M. Vetto, and A. I. Swann: Transfer of keyhole limpet hemocyanin dermal reactivity to man with bovine TF. Cell. Immunol. 43, 192 (1979).

154b J. F. Jones, M. J. Schumacher, W. S. Jeter, and M. J. Hicks: Oral bovine transfer factor (OTF) use in the hyper-IgE syndrome in Immunobiology of

Transfer Factor, ed. C. H. Kirkpatrick, H. S. Lawrence, D. R. Burger. Academic Press; New York.

155 G. B. Wilson, T. M. Welch, and H. H. Fudenberg: Human transfer factor in guinea pigs: Partial purification of the active component in Transfer Factor: Basic Properties and Clinical Applications, p. 409, ed. M. S. Ascher, A. A. Gottlieb, and C. H. Kirkpatrick. Academic Press; New York (1976).

156 P. Klesius: Unpublished observations (1983).

157 R. W. Steel, J. W. Eichberg, R. L. Heberling, J. J. Eller, S. S. Kalter, W. T. Kniker: Transfer of cellular reactivity to three nonhuman species with human and baboon transfer factor. Cell. Immun., 22, 110–20 (1976).

158a Y. Zhan, P. Wang, D. Li: Transfer of Taekypleus Triclententus Hemocyanin and DNP-BSA Dermal Reactivity to Human with Goose Derived Transfer Factor in Research and Application of Transfer Factor and DLE, p. 60–66, ed. Huo Bao-lai, Wang Ru-zhang, Zou Zhao-fen. Xueyuan Press; Beijing, China (1989).

158b C. L. Boucheix, J. Phillips, C. Piza, G. Sartorio, D. Viza: Activity of animal transfer factor in men. Lancet, 1, 198–9 (1977).

158c S. Tsugi, S. Oshima, M. Oshiro, T. Izumi: Studies on the "transfer factor" of tuberculin sensitivity in animals. J. Immun., 93, 838–49 (1964).

159 D. Viza, G. Pizza: In preparation (1993).

160 G. Pizza, C. Pizza, H. H. Fudenberg: In preparation (1993).

161 H. H. Fudenberg, G. B. Wilson, J. M. Goust, K. Nekam, and C. L. Smith: Dialyzable leukocyte extracts (transfer factor): A review of clinical results and immunologic methods for donor selection, evaluation of activities, and patient monitoring. Thymus, Thymic Hormones and T Lymphocytes. Eds. F. Aiuti and H. Wigzell, Proc. Sereno Symp. 38, 391 (1980).

162 S. J. Rozzo, C. F. Merryman, C. H. Kirkpatrick: Murine transfer factor: studies with genetically regulated immune responses in Research and Application of Transfer Factor and DLE, p. 140–164, ed. Huo Bao-lai, Wang Ru-zhang, Zou Zhao-fen. Xueyuan Press; Beijing, China (1989).

163 H. H. Fudenberg: Influence of per cent granulocytes and degree of donor-patient contact on clinical efficacy of transfer factor. Submitted.

164 M. P. Arala-Chaves, H. H. Fudenberg, unpublished observations (1980).

165 H. H. Fudenberg: Florence Nightingale Disease (FND): A multisystem experiment of nature: Observations and speculations on etiology and pathogenesis. Submitted.

166 W. Jeffries: Personal communication (1987).

167 J. Von Hertog: Personal communication (1987).

168 M. Demitrack, J. Dale, E. Straus, et al.: Evidence for impaired activation of the hypothalamic-pituitary-adrenal axis in patients with chronic fatigue syndrome. J. Clin. Endocrinology and Metabolism, 73, 1224–34 (1992).

169 J. G. Goldstein. Chronic Fatigue Syndrome Humana Press (1992) ??

170 L. M. Pachman, C. H. Kirkpatrick, D. B. Kaufman, R. M. Rothberg: The lack of effect of transfer factor in thymic dysplasia with immunoglobulin synthesis. J. Pediat., 84, 681–8 (1974).

171 M. Coleman: Personal communication (1986).

172 H. H. Fudenberg, N. Carrigg: Unpublished observations (1974).

173 H. H. Fudenberg, G. B. Wilson, and K. Y. Tsang: Evaluation of "transfer factor" potency and prediction of clinical response in Immunomodulation: New Frontiers and Advances, p. 115–30, ed. H. H. Fudenberg, H. Whitten, F. Ambrogi. Plenum; New York (1984).

174 D. Viza, F. Rosenfeld, J. Phillips, J. M. Vich, J. Denis, et al.: Specific bovine transfer factor for the treatment of herpes infections in Immunobiology of Transfer Factor, p. 245–59, ed. C. H. Kirkpatrick, H. S. Lawrence, D. R. Burger. Academic Press; New York (1983).

175 P. H. Klesius and C. H. Kirkpatrick: Dialyzable leukocyte extract contai-
     ning transfer factor – its future in veterinary medicine in Immunobiology
     of Transfer Factor; p. 129–42, ed. C. H. Kirkpatrick, H. S. Lawrence, D. R.
     Burger. Academic Press; New York (1983).

176 G. B. Wilson, R. R. Shuler: Swine transmissible gastroenteritis specific
     immunity inducer (TF); clinical efficacy and licensing by the United States
     Department of Agriculture in Research and Application of Transfer
     Factor and DLE, p. 259–277, ed. Huo Bao-lai, Wang Ru-zhang, Zou
     Zhao-fen. Xueyuan Press; Beijing, China (1989).

177 G. B. Wilson, C. Poindexter, J. D. Fort, K. D. Ludden: De novo initiation
     of specific-cell-mediated immune responsiveness in chickens by transfer
     factor (specific immunity inducer) obtained from bovine colostrum and
     milk. Acta Virol., 32, 6 (1988).

178 Texas Cattle Breeders Association; Houston, Texas: Personal communica-
     tion; (1983).

179 B. Guo, X. Guo, S. Gao: The effect of transfer factor curing mastitis of 159
     cows in Research and Application of Transfer Factor and DLE, p. 520–25,
     ed. Huo Bao-lai, Wang-Ru-zhang, Zou Zhao-fen. Xueyuan Press; Beijing,
     China (1989).

180 M. Cerhova, V. Podlaha, K. Cech, J. Pekárek: The use of DLE for the
     protection of weaning calves in Research and Application of Transfer
     Factor and DLE, p. 530–2, ed. Huo Bao-lai, Wang Ru-zhang, Zou Zhao-
     fen. Xueyuan Press; Beijing, China (1989).

181 W. S. Jeter, R. Kibler, T. C. Soli, and C. A. L. Stephens: Oral administra-
     tion of bovine and human dialyzable transfer factor to human volunteers
     in Immune Regulators in Transfer Factor, p. 451. New York: Academic ed.
     by A. Khan, C. H. Kirkpatrick, N. O. Hill.

182 J. Goldstein, P. H. Klesius, H. H. Fudenberg: Unpublished observations
     (1988).

183 C. H. Rossi, P. H. Klesius, H. H. Fudenberg: Unpublished observations
     (1979).

184 J. A. Mohr: The possible induction and/or acquisition of cellular hyper-
     sensitivity associated with ingestion of colostrum. J. Pediat., 82, 1062–4
     (1973).

185 D. Viza, Cl. Boucheix, J. P. Cesarini, D. V. Ablashi, G. Armstrong, P. Levi-
     ne, and G. Pizza: Characterization of a human lymphoblastoid cell line,
     LDV/7, used to replicate transfer factor and immune RNA. Bio. Cell, 46,
     1–10 (1982).

186 Discussion in Research and Application of Transfer Factor and DLE, ed.
     Huo Bao-lai, Wang Ru-zhang, Zou Zhao-fen. Xueyuan Press; Beijing,
     China (1989).

187 Deleted in proof.

188 G. Tarro, H. H. Fudenberg: In preparation.

189 Deleted in proof.

190 G. V. Paddock, G. B. Wilson, F. K. Lin, N. O'Leary, H. H. Fudenberg:
     Effects of dialyzable leukocyte extracts with transfer factor activity on
     leukocyte migration in vitro. VI. studies on the primary structure of
     transfer factor in Electrophoresis 81, p. 479–85, ed. R. C. Allen, P. Arnaud.
     Walter de Gruyter; Berlin, Germany (1981).

191 G. V. Paddock, G. B. Wilson, A. M. Williams, and H. H. Fudenberg:
     Human Transfer Factor: Exogenous labelling, purification, and role of
     ribonucleic acid segment in Immunobiology of Transfer Factor, ed. C. H.
     Kirkpatrick, H. S. Lawrence, D. R. Burger. Academic Press; New York,
     NY (1979).

192 G. B. Wilson, G. V. Paddock, and H. H. Fudenberg: Effects of dialyzable
     leukocyte extracts with transfer factor activity on leukocyte migration in

vitro. V. Antigen-specific lymphocyte responsiveness can be initiated by two structurally distinct polyribonucleotides. Thymus, *2*, 257 (1981).

193   G. B. Wilson, H. H. Fudenberg, G. V. Paddock, K. Y. Tsang, A. M. Williams, and E. Floyd: Mechanism(s) of action of human transfer factor: Insights obtained from studying "antigen liberated transfer factor" specific for tuberculin in Immunobiology of Transfer Factor, p. 331–46, ed. C. H. Kirkpatrick, H. S. Lawrence, D. R. Burger. Academic Press; New York (1983).

194   D. R. Burger, A. A. Vandenbark, R. M. Vetto, and P. H. Klesius: Human Transfer Factor: Specificity and structural models, p. 33–49, in Immunobiology of Transfer Factor, ed. C. H. Kirkpatrick, H. S. Lawrence, D. R. Burger. Academic Press; New York (1983).

195   G. V. Paddock, G. B. Wilson, H. H. Fudenberg, A. C. Wang, and R. E. Lovins: Purification and structural analysis of the Transfer Factor-like activity detected in vitro by leukocyte migration inhibition in Immune Regulators in Transfer Factor, p. 419–32, ed. A. Khan, C. H. Kirkpatrick, N. O. Hill. Academic Press; New York (1979).

196   C. A. Dinarello: Biology of interleukin-1. FASEB J., *2*(2), 108 (1988).

197   I. I. Singer, S. Scott, G. L. Hall, G. Limjuco, J. Chin, and J. A. Schmidt: Interleukin 1-beta is localized in the cytoplasmic ground substance but is largely absent from the golgi apparatus and plasma membranes of stimulated human monocytes. J. Exp. Med., *167*, 389 (1988).

198   J. D. Ashwell: Are B-lymphocytes the principal antigen-presenting cells in vivo? J. Immunol., *140*(11), 3697 (1988).

199   H. H. Fudenberg, J. R. L. Pink, A. C. Wang, and G. B. Ferrara: Basic Immunogenetics, 3rd ed. Oxford Univ. Press; New York (1984).

200   D. C. Gadjusek: Plenary lecture at U. of Göteborg International Symposium on Neurodegenerative Disorders, Jamaica (1993).

201   T. R. Cech: The chemistry of cell splicing of RNA and RNA enzymes. Science, *235*, 1531 (1987).

202   R. M. Bennett, G. T. Gabor, and M. M. Merritt: DNA binding to human leukocytes; evidence for a receptor-mediated association, internalization, and degradation of DNA. J. Clin. Invest., *76*, 1 (1985).

203   R. M. Bennett, S. H. Hefeneider, A. Bakke, M. Merritt, C. A. Smith, et al.: The production and characterization of murine monoclonal antibodies to a DNA receptor on human leukocytes. J. Immunol., *140*, 2937 (1988).

204   S. Saito, K. Takenouchi, S. Sasakawa: Inhibitory effects of dialyzable leukocyte extracts on cell functions of lymphocytes and other cell lines in Recent Advances in Transfer Factor and Dialyzable Leucocyte Extracts, p. 117–24, ed. T. Fujisawa, S. Sasakawa, Y. Iikura, F.Komatsu, Y. Yamaguchi. Maruzen Co., Ltd.; Tokyo, Japan (1992).

205   McFarlane Burnett: Personal communications (1974).

206   M. P. Arala-Chavez: Unpublished observations (1978).

207   V. Meyer: Personal communications (1987).

208   S. Sasakawa, K. Takenouchi, C. Matsumoto, T. Mura, S. Saito, et al.: Clinical trials of dialyzable leukocyte extract (RCTF-1) in Japan in Leukocyte Dialysates and Transfer Factor, p. 419–35 ed. V. Mayer, J. Borvak, Inst. Virol., Slovak Acad. Sci. (1987).

Progress in Drug Research, Vol. 42
Edited by Ernst Jucker
© 1994 Birkhäuser Verlag Basel (Switzerland)

Transfer factor in malignancy

By Giancarlo Pizza[1], Caterina De Vinci[1] and H. Hugh Fudenberg[2]

S. Orsola-Malpighi Hospital, Bologna, Italy, and[2] NeuroImmuno Therapeutics Research Foundation Spartanburg, SC, USA

1   Introduction

Cell-mediated immunity (CMI) plays an important role in controlling the proliferation of tumor cells. Since transfer factor (TF) is reportedly able to increase CMI, it was tempting to plan clinical trials whereby transfer factor could be used to increase cancer patients' cellular immune response to their tumor cells.

The first such clinical study was published by Thompson in 1971 [1]. Numerous reports have followed since, but most studies, like the original one, are criticizable on several accounts: they were uncontrolled, the number of subjects involved was small, more often than not the patients were in a stage of advanced disease and their tumor load was important, the follow-up period was short. Furthermore, it is impossible to draw any, even preliminary, conclusion when results of different centers pertaining to the same tumor type are contradictory. The lack of a product whose activity is known and can be standardized makes it difficult to decide whether the reported failures are due to the lack of activity of the transfer factor used, to the protocol of its administration, or to the ineffectiveness of this kind of immunotherapy for the type of tumor treated.

Nonetheless, and despite these criticisms, several studies produced encouraging and sometimes unequivocal results which prompted further clinical trials for other types of cancer [2–6]. Furthermore, some laboratory studies were showing that incubation of unreactive lymphocytes with TF was able to induce recognition of TAA.

In 1976, Byers et al. [7] were among the first to produce evidence for such in vitro transfer of reactivity to tumor cells. They extracted transfer factor from osteosarcoma patients whose lymphocytes were showing cytotoxicity against osteosarcoma cells. The dialysate was then used to inject osteosarcoma patients whose lymphocytes became subsequently cytotoxic and able to kill autologous tumor cells.

At that time, we have also shown that specific transfer factor, obtained from patients with high levels of CMI to tumor-associated antigens (TAA) of bladder carcinoma – as assessed by the leucocyte migration inhibition test (LMT) – was able to transfer to the leucocytes of the recipient, by in vitro incubation or by in vivo injection, the reactivity observed in the TF donor [8–10].

Such observations encouraged tumor immunologists to treat cancer patients with transfer factor in the hope that the modulation of their immune response against TAA could counter the tumor growth.

However, the distinction between specific and non-specific transfer factor was not always made at the time and clinicians would use the so-called non-specific transfer factor obtained from pools of buffy coats from blood donors. But even when it was accepted that specific transfer factor was more desirable than non-specific, its scarcity-obliged investigators to use dialysates from pools of leucocytes.

Some investigators would nonetheless argue that the clinical benefit of transfer factor may be related to the non-antigen-specific immuno-potentiating effects of the leucocyte dialysate, rather than to the specific transfer of cellular immunity. Furthermore, one cannot exclude that the so-called non-specific transfer factor may, by chance, contain information for tumor specificities relevant to the tumor type of the recipient.

Indeed, using such "non-specific" transfer factor, Krown and co-workers reported in 1978 two tumor regressions in 18 patients with advanced cancer and they also observed that the treatment was associated with at least a temporary increase of delayed hypersensitivity reactions in 12/17 patients tested. They concluded that lymphocyte dialysates may augment delayed hypersensitivity in patients with advanced cancer, and that some of the observed effects may be non-specific, i.e. unrelated to transfer of information pertaining to TAA [11].

Results of clinical trials using transfer factor therapy in various malignancies have been extremely variable. In non-randomized trials, more than 300 patients have been enrolled, and clinical benefit has been reported in about 1/3 of them. Results of randomized studies also vary: in some, beneficial clinical effects, measured by increased disease-free interval and prolonged survival, have been claimed, whereas in other studies, transfer factor has been reported to be of no clinical benefit. Finally, some reports suggest that certain patients receiving transfer factor do not do as well as those receiving placebo, although this type of observation has never reached statistical significance.

Since there are many variables in the design of transfer factor clinical trials, it is impossible from their analysis to identify the key factors responsible for the observed success or failure. For instance, the state of disease, previous and/or concomitant chemotherapy and/or radiotherapy vary widely and their impact in the clinical and immunological response is unclear. Obviously, the source, but also more often than not the dose of transfer factor used vary from one clinical study to another, and this is another serious handicap for establishing valid comparisons and overall evaluations of efficacy.

Finally, it should be reminded here that the methods of preparation of transfer factor also vary and the products used in the different studies are not a priori comparable nor are there reliable tests allowing measurements of specific activity and thus making comparisons between laboratories possible.

Several tumor types have been treated with transfer factor, but because of the uncertainties mentioned above, it is not established which tumors only partially respond to this therapy and which are totally unresponsive.

The results obtained in the most important clinical studies in the last twenty years are briefly described hereafter.

2   Lung cancer

One of the most important studies on lung cancer was published by Whyte et al. who, between 1976 and 1982, treated sixty-three patients with bronchogenic carcinoma with TF obtained from apparently healthy blood donors. These patients had previously undergone pulmonary resection, mediastinal lymph node dissection, and, when it was necessary because of mediastinal lymph node involvement, mediastinal irradiation. Patients were randomized into two groups. A group of 28 patients received pooled TF 3 months after surgery, whereas 35 patients of the control group received saline injections. Follow-up was completed in 1990. In the transfer factor group, the 2-, 5-, and 10-year survival rates were 82%, 64%, and 43% respectively, whereas in the control group they were 63%, 43%, and 23%. Survival in patients receiving TF was consistently better than in the placebo group for both adenocarcinoma and squamous cell carcinoma.

Although these long-term results were not statistically significant, using survival analysis (p = 0.08), the authors were able to confirm their previous observations in a smaller number of lung cancer patients treated for a short-time period suggesting that administration of TF can enhance CMI and improve survival in patients with bronchogenic carcinoma [12].

In a different study, Busutti et al. also reported a beneficial effect of TF administration in a series of 26 non small cell lung carcinoma patients (NSCLC) [13].

In order to evaluate the efficacy of adjuvant TF immunotherapy after surgery, Fujisawa and coworkers treated, from March 1978 to October 1984, 263 primary NSCLC cancer patients who had undergone pulmonary resection. They showed that in patients in stage I of the disease (but not in stages II, III and IV), the effect of TF was statistically significant, thus suggesting that TF can only suppress "micrometastases" existing at the time of surgery. The authors also immunized in vitro lymphocytes from household contacts (i. e. family members) with IL-2 and mitomycin-treated lung cancer cells. These T-lymphocytes showed considerable cytotoxic activity against the target cells, which were used for in vitro sensitization, and their dialysate showed capability to transfer specific cytotoxic activity against lung cancer cells [14–16].

In another controlled trial on 102 lung cancer patients, randomized after surgery, the TF group of 44 patients was compared to a control group of 47. Again, the survival of the TF group was significantly better than that of the control in patients of stage I (p<0.05). However, there was no significant difference in patients of stage II, III or IV. Furthermore, significant differences were found between the TF and control groups in patients who had undergone curative resection (p<0.05). The authors concluded that TF seems to inhibit postoperative recurrence and appears to be an effective post-operative adjuvant immunotherapeutic tool for primary resected adenocarcinoma of the lung patients, especially at the early stage [16–23].

In contrast to the work cited above, Kirsh and coworkers observed good clinical results also in patients of advanced stages. In 28 patients with lung cancer (treated with 1 ml of TF extracted from the blood of normal individuals of 3-month intervals), they showed a significant increase of survival, when the TF-treated group was compared with 35 randomized control patients. The 2-year survival was 78% for the TF-treated patients and 46% for the control group (p<0.04) [24–25].

3   Osteosarcoma

The work of Fudenberg's team produced solid evidence concerning the ability of TF from selected donors to increase the CMI responses in human osteogenic sarcoma patients [7, 26–28]. An animal Osteosarcoma Tumor model using TF has also been reported by the same team [29]. In addition, in another section of the present volume, very important results are also reported by Fudenberg, regarding the prevention of human osteosarcoma lung metastases in hamsters pretreated with specific TF.

Levin et al. administered specific TF after surgical removal of the primary tumor to patients without apparent metastases. Five out of 6 patients were still alive 5 years later, after 2 years of TF administration. This survival was significantly better than no treatment or other treatment, when compared to historical controls ($p<0.008$) and it was attributed to the prevention of lung metastases [30]. Their results were confirmed by others [31–33]. Similar results were obtained in an animal model [34].

The first report of a randomized postsurgical clinical trial with TF versus combination chemotherapy in osteogenic sarcoma was published by Ivins and coworkers in 1976 [35]. Twenty-six patients with osteosarcoma were randomized to receive either TF or combination chemotherapy. Eight of 14 patients who received transfer factor converted their skin test markers demonstrating biological activity of the TF. Of these eight patients, all were alive and four free of disease, in a 6-month follow-up. Of the 18 patients who received combination chemotherapy, 14 were alive and 12 free of disease, during the same observation period. Laboratory tests subsequently showed that transfer factor appeared to enhance CMI, although no predictive correlation could be established between laboratory results for each patient and his clinical response to TF treatment. However, the limited number of patients and the short duration of the study did not allow to draw definitive conclusions [35].

Gilchrist and coworkers [36] proposed an adjuvant TF therapy for the treatment of non-metastatic osteogenic sarcoma after apparent complete surgical ablation of the primary tumor compared to combination chemotherapy. From a total of 32 patients assessed, 22 received chemotherapy; in this group three died of drug-related complications and six were alive without disease recurrence between 260 and 673 days after operation. The ten patients in the transfer factor group all converted their skin tests, and five were alive without recurrence 420–753 days after operation. No significant difference was seen between the two groups with respect to disease-free survival [36].

4   **Melanoma**

Several clinical trials have been carried out in patients with malignant melanoma. The results have been inconclusive and sometimes contradictory. Thus, in one of these studies, performed in double blind on 68 patients of stage I and II as adjuvant therapy after surgery and having as end-point the time of stage III metastases, a trend in favor of the placebo group was observed [37].

In contrast, in a non-randomized clinical trial with a control group of 46 patients, the results were more encouraging. One hundred patients at stage I melanoma were treated with transfer factor and monitored with a median follow-up period of 30 months. The survival rate was 99% at five years compared to 69% in the control group. These results suggest that TF immunotherapy may be a valuable adjunct in the treatment of patients with high risk stage I melanoma [38].

Gonzalez and Spitler treated with surgery and TF nine patients with resectable pulmonary metastases of malignant melanoma. Twelve months after thoracotomy, they were all alive and after a median follow-up of 20 months, only one patient had died. Historic controls of patients from other centers treated with surgery alone showed a significantly lower survival rate ($p < 0.025$). Recurrence rates tended to be lower in the TF group, but no significant difference was found with historic controls. The data seem to suggest that transfer factor may prolong survival in patients with a small residual tumor burden and furthermore, this type of immunotherapy produces better results in lung metastases [39]. In a randomized controlled trial of stage II malignant melanoma, Bukowski et al. were unable to find any statistical difference in survival between the 18 patients treated with TF compared to the 18 patients of the control group, despite the fact that the median disease-free intervals were respectively 12.0 and 10.0 months, and survival 40.8 and 27.0 months. Nine TF-treated patients and four control patients remained alive 68 months after the end of the treatment [40].

However, no improvement was seen when TF was added to the protocol of chemotherapy and BCG immunotherapy used for the treatment of disseminated malignant melanoma [41].

In conclusion, although some encouraging results have been observed in certain clinical studies when TF was used for the treatment of melanoma patients, further clinical trials should be planned using selected specific TF, covering several melanoma antigenic specificities before any meaningful conclusion can be drawn.

5   Papillomatosis of larynx

Although some anecdotal encouraging responses were observed in some patients [42–45], no controlled clinical trials have been carried out on papillomatosis of the larynx. Borkowsky reported complete remission of pulmonary metastatic lesions in a 6-years-old girl after 2 years of treatment with TF prepared from her mother. A computer tomographic scan performed after four months of therapy revealed almost complete resolution of her pulmonary lesions [42]. Two other cases have been reported by Ortiz and coworkers [43].

6   Nasopharyngeal cancer (NPC)

Numerous studies substantiate the hypothesis of the role EBV in the pathogenesis of BL and NPC, thus making the idea of potentiating the CMI against the EBV antigens in these patients in order to prevent relapses a plausible one [46–48].

However, the difficulties in the choice of the best TF donor should be underlined. In view of the preparation of an active anti-EBV TF for in vitro replication by the LDV/7 lymphoblastoid cell line, we used different sources: a) nude mice immunized with EBV, b) a patient who had recovered from infectious mononucleosis and c) a NPC patient in remission showing a very strong CMI, as assessed by lymphocyte stimulation and leucocytes migration inhibition in presence of EBV-superinfected Raji cells. Transfer factor extracted from PBL of the NPC patient was the most active in transferring both in vitro and in vivo reactivity to EBV antigens. These data suggest that negative results obtained in clinical trials of NPC using TF from other sources might be artifactual because of the lack of TF reactivity [46]. The clinical results obtained with an active anti-EBV TF in Burkitt's Lymphoma [47] makes this assertion so much more credible.

Goldenberg et al. treated 100 NPC patients in a cooperative trial with EBV-specific transfer factor [48]. The prospectively randomized, double-blind clinical trial was planned to evaluate the effect of immunotherapy with transfer factor as an adjunct to radiotherapy on patients with stage III NPC. The TF was obtained from healthy young adult volunteers with a proven history of infectious mononucleosis and from healthy blood donors with elevated anti-EBV-capsid-antigen antibody titers. TF thus prepared was previously to its clinical use shown (by the leucocyte adherence inhibition test) to convert in vitro NPC patients' leucocytes. When it was administered to NPC patients *in vivo,* it seemed to slow tumor growth, and this was associated with lymphocyte infiltration of the tumor, and recovery of delayed cutaneous hyper-sensitivity reactions [49]. From 1974 to 1977, 100 patients with NPC were entered in the study; one-half of the patients were treated with radiotherapy alone, whereas the other half received radiotherapy and an 18-month course of TF immunotherapy. The patients were followed for at least 5 years. No significant difference in survival or disease-free interval was noted between the two groups. One may conclude that this particular TF preparation and/or the schedule of administration was devoid of any anti-tumor activity [48].

7   Burkitt's lymphoma (BL)

Because in endemic areas BL seems to be reinduced by the persistence of the Epstein-Barr virus (EBV) infection, we thought that the reinforcement of the CMI against EBV in BL patients in remission could prevent late relapses, early relapses being considered as relapses of the primary tumor not eradicated by chemotherapy. Prior to the clinical study we had shown that a specific TF replicated in vitro was able to transfer in rhesus monkeys, both in vitro and in vivo, cell-mediated immune reactivity against membrane antigens induced on Raji cells superinfected with the EBV marmoset strain [46, 50].

Twenty-seven children with abdominal Burkitt's lymphoma (stage III), who had achieved complete remission by standard chemotherapy, entered into a prospective controlled randomized trial of adjunct treatment with EBV-specific TF [46]. Two out of 12 TF-treated patients and 5 out of 11 controls suffered relapses. Time to first late relapse was longer among TF-treated patients ($p = 0.08$), and no late relapses occurred while patients were receiving TF treatment. It thus seems that EBV-specific TF might be useful in the management of endemic Burkitt's lymphoma and also in the treatment of other virus-associated cancers [47].

8   Cervical cancer and household contacts TF

In a prospective randomized double-blind study on 60 patients with invasive cervical cancer, Wagner and coworkers treated 32 women with TF derived from the leucocytes of their husbands, and 28 with placebo. Within the first 2 years after radical hysterectomy, 11 out of 28 placebo and five out of 32 TF-treated patients developed recurrence of malignancy. These data are statistically significant ($p < 0.05$) [51–53]. Vetto et al. also treated 35 patients with various tumor types (viz. melanoma, osteogenic sarcoma, rhabdomyosarcoma, Wilms tumor, renal cell carcinoma, epidermoid carcinoma, colon adenocarcinoma, lymphosarcoma) using TF obtained from donors selected among family members living in cohabitation. The objective of this study was to stimulate CMI to specific tumor antigens by specific TF. Cancer patients not suitable for further conventional therapy were selected for this protocol and TF was administered at 2-week intervals. The TF immunotherapy produced tumor regression in 13 patients, and arrest of metastatic disease and pain relief in 14 patients. Conversion of dermal reactivity to specific TAA was observed during periods of clinical improvement. Despite continued immunotherapy, the duration of clinical improvement was short (2 weeks to 12 months). Seven of the 11 patients not responding to therapy exhibited serum blocking of lymphocyte responsiveness. The results suggest that TF from household contacts can effectively stimulate specific CMI in cancer patients and produce in some cases an inhibition of tumor growth [54].

9   Hodgkin's disease (HD)

Several investigators claimed increase of CMI in patients with Hodgkin's lymphoma. It was assessed by the increase of patients' dermal reactivity to various antigens and/or increase of circulating total T and CD4 + lymphocytes. In contrast the number of NK cells in the peripheral blood does not appear markedly affected [55–58].
Furthermore, a beneficial effect on the impaired functions of mononuclear leucocytes was observed, whereas the decreased phagocytosis and chemotaxis of monocytes was increased almost to the values of healthy controls [56]. The number of T cells bearing histamine and IgG Fc receptors was reduced initially and increased during TF therapy, but this effect was only temporary. Furthermore, non-specific

TF injections in children with Hodgkin's disease seem to produce an increase in B-lymphocytes, both in percentage and absolute number [59].

Only one randomized clinical trial has been reported by Hancock and coworkers [60]. They prepared TF from 493 buffy coats obtained from healthy donors including individuals convalescent from miscellaneous viral infections. Twenty-two Hodgkin's patients were randomized and subcutaneously injected every 3 months with 1 ml of TF (3×10^8 mononuclear cell equivalent); 25 patients, injected with 1 ml of saline, served as controls. The authors confirmed the increase of skin reactions in anergic patients, but did not show augmentation of other immune parameters neither noticed reduction of the incidence of viral infections [60].

10   Renal cancer

In 1978, in a prospective but not randomized trial on 27 metastatic renal cell cancer patients (MRCC), Bukowski et al. reported some benefit when TF was used for treatment alone or in combination with BCG or chemotherapy [61]. Previously they had treated with TF 5 MRCC patients and observed temporary stabilization of the disease [62]. Two additional patients, without clinically evident metastases, but at a high risk for recurrent disease, were also treated and remained disease-free.

A critical review of immunotherapy of disseminated renal adenocarcinoma was published in 1982 by Montie et al. [63]. Sixty patients with renal adenocarcinoma had been treated in five different immunotherapy protocols consisting of 1) transfer factor, 2) association of TF and BCG, 3) association of TF, BCG, Chloroethylcyclohexy-nitrosurea (CCNU) and megestrol acetate (Megase), 4) association of BCG, CCNU, and Megase, and 5) BCG alone. While this non-specific immunotherapy of renal adenocarcinoma has been associated with documented regression of metastases, response rates were similar to those obtained with hormonal therapy alone. However, because of these results, further clinical studies were undertaken [63].

Thirty-seven MRCC patients, compared to 27 historical controls, were treated with combined immunotherapy including direct lymphatic injection of IL-2 and Lak cells, intramuscular injection of alpha-2a-interferon (10^6 units biweekly) and TF (bimonthly injections of 4×10^8

mononuclear cell equivalent obtained from pooled buffy coats of healthy blood donor). This regimen produced complete and partial remissions of metastases in 34% of the patients treated and stabilized progression of the disease in an additional 8%. The median survival is, respectively, 26 and 27 months for synchronous and metachronous metastatic treated patients against 8 and 14 months for the control group (p <0.001) [64]. While no side effects were noticed in the treated patients, the observed results are comparable to those obtained by intravenous injections of large amounts of IL-2 and Lak cells, a protocol which produced severe adverse side effects [65].

11   Bladder cancer

TF was extracted from lymphocytes of patients with transitional cell carcinoma of bladder (TCCB) and replicated in culture using the LDV/7 lymphoblastoid cell line [66]. The ability of the in vitro replicated TF in transferring sensitivity to TCCB was assessed in LMT using formalin-treated TCCB cells as antigen. It was shown that it was able to transfer not only to leucocytes of healthy blood donors but also to leucocytes of TCCB patients [9].

When TCCB patients were injected with this TF, we observed transfer of reactivity against autologous tumor cells in 6 out of 8 patients and in 11 out of 14 for allogeneic bladder tumor cells [8, 10, 67]. Increase of total number of lymphocytes and T cells was also noticed when their values were low before TF injection, whereas responses to PHA and Con-A appeared also increased after the TF injections [9].

In certain patients evaluation of antibodies against TCCB antigens showed a drop of the antibody titer immediately after the TF injection. This was attributed to the increase of the number of cytotoxic lymphocytes and the subsequent destruction of tumor cells, thus liberating TAA reacting with the circulating antibodies [68]. We must remind, in fact, that 80% of TCCB patients show the bloodstream complement fixing antibodies against their own tumor as assessed by indirect immunofluorescence test on fresh or fixed tumor cells [69]. The same antibodies, harvested by plasmapheresis or produced in vitro, are now used in passive immunoprophylaxis of the tumor [70] and the results on the first 114 TCCB patients appear encouraging. In fact we notice significant reduction of tumor relapse index without noticing any side effect (p <0.01). It is worth mentioning here that we also administer, to our patients, TF at monthly intervals $(4 \times 10^8$ mononuclear cells) because it seems able to induce a better antibody anti-tumoral response against the autologous tumor with respect to non-injected patients (G. Pizza, C. De Vinci, unpublished observations).

Immunotherapy of recurrent, superficial papillary TCCB, using non-specific TF as sole therapy, was also attempted. Only one controlled study was published which fails to show any difference between the TF treated patients and those of the control group [71].

12   Prostate cancer

In a preliminary trial, 7 patients with hormone-resistant metastatic adenocarcinoma (stage D3) were treated monthly with the in vitro replicated TF, used for the treatment of TCCB. In one patient, a complete regression of multiple bone metastases as well as the primary tumor was noticed [72]. These observations were confirmed in a study of 56 same stage prostate cancer patients. The patients received monthly an intramuscular injection of in vitro produced TCCB-specific TF. Follow-up, ranging from 1 to 8 years, showed that complete remission was achieved in 2 patients, partial remission in 6, and there was no progression of metastatic disease in 14. The median survival was 17 months, higher than the survival rates reported elsewhere [73].

Effect of transfer factor on tumor-associated immunity and tumor growth of the Dunning R-3327G rat prostate adenocarcinoma was reported by Shaw and coworkers [74]. Dunning R-3327 rat prostate adenocarcinoma, and its sublines, represent an experimental tumor model of its human counterpart. In a preliminary study, the effect of TF on tumor-associated immunity and tumor growth and histology of the G subline (a poorly differentiated, fast-growing, androgen sensitive, and poorly metastatic cell-line) was evaluated. TF was prepared from the leucocytes of tumor-bearing animals and non-tumor-bearing animals. Its administration showed no significant effect on the tumor size. The only noticeable effect of TF was the presence of variable and moderate lymphocyte infiltration, necrosis, and degenerative-type cells in tumors of animals receiving TF from immunized animals. The authors conclude that additional evaluation of the effect of TF on other, more immunogenic, cell sublines is needed [74].

13   Epidermodysplasia verruciforme

Vasily and coworkers treated 2 patients with epidermodysplasia verruciformis, a chronic cutaneous infection with a variety of human papilloma viruses using TF obtained from household contacts. One patient with longstanding (30-year) disease and no response to previous therapy, showed gradual and definite resolution of extensive tinea-versicolor-like verrucae planae plaques, as well as tumor lesions scattered over his entire integument. Cessation of TF therapy for a short time resulted in recurrence of partially regressed lesions and also in the development of new tumors. The second patient (grandson of the first) with minimal disease showed no worsening of his condition during TF prophylaxis. Patients showed low numbers of T suppressor lymphocytes, a defect in cell-mediated immunity not previously reported in patients with this disease [75].

14   Childhood leukemia

Few studies were performed on childhood leukemia. De Bruyere and coworkers found an association between long survival in childhood acute lymphoblastic leukemia treated with transfer factor and certain HLA haplotypes. The study was carried out in 116 children. Patients with A2 B12 and/or A2 B40 haplotypes survived longer than patients without these two haplotypes. Since all children were treated with TF obtained from their relatives, it is suggested that children with A2 B12 or A2 B40 haplotypes may respond better to this type of immunotherapy [76]. Unfortunately no other studies to further investigate and confirm this interesting hypothesis have been published.

15   Mycosis fungoides (MF)

In a controlled study, Thestrup and coworkers treated 16 patients with mycosis fungoides with non-specific TF obtained from healthy blood donors as adjuvant therapy to topical nitrogen mustard or PUVA. The clinical evaluation after 2 years of therapy failed to show any effectiveness of the treatment in the control of the disease [77].
In another non-randomized study, TF was associated to oral retinoids in combination with chemotherapy [78]. The patients were divided into two groups, only one received retinoids, whilst both groups

received a 3-drug combination chemotherapy consisting of bleomycin, cyclophosphamide and prednisone. Complete remission, including regression of all signs of lymph-node involvement was observed in 8 of 10 patients of the group treated with retinoids, while none went into complete remission in the control group. All patients in the control group died between 3 and 12 months after the end of therapy, whereas all but one in the group treated with retinoids remained alive. These results suggest that TF in the absence of retinoids has no beneficial effect [78]. Nonetheless, it would be of interest to compare a group of patients receiving TF immunotherapy with a group not receiving this treatment, both groups receiving chemotherapy and retinoids.

Promising results were also reported by Zachariae and coworkers. They treated, using TF as additional therapy to conventional treatment, after the latter had failed, 13 patients with clinically and histologically confirmed MF. Approximately 3 years later, 3 patients were in complete remission, 4 patients were significantly improved and considered as being in partial remission, whereas no change was noticed in 3 patients. The condition of one patient was worse, 1 patient died after discontinuation of the therapy and 1 patient opted out of the study. The number of T lymphocytes, which was low prior to treatment, increased to normal values during TF administration. During the first year a decrease in serum IgE was noticed. The results of the clinical evaluation seem to indicate that TF could be of value as an adjuvant therapeutic agent in MF, although further controlled clinical trials are needed to corroborate this assumption [79].

16   Miscellaneous

Ten patients with breast cancer were treated with TF. Clinical improvement was observed in 2 of 10 patients, whereas increase of skin reactivity was noticed in 3/10 [80–81].

Some encouraging results of transfer factor therapy in Waldenstrom's macroglobulinemia and multiple myeloma were observed by Silverman et al. [82].

Pain relief was observed by Vetto et al. in one patient with epidermoid carcinoma and 75% tumor regression for 3 months in one colon carcinoma patient [83].

Vetto et al. also treated patients with head and neck cancer. The

T-lymphocyte levels increased in 8/38 patients who received non-specific TF, although leucocyte adherence inhibition (a test used to determine tumor immunity) did not occur. No clinical results were reported [83].

17   Conclusions and perspectives

The results of the clinical trials reported here clearly suggest that transfer factor cannot be used as sole treatment of cancer, despite the reported cases of remission. It remains nevertheless that transfer factor can play an important role as an adjuvant to other treatments (i.e. surgery, irradiation, chemotherapy) or in combination with other lymphokines. For instance, we are now using immunotherapy for metastatic renal carcinoma which combines intralymphatic injections of IL-2, [64, 84] α-interferon and specific transfer factor. Our results show that this regimen is at least as efficacious as I.V.IL-2 injections and far less toxic.

Controlled studies are of the essence for future evaluation of the clinical activity of transfer factor. Obviously, a prerequisite for such studies is to dispose of adequate amounts of an active product. Furthermore, for the comparison of studies carried out in different centers using dialysates from various origins, it is essential to adopt the same criteria for measuring in vitro activity. Only one such in vitro test, the leucocyte migration inhibition, has so far been widely used but the results are not always transposable from one laboratory to another.

Furthermore, the choice of the target antigen to determine the activity of the dialysate is important. In our studies with bladder carcinoma, we have been using formalin-treated autologous and/or allogeneic tumor cells, whereas for Burkitt's lymphoma, AIDS and herpes studies, formalin-fixed virus-infected cells have been utilized.

It should be reminded here that for several decades, one of the main curtailments for the clinical use of transfer factor has been the lack of adequate supplies of active material. Indeed, twenty years ago, the only source of transfer factor was human leucocytes. Buffy coats from healthy blood donors were thus used to prepare large amounts of material whose specific activity was unknown. The possibility of encountering the appropriate specificity in a given batch for a given patient was amounted to a lottery draw. At that time (1974), some of us proposed the use of a lymphoblastoid cell line to replicate transfer factors of known specificity [85]. Multiple reports have now confirmed that such replicated transfer factor carries the original specificity and it is able to transfer it not only in vitro but also in vivo [8–10, 47, 57, 86, 87].

A few years later, the same laboratory showed that animal transfer factor is active in humans [88]. Several studies have subsequently shown that transfer factor from animal origin can be replicated in vitro and that both the in vitro replicated or the animal transfer factor retain their activity even when they are orally administered.

For instance, in an important clinical trial, more than 200 patients suffering from genital, labial or ocular herpes were orally treated using specific anti-HSV transfer factor from bovine origin [89–93, and Pizza et al., unpublished].

Thus, the problem of the preparation of large amounts of active material seemed to be solved. Unfortunately, at that time, transfer factor became compound non grata in the scientific community who is dominated by what some call hard science which denies the right of existence to unexplained phenomena in biology which seem to challenge the day's paradigm and disturb the consensus.

The logical approach to produce sufficient amounts of TF when the antigen is known and readily available, is animal immunization, whereas when the involved antigen(s) is (are) unknown, one can use transfer factor obtained from the patient's lymphocytes and/or those of household contacts. This transfer factor can be subsequently replicated in tissue culture. The in vitro replication allows to replenish the stocks indefinitely when an active transfer factor is found.

Acknowledgments: We are indebted to the „FONDATION ASCLE-PIOS" for its support to some of the originaol studies described in this paper.

Acknowledgment

We are indebted to the FONDATION ASCLEPIOS for its support to some of the original studies described in this paper.

References

1   R. B. Thompson: Rev. Eur. Et. Clin. Biol. 16, 201 (1971).
2   L. E. Spitler: Prog. Exp. Tumor. Res., 25: 178 (1978).
3   R. M. Bukowski, S. Deodhar, J. S. Hewlett: In: Ascher MS, et al., ed. Transfer factor: basic properties and clinical applications. New York, Academic Press, p. 543 (1976).
4   A. S. Levin, V. S. Byers, L. LeCam, J. O. Johnston: In: M. S. Ascher, et. al., ed. Transfer factor: basic properties and clinical applications, NY, Ac. Press, p. 537 (1976).
5   J. D. III Bearden, D. E. Thor, C. A. Jr Coltman: In: Ascher MS, et al., ed. Transfer factor: basic properties and clinical applications. NY, Ac. Press, p. 553 (1976).
6   J. U. Gutterman, G. Mavligit, R. Reed, S. Richman, C. E. McBride, E. M. Hersh: Semin, Oncol. 2(2), 155 (1975).
7   V. S. Byers, A. S. Levin, L. LeCam, J. O. Johnston, A. J. Hackett: Ann. NY Acad. Sci. 277, 621 (1976).
8   G. Pizza, D. Viza, C. Boucheix, F. Corrado: Br. J. Cancer 33(6): 606 (1976).
9   G. Pizza, D. Viza, C. Boucheix, F. Corrado: Eur. J. Cancer. 13(9), 917 (1977).
10 G. Pizza, D. Viza, C. Boucheix, F. Corrado In: Ascher MS, et al., ed. Transfer factor: basic properties and clinical applications. New York, Ac. Press, pp. 173 (1976).
11 S. E. Krown, C. M. Pinsky, Y. Hirshaut, J. A. Hansen, H. F. Oettgen: Isr. J. Med. Sci. 14(10), 1026 (1978).
12 R. I. Whyte, M. A. Schork, H. Sloan, M. B. Orringer, M. M. Kirsh: Ann. Thorac. Surg. 53(3), 391 (1992).
13 L. Busutti, A. Blotta, M. Mastrorilli, G. Savorani, G. Pizza, C. De Vinci: J. Exp. Pathol. 3(4), 565 (1987).
14 T. Fujisawa: Nippon Kyobu Shikkan Gakkai Zasshi. 23(1): 68 (1985).
15 T. Fujisawa: Nippon Geka. Gakkai. Zasshi. 86(9), 1055 (1985).
16 T. Fujisawa, Y. Yamaguchi, H. Kimura, M. Arita, M. Shiba, M. Baba: Jpn. J. Surg. 14(6), 452 (1984).
17 T. Fujisawa, Y. Yamaguchi, H. Kimura, M. Arita, M. Baba, M. Shiba: Cancer. 54(4), 663 (1984).
18 T. Fujisawa, Y. Yamaguchi: Gan. No. Rinsho. 29(12), 1409 (1983).
19 T. Fujisawa, Y. Yamaguchi, H. Kimura: Jpn. J Surg. 13(4), 304 (1983).
20 Y. Yamaguchi: Rinsho. Kyobu. Geka. 1(3): 397 (1981).
21 W. W. Deng: Chung. Hua.hie: Chi.Ping.Tsa.Chih. 3(4): 199 (1980).
22 A. Slowik Gabryelska, R. Krzysko: Pneumonol. Pol. 48(3), 187 (1980).
23 J. Hainaut, P. Challan-Belval, G. Haguenauer, J. Pellegrin, P. Allard, J. Kermarec: Ann. Med. Interne. Paris 130 (11), 517 (1979).
24 M. A. Kirsh, M. B. Orringer, S. McAuliffe, M. A. Schork, B. Katz, J. Jr. Silva: Ann. Thorac. Surg. 38(2), 140 (1984).
25 M. M. Kirsh, J. Tashian, H. Sloan: J. Fam. Pract. 8(6): 1127 (1979).
26 H. H. Fudenberg: Ann. NY Acad Sci. 277, 545 (1976).
27 A. S. Levin, V. S. Byers, H. H. Fudenberg, J. Wybran, A. J. Hackett, J. O. Johnston: Trans. Assoc. Am. Physicians. 87: 153 (1974).
28 A. S. Levin, V. S. Byers, H. H. Fudenberg, J. Wybran, A. J. Hackett, J. O. Johnston, L. E. Spitler: J. Clin. Invest. 55, 487, (1975).
29 H. H. Fudenberg, K. Y. Tsang, Theories and Models in Cellular Transformation, ed. Santi et al., London Academic, 23, (1985).
30 H. H. Fudenberg and H. H. Fudenberg: Ann. Rev. Pharmacol. Toxicol. 29, 475 (1989).
31 G. D. Novelli In: Ascher MS, et al., ed. Transfer factor: basic properties and clinical applications. New York, Academic Press. p. 723, (1976).

32 M. Fazio, L. Negri, V. Mastromatteo, D. Pacchioni, F. Calabrese, S. Giacomasso: J. Exp. Pathol. 3(4), 569 (1987).

33 F. Franchi, V. Russo, G. Luzi, F. S. Santori, N. De Chiara, F. Aiuti: Minerva Med. 71(25), 1815 (1980).

34 K. Y. Tsang, H. H. Fudenberg, J. F. Pan: Cell. Immunol., 90, 295 (1985).

35 J. C. Ivins, R. E. Ritts, D. J. Pritchard, G.S. Gilchrist, G. C. Miller, W. F. Taylor: Ann. NY Acad. Sci. 277, 558 (1976).

36 G. S. Gilchrist, J. C. Ivins, R. E. Ritts Jr, D. J. Pritchard, W. F. Taylor, J. M. Edmonson: Cancer Treat. Rep. 62(2), 289 (1978).

37 L. E. Spitler, R. E. Allen, D. R. Minor: Cancer. 61(8): 1543 (1988).

38 M. R. Blume, E. H. Rosenbaum, R. J. Cohen, J. Gershow, Glassberg AB, E. Shepley: Cancer. 47(5), 882 (1981).

39 R. L. Gonzalez, P. Wong, L. E. Spitler: Cancer, 45(1): 57 (1980).

40 R. M. Bukowski, S. Deodhar, J. S. Hewlett, R. Greenstreet: Cancer 51(2), 269 (1983).

41 M. A. Schwarz, J. U. Gutterman, M. A. Burgess, L. K. Heilbrun, W. K. Murphy, G. P. Bodey, E. Stone, V. Turner-Chism, E. M. Hersh: Cancer. 45(10): 2506 (1980).

42 W. Borkowsky, D. Martin, H. S. Lawrence: Am. J. Dis. Child. 138(7), 667 (1984).

43 A. Ortiz, O. Delgado, Z. Rojas: An. Otorrinolaringol. Ibero. Am. 8(4), 289 (1981).

44 C. A. Quick, H. W. Behrens, M. Brinton-Darnell, R. A. Good: Ann. Otol. Rhinol. Laryngol. 84(5 Pt 1): 607 (1975).

45 J. A. Neidhart, A. F. LoBuglio: Arch. Otolaryngol. 101(11): 664 (1975).

46 G. Pizza, D. Viza, D. V. Ablashi, L. Jerome, G. Armstrong, P. H. Levine: idem, 301 (1981). See ref. 50.

47 J. Neequaye, D. Viza, G. Pizza, P. H. Levine, C. De Vinci, D. V. Ablashi, R. J. Biggar, F. K. Nkrumah: Anticancer Res. 10(52 A), 1183 (1990).

48 G. J. Goldenberg, L. J. Brandes, W. H. Lau, A. B. Miller, C. Wall, J. H. C. Ho: Cancer. Treat. Rep. 69(7–8), 761 (1985).

49 G. J. Goldenberg, L. J. Brandes: Cancer Res. 36(2 pt 2), 720 (1976).

50 P. H. Levine, G. Pizza, G. Cannon, D. Ablashi, G. Armstrong, D. Viza: In: Cancer Campaign, Vol. 5 Nasopharyngeal Carcinoma: Grundmann et al., Eds. Fisher-Verlag Publ. Stuttgart–New York, 137 (1981).

51 G. Wagner, W. Knapp, E. Gitsch, S. Selander: Cancer Detect, Prev. Suppl. 1: 373 (1987).

52 G. Wagner, E. Gitsch, L. Havelec, W. Knapp, H. Rainer, S. Selander: Wien. Klin. Wochenschr. 95(20), 738 (1983).

53 R. S. Freedman, J. T. Wharton, F. Rutledge, J. G. Sinkovics: Am. J. Obstet. Gynecol. 130 (5), 572 (1978).

54 R. M. Vetto, D. R. Burger, J. E. Nolte, A. A. Vandenbark, H. W. Baker: Cancer 37(1), 90 (1976).

55 J. Mydill: Cesk. Pediatr. 46(5), 266 (1991).

56 K. Lukacs, M. Kavai, E. Berenyi, G. Frendl, I. Schroder, S. O. Szegedi: Haematologia Budap. 18(2), 105 (1985).

57 J. Phillips, C. Boucheix, G. Pizza, C. Satorio, D. Viza: B. J. Haematol., 38(3), 430 (1978).

58 Heinonen E., Gröhn P., Tarkkanen J., Maiche A., Wasenius V. M.: Cancer Immu. 11, 73 (1981).

59 M. Pasino, C. R. Vadala, G. P. Tonini, A. Comelli, P. Perutelli: Boll. Ist. Sieroter. Milan. 55(2): 168 (1976).

60 B. W. Hancock, L. Bruce, R. J. Sokal, A. Clark: Eur. J. Cancer Clin. Oncol. 24, 929 (1988).

61 R. M. Bukowski, J. S. Hewlett, S. H. Deodhar: J. Clin. Hematol: Oncology 8, 129 (1978).

62   J. E. Montie, R. M. Bukowski, S. H. Deodhar, J. S. Hewlett, B. H. Stewart, R. A. Straffon: J. Urol., 117(51), 553 (1977).

63   J. E. Montie, R. M. Bukowski, R. E. James, R. A. Straffon, B. H. Stewart: J. Surg. Oncol. 21(1), 5 (1982).

64   F. Corrado, C. De Vinci, G. Corrado, G. Pizza: In: Immunotherapy of Renal Cell Carcinoma. Clinical and Experimental Developments. F. M. J. Debruyne, R. M. Bukowski, J. E. Pontes, P. H. M. De Mulder Eds., Springer Verlag, Berlin, p. 105 (1991).

65   A. S. Rosenberg, M. Lotze, L. M. Muul et al.: NEJM, 313, 1485 (1985).

66   D. Viza, Cl. Boucheix, J. P. Césarini, D. V. Ablashi, G. Armstrong, P. Levine, G. Pizza: Bio. Cell 46: 1–10 (1982).

67   G. Pizza, D. Viza, J. Wood, C. Boucheix, C. Ortolani, F. Corrado: In: Immune Regulators in Transfer Factor. A. Khan, C. H. Kirkpatrick, N. O. Hill Eds., Ac. Press NY, 323 (1979).

68   T. M. Philips, G. Pizza, D. Viza et al.: idem. 331, (1979).

69   G. Pizza, C. De Vinci: J. Exp. Pathol., 3, 335 (1987).

70   C. Corrado, G. Pizza et al.: J. Exp. Pathol., 3, 347 (1987).

71   J. Tarkkanen, P. Grohn, E. Heinonen, O. Alfthan, S. Pyrhonen: Cancer Immunol. Immunother. 10, 251 (1981).

72   F. Corrado, G. Pizza: Arch. Esp. Urol. 37 Suppl. 2: 659 (1984).

73   F. Corrado, G. Pizza, C. De Vinci, G. Corrado: Arch. Esp. Urol., 42 Suppl. 2, 191 (1989).

74   M. W. Shaw, R. J. Ablin, P. D. Guinan, R. A. Bhatti Am. J. Reprod. Immunol. Microbiol. 3, 80 (1985).

75   D. B. Vasily, O. F. Miller, H. H. Fudenberg, J. M. Goust, G. B. Wilson J. Clin. Lab. Immunol. 14(1) 49 (1984).

76   M. De Bruyere, G. Cornu, T. Heremans-Bracke, J. Malchaire, G. Sokal: Br. J. Haematol. 44 (2), 243 (1980).

77   K. Thestrup-Pedersen, E. Grunnet, H. Zachariae. Acta Derm. Venereo. Stockh. 62 (1), 47 (1982).

78   H. Zachariae, E. Grunnet, K. Thestrup-Pedersen, L. Molin, H. Schmidt, F. Starfelt, K. Thomsen: Acta Der. Venereol. Stockh., 62, 162 (1982).

79   H. Zachariae, J. Ellegaard, E. Grunnet, K. Thestrup, K. Pedersen: Dermatologica. 160(1), 1, (1980).

80   H. F. Oettgen, L. J. Old, J. Farrow et al.: J. Clin. Invest. 50, 71a (1971).

81   G. V. Smith, P. A. Morse, G. D. Deraps et al.: Surgery, 74, 59 (1973).

82   M. A. Silverman, S. Meltz, C. Sorokon, P. R. Glade: In: Ascher MS, et al., eds. Transfer factor: basic properties and clinical applications. New York, Ac. Press, 633 (1976).

83   R. M. Vetto, D. R. Burger, J. E. Nolte, A. A. Vandenbark: In: Ascher MS, et al., eds. Transfer factor: basic properties and clinical applications. New York, Ac. Press. 523 (1976).

84   A. Lefesvre, D. Viza, M. Patrasco, J. Phillips, C. De Vinci, G. Pizza: J. Exp. Path. 3, 533 (1987)

85   D. Viza, J. M. Goust, R. Moulias, L. K. Trejdosiewicz, A. Collard, N. Müller-Bérat: Transplan. P. VII (suppl. 1), 329 (1975).

86   G. Pizza, D. Viza, Cl. Boucheix, F. Corrado: In: Immunotherapy of Malignant Diseases, H. Rainer (ed.), F. K. Schattauer Verlag, Stuttgart, 1978, pp. 356.

87   G. Pizza D. Viza, A. Roda, R. Aldini, E. Roda, L. Barbara: N. Eng. J. Med. 300, 1332 (1979).

88   Cl. Boucheix, J. Phillips, G. Pizza, Sartorio C., D. Viza: Lancet i: 198 (1977).

89   D. Viza, F. Rosenfeld, J. Phillips, J. M. Vich, J. Denis, J. F. Bonissent, K. Dobge: In: Immunobiology of Transfer Factor, C. H. Kirkpatrick et al., (eds.), Academic Press, New York. 245 (1983).

90 F. Rosenfeld, D. Viza, H. Phillips, J. M. Vich, O. Binet, R. Aron-Brune-
    tière: Presse Méd 13, 537 (1984).
91 J. Denis, T. Hoang-Xuan, J. F. Bonissent, K. Dogbe, C. Clay, D. Viza,
    F. Rosenfeld, J. Phillips, J. M. Vich: In: Herpetic Eye Diseases, P. C.
    Maudgal, L. Missotten (eds.), Dr. W. Junk Publishers, Dordrecht, 111 (85).
92 D. Viza, J. M. Vich, J. Phillips, F. Rosenfeld: Lymphok. Res. 4, 27 (1985).
93 D. Viza, J. M. Vich, J. Phillips, D. A. L. Davies: J. Exp. Path. 3, 407 (1987).

Index Vol. 42

The references of the Subject Index are given in the language of the respective contribution.
Die Stichworte des Sachregisters sind in der jeweiligen Sprache der einzelnen Beiträge aufgeführt.
Les termes repris dans la Table des Matières sont donnés selon la langue dans laquelle l'ouvrage est écrit.

Index of titles
Verzeichnis der Titel
Index des titres
Vol. 1–42 (1959–1994)

Author and paper index
Autoren- und Artikelindex
Index des auteurs et des articles
Vol. 1–42 (1959–1994)